Genetics for Health Professionals in Cancer Care

D1448420

Preface

This book is based on an established and popular course run by King's College London and St George's, University of London in partnership with the London regional genetics centres. The book, like the course, is aimed at health professionals in the UK and Europe who do not specialise in cancer genetics but who, in their day-to-day clinical practice, come across patients with hereditary cancer or with a family history of cancer and/or concerns about their risk of developing cancer.

There is rising awareness of the significance of genes in the development of cancer and growing demand for genetic testing and cancer screening. Alongside this advances in technology are reducing the costs and increasing the availability of genetic tests. As a result there is a global move towards greater integration of genetics/genomics into mainstream healthcare, highlighting the importance of a sound knowledge base in cancer genetics for health professionals working with patients who have cancer or who have a family history of cancer.

This book includes contributions from specialists in genetics and cancer care with a background in clinical practice and research or education. It aims to equip non-genetics health professionals with the knowledge and skills required for all aspects of managing cancer family history, including: taking an accurate cancer family history and drawing a family tree; understanding basic cancer biology and genetics and the genes involved in hereditary breast, ovarian, prostate, colorectal, gastric and related gynaecological cancers and rare cancer-predisposing syndromes; assessing cancer risk and communicating risk information; early detection and risk-reducing measures available for those at increased risk; and managing individuals with hereditary cancer. In addition, this book provides insight into what happens when a patient is referred for genetic counselling and genetic testing, including the psychological, social and ethical issues faced by individuals and families with and at risk of hereditary cancer. The final section draws on the experiences of health professionals who have managed cancer family history in primary, secondary and palliative care, identifying the particular challenges raised and strategies to overcome these and providing practical guidance on setting up a cancer family history clinic in primary or secondary care.

The book is divided into nine sections. In each section an introductory chapter sets the context and outlines the basic principles and key elements. This is followed by a number of chapters written by invited authors who are specialists in their fields, providing the details for particular cancer types or areas of expertise. Finally, for each section there is a summary chapter which draws together the key learning points across the whole section, providing suggestions for further reading and exercises aimed to consolidate learning.

Acknowledgements

With grateful thanks to all those who have contributed to this book and to our colleagues, families and friends for their understanding, patience and support.

Contents

Section 4 **Cancer risk assessment and communicating risk**

Section 5 **Early detection of hereditary cancer**

Section 6 **Reducing the risk of cancer**

Section 7 **Managing hereditary cancer**

List of Abbreviations

ACMG	American College of Medical Genetics and Genomics		DALM	dysplasia-associated lesion or mass
ACPGBI	Association of Coloproctology of Great Britain and Ireland		DCIS	ductal carcinoma *in situ*
			DIEP	deep inferior epigastric perforator
ACTH	adrenocorticotropic hormone		DRE	digital rectal examination
ACU	assisted conception unit		DSB	double-strand break
ADM	acellular dermal matrix		EBMG	European Board of Medical Genetics
A-T	ataxia telangiectasia		EC	endometrial cancer
BCC	basal cell carcinoma		ER	oestrogen receptor
BCLC	Breast Cancer Linkage Consortium		ESHG	European Society of Human Genetics
BCRAS	Breast Cancer Risk Assessment Service		FAMM	familial atypical mole and melanoma
			FAP	familial adenomatous polyposis
BCS	breast-conserving surgery		ffDNA	free foetal DNA
BCSP	[UK] Bowel Cancer Screening Programme		FGF	fibroblast growth factor
			FHQ	family history questionnaire
BHDS	Birt–Hogg–Dubé syndrome		FOBT	faecal occult blood testing
BME	black and minority ethnic		FTC	fallopian tube cancer
BRRS	Bannayan–Riley–Ruvalcaba syndrome		5FU	5-fluorouracil
			GC	gastric cancer
BSG	British Society of Gastroenterology		GCRB	Genetic Counsellor Registration Board
BSGM	British Society for Genetic Medicine			
BSO	bilateral salpingo-oophorectomy		GI	gastrointestinal
CA125	cancer antigen 125		GOG	Gynecologic Oncology Group
CBC	contralateral breast cancer		GP	general practitioner
CBT	cognitive behavioural therapy		GWAS	genome-wide association studies
CCC	clear cell carcinoma		HBOC	hereditary breast and ovarian cancer
CDK	cyclin-dependent kinase		HDGC	hereditary diffuse gastric cancer
CDKI	cyclin-dependent kinase inhibitor		HE4	human epididymis protein 4
CGN	Cancer Genetics Network		HER2	human epidermal growth factor receptor
CHRPE	congenital hypertrophy of the retinal pigment epithelium			
			HGSC	high-grade serous carcinoma
CIN	chromosomal instability		HIF	hypoxia-inducible factor
CMMR-D	constitutional mismatch repair-deficiency syndrome		HLRCC	hereditary leiomyomatosis and renal cell cancer
			HR	homologous recombination
CNS	clinical nurse specialist(s)		HRT	hormone replacement therapy
CRC	colorectal cancer		IBD	inflammatory bowel disease
CRRM	contralateral risk-reducing mastectomy		IGF	insulin growth factor
			IHC	immunohistochemical
CT	computed tomography		IUS	intrauterine system
CVS	chorionic villous sampling			

IVF	*in vitro* fertilisation	PR	progesterone receptor
KSF	knowledge and skills framework	PSA	prostate-specific antigen
LD	latissimus dorsi	QA	quality assurance
LFS	Li–Fraumeni syndrome	RGC	regional genetics centre
LS	Lynch syndrome	RMI	risk of malignancy index
MAP	*MUTYH*-associated polyposis	ROC	risk of ovarian cancer
MDT	multidisciplinary team	RRM	risk-reducing mastectomy
MEN1	multiple endocrine neoplasia type 1	RRSO	risk-reducing salpingo-oophorectomy
MEN2	multiple endocrine neoplasia type 2	RR-THBSO	risk-reducing total hysterectomy and bilateral salpingo-oophorectomy
MMR	mismatch repair		
MRI	magnetic resonance imaging	SCM	subcutaneous mastectomy
MSI	microsatellite instability	SDH	succinate dehydrogenase
MTC	medullary thyroid cancer	SERM	selective oestrogen receptor modulator
MTS	Muir–Torre syndrome		
NF1	neurofibromatosis type 1	SFT	solution-focused therapy
NGS	next generation sequencing	SGAP	superior gluteal artery perforator
NHS	National Health Service	SHH	sonic hedgehog
NHSBSP	NHS Breast Screening Programme	SNP	single nucleotide polymorphism
NICE	National Institute for Health and Care Excellence	SSA	sessile serrated adenoma
		SSM	skin-sparing mastectomy
NMC	Nursing and Midwifery Council	TGFα	transforming growth factor-α
NPV	negative predictive value	TIC	tubal intra-epithelial carcinoma
NSAIDs	non-steroidal anti-inflammatory drugs	TMG	transverse myocutaneous gracilis
		TNBC	triple-negative breast cancer
OC	ovarian cancer	TRAM	transverse rectus abdominis myocutaneous
PAP	profunda artery perforator		
PARP	poly ADP-ribose polymerase	TVS	transvaginal ultrasound
PCC	phaeochromocytoma	UC	ulcerative colitis
PDGF	platelet-derived growth factor	UKCTOCS	United Kingdom Collaborative Trial of Ovarian Cancer Screening
PFS	progression free survival		
PGD	pre-implantation genetic diagnosis	UKFOCSS	UK Familial Ovarian Cancer Screening Study
PGL	paraganglioma		
PJS	Peutz–Jeghers syndrome	UV	unclassified variants
pCR	pathological complete response	VEGF	vascular endothelial growth factor
PND	prenatal diagnosis	VHL	Von Hippel–Lindau disease
PPC	primary peritoneal cancer	VMA	vanillylmandelic acid
PPNAD	primary pigmented nodular adrenocortical disease	VUS	variant(s) of uncertain significance
		XRM	X-ray mammography
PPV	positive predictive value		

List of Contributors

Editors

Chris Jacobs MSc, BSc (Hons), DPSN, RN (GCRB registered 159),
NIHR Doctoral Research Fellow,
University College London (UCL),
Consultant Genetic Counsellor
in Cancer Genetics,
Guy's Regional Genetics Service,
Guy's and St Thomas' NHS Foundation Trust,
London, UK

Patricia Webb MPhil, RN,
Principal Lecturer,
Faculty of Health, Social Care and Education,
St George's, University of London,
London, UK

Lorraine Robinson MSc, PGDE, BSc, RN, RNT,
Principal Lecturer,
Department of Adult Nursing,
Florence Nightingale School of Nursing and Midwifery,
King's College London,
London, UK

Contributing authors

Mahmoud Ali Zohree Ali MRCP
Clinical Oncology Fellow,
Guy's and St Thomas' NHS Foundation Trust,
London, UK

Audrey Ardern-Jones MSc, RN, Dip N (Lon) Genetics Cert,
Associate Lecturer/Nurse Specialist in Cancer Genetics,
The Royal Marsden Hospital,
London, UK

Elizabeth Bancroft PhD, RN,
Senior Research Nurse in Oncogenetics,
Royal Marsden NHS Foundation Trust
and Institute of Cancer Research,
London, UK

Gillian Bowman MSc, BSc, RN,
Lead Nurse,
South East London Breast Screening Programme,
King's College Hospital NHS Foundation Trust,
London, UK

Eric Alexandre Chung MD, FRCS,
Consultant Colorectal Surgeon,
St George's Healthcare NHS Trust,
London, UK

Emma Crosbie BSc, MBChB (Hons), PhD, MRCOG,
NIHR Clinician Scientist, Senior Lecturer and Honorary Consultant in Gynaecological Oncology,
Institute of Cancer Sciences, University of Manchester, St Mary's Hospital,
Manchester, UK

Claire Coughlan MA, BA, RN,
Consultant Nurse, Colorectal,
Lewisham Hospital NHS Trust,
London, UK

Linda Dyer RN,
Family History Specialist Nurse Digestive Diseases, Inflammatory Bowel Disease Nurse Specialist and Nurse Endoscopist,
Royal Sussex County Hospital,
Brighton, UK

Charlotte Eddy MSc (GCRB registered no 233),
Genetic Counsellor,
South West Thames Regional Genetics Service,
St George's Healthcare NHS Trust,
Honorary Senior Lecturer,
Kingston University, UK

Rosalind Eeles PhD, MBBS, FMedSci, FRCP, FRCR,
The Institute of Cancer Research and
Royal Marsden NHS Foundation Trust,
London and Surrey, UK

Jian Farhadi MD, PD, FMH(Plast), EBOPRAS,
Consultant Plastic Surgeon and
Director Department of Plastic Surgery,
Guy's and St Thomas' NHS Foundation Trust,
London, UK

Clare Firth DClinPsych,
Clinical Psychologist (HCPC Registered Practitioner Psychologist),
Guy's and St Thomas' NHS Foundation Trust,
London, UK

Aleksandra Gentry-Maharaj PhD, MSc, BSc (Hons)
Senior Research Associate,
Gynaecological Cancer Research Centre,
Institute for Women's Health,
University College London (UCL),
London, UK

Jennifer Glendenning MRCP, FRCR,
Clinical Oncology Fellow,
Guy's and St Thomas' NHS Foundation Trust and King's College London (KCL),
London, UK

Mark George BSc, MS, FRCS (Gen),
Consultant Colorectal and General Surgeon,
Guy's and St Thomas' NHS Foundation Trust,
London, UK

Sheila Goff MSc, RN,
Clinical Nurse Specialist in Palliative Care,
St Joseph's Hospice,
London, UK

Hisham Hamed MBBCh, PhD, FRCS,
Consultant Oncoplastic Breast Surgeon,
Guy's and St Thomas' NHS Foundation Trust,
London, UK

Kati Harris RN, PG Cert Genetics,
Clinical Nurse Specialist, Cancer Family History, Breast Cancer Risk Assessment Service
Guy's and St Thomas' NHS Foundation Trust,
London, UK

Eshika Haque MSc, BSc (GCRB registered no 286),
Genetic Counsellor, Guy's Regional Genetics Service,
Guy's and St Thomas' NHS Foundation Trust, London, UK

Vicki Kiesel MSc, BSc (GCRB registered no 237),
Lead Genetic Counsellor,
North West Thames Regional Genetics Service at the Kennedy Galton Centre,
Northwick Park NHS Trust,
London, UK

Ashutosh Kothari MS, DNB, MNAMS,
Breast Surgeon,
Guy's and St Thomas' NHS Foundation Trust,
London, UK

Belinda Lötter RN, PG Cert Genetics,
Clinical Nurse Specialist, Cancer Family History, Breast Cancer Risk Assessment Service,

Guy's and St Thomas' NHS Foundation Trust,
London, UK

Michael Michell MB, BChir, DMRD, FRCR,
Consultant Radiologist and Director,
South East London Breast Screening Programme,
King's College Hospital NHS Foundation Trust,
London, UK

Athalie Melville MSc, BSc (GCRB registered no 264),
Genetic Counsellor,
North West Thames Regional Genetics Service at the Kennedy Galton Centre,
London, UK

Usha Menon MBBS, DGO, MD (Obs & Gynae), MD (Res), FRCOG,
Head, Gynaecological Cancer Research Centre,
Consultant Gynaecologist,
University College London (UCL),
London, UK

Kevin John Monahan MRCP, PhD,
Consultant Gastroenterologist and General Physician,
Family History of Bowel Cancer Clinic,
West Middlesex University Hospital,
London, UK

Ana Montes LMS, PhD,
Consultant Medical Oncologist,
Guy's and St Thomas' NHS Foundation Trust,
London, UK

Charlotte Moss MRCP, PhD,
Consultant in Medical Oncology,
Brighton and Sussex University Hospitals,
Brighton, UK

Christine Patch PhD, RN (GCRB registered 182),
Reader in Clinical Genetics King's College London,
Consultant Genetic Counsellor/Manager,
Guy's Regional Genetics Service,
Guy's and St Thomas' NHS Foundation Trust,
London, UK

Gabriella Pichert MD, FMH, VENIA LEGENDI,
Consultant in Cancer Genetics,
London Bridge Hospital,
London, UK

Sarah Rose MSc, BSc (GCRB registered no 238),
Genetic Counsellor,
Guy's Regional Genetics Service,
Guy's and St Thomas' NHS Foundation Trust,
London, UK

Adam Rosenthal MBBS, BSc (Hons), PhD, MRCOG,
Senior Lecturer and Honorary Consultant Gynaecological Oncologist,
Barts Cancer Institute and Barts Health NHS Trust,
London, UK

Paul Ross PhD, FRCP
Consultant Clinical Oncologist,
Guy's and St Thomas' NHS Foundation Trust,
London, UK

Deborah Ruddy PhD, MBBS,
Consultant Clinical Geneticist,
Guy's Regional Genetics Service,
Guy's and St Thomas' NHS Foundation Trust,
London, UK

Gillian Scott MSc, MBA, BSc (GCRB registered no 146),
Genetic Counsellor,
Southern General Hospital,
Glasgow, UK

Adam Shaw BM, MD, FRCP,
Consultant in Clinical Genetics,
Guy's Regional Genetics Service,
Guy's and St Thomas' NHS Foundation Trust,
London, UK

Amanda Shewbridge MSc, BSc (Hons), RN,
Consultant Nurse Breast Cancer,
Guy's and St Thomas' NHS Foundation Trust,
London, UK

Kiruthikah Thillai MRCP, BSc
Specialist Registrar in Medical Oncology,
Guy's and St Thomas' NHS Foundation Trust,
London, UK

Vishakha Tripathi MBBS, MSc, MSc (GCRB registered no 212),
Principal Genetic Counsellor,
South West Thames Regional Genetics Service,
St George's Healthcare NHS Trust,
Honorary Senior Lecturer,
Kingston University, UK

Andrew Tutt PhD, FRCR, MRCP, MB ChB,
Consultant Clinical Oncologist,
Guy's and St Thomas' NHS Foundation Trust,
Director Breakthrough for Breast Cancer,
Institute of Cancer Research,
London, UK

Sally Watts MSc, BSc (Hons), RGN (GCRB registered no 110),
Lead Genetic Counsellor,
Guy's Regional Genetics Service,
Guy's and St Thomas' NHS Foundation Trust,
London, UK

Emma Williams MSc (Dist), BSc (Hons) (GCRB registered no 245),
Genetic Counsellor,
North East Thames Regional Genetics Service,
Great Ormond Street Hospital for Children NHS Foundation Trust,
London, UK

Audrey Yandle BA, MSc, RN, PGCEA, Cert Biomedicine,
Lecturer,
Florence Nightingale School of Nursing and Midwifery,
King's College London,
London, UK

Abdulkani Yusuf MRCP-UK,
Gastroenterology Specialist Registrar,
Family History of Bowel Cancer Clinic,
West Middlesex University Hospital,
London, UK

Section 1

Putting cancer genetics into context

Chapter 1

Putting cancer genetics into context

Chris Jacobs

Introduction to putting cancer genetics into context

The role of genes is becoming increasingly important in all aspects of medicine, not least in the field of cancer care. Advances in genetics knowledge are being incorporated into clinical practice, impacting on diagnosis, risk stratification, prevention and treatment. A rising awareness amongst the general public of the importance of family history in determining the risk of cancer and a growing demand for screening and genetic testing, highlight the importance for all health professionals of identifying a significant cancer family history in order that services can be targeted appropriately. While most cancers are explained by the interaction between genes and environment, a small proportion are due to a highly penetrant inherited single gene mutation. As advances in technology increase the effectiveness and reduce the cost of genetic testing, new genetic variants are being discovered and rapid genetic testing is enabling targeting of chemotherapy and surgery close to cancer diagnosis; it will therefore become increasingly important for healthcare professionals working in the field of cancer to have a sound basic knowledge of cancer genetics and an awareness of the implications of a cancer family history.

This chapter aims to put the developments in genetics into context for health professionals specialising in cancer care. The learning objectives are:

+ to understand the impact of scientific advances in genetic/genomic medicine on cancer patients and health professionals in cancer care;

+ to be aware of developments in government policy and in public health that relate to genetic/genomic medicine and relate these to cancer patients and health professionals in cancer care.

Genetics/genomics

The terms 'genetics' and 'genomics' are often used interchangeably. The accepted definition of genetics is 'the study of heredity' (World Health Organization, 2002), whereas genomics is defined as 'the study of genes and their functions, and related techniques' (World Health Organization, 2004). The use of genetic information and technologies to determine disease risk and diagnose and treat disease is termed 'genomic medicine'. The rapid advances in this field of medicine are rapidly changing the face of healthcare and there is an urgent need for health professionals to keep abreast of these changes in order to meet the needs of their patients.

Scientific advances in understanding of the human genome

The impact of the discovery of the structure of DNA in 1953 was far-reaching and hugely significant for understanding how the human body functions. In the late 1970s, DNA sequencing was developed, enabling the techniques that six decades later, in 2003, led to decoding of the complete human genome. This made way for the identification of hundreds of genes that contribute to human disease and has had a profound impact on the potential for improving the prevention, diagnosis and treatment of common diseases.

Labour-intensive and costly methods of DNA sequencing are being replaced by highly automated robotics, driving down the cost and lowering the threshold for offering genetic testing. However, even with increased capacity, it is important to acknowledge that most common diseases are not due to the inheritance of high-risk single gene mutations, and therefore the genetic testing that is currently available will not be helpful in explaining most diseases, including cancer. The great majority of cancers are caused by a combination of genetic and environmental factors. However, for a small proportion of individuals, genetic testing for cancer susceptibility may be extremely helpful and important in prevention, diagnosis or treatment of the disease.

Organisation of genetics services

In the UK, parts of Europe, North America and Australasia, genetic counselling is provided by clinical geneticists (doctors) and genetic counsellors (non-medical health professionals with a nursing and/or science background). Genetics health professionals have training and expertise in clinical genetics and in counselling. In the UK, genetics services are organised regionally serving large populations. Specialist clinical scientists provide molecular and cytogenetic testing and bioinformatic analyses of genetic data. Through a UK network of laboratories, tests are available for an increasingly wide range of syndromes predisposing to cancer.

Developments in government policy and public health that relate to genomics

The speed and significance of the scientific advances in understanding the human genome and the implications of this for healthcare in general and for cancer care specifically are only just beginning to emerge. The impact of these advances has been highlighted in several policy documents over the last 10 years. The government White Paper, *Our inheritance, our future* (Department of Health, 2003), was the first to set out explicit policy commitments in the field of human genetics and a vision of the way in which advances in genetics could benefit patients in the future. The policy served to raise awareness of genetics in healthcare and build genetics into mainstream services. Investment in clinical genetic testing, service development, education and training and pharmacogenetics research enabled advances in the development of a system for evidence-based evaluation of clinical DNA tests through the UK Genetic Testing Network (<http://www.ukgtn.nhs.uk>) and in education and training for health professionals through the establishment of the National Genetics and Genomics Education Centre (<http://www.geneticseducation.nhs.uk>).

In 2009, the Science and Technology Committee on Genomic Medicine further investigated how scientific advances in genomic medicine might improve public healthcare and the quality of life (House of Lords Science and Technology Committee, 2009). The aim of the committee was to investigate whether health services were in a position to take advantage of scientific advances, to review the ethical and regulatory frameworks that would need to be put in place and the impact of these, and the new economic opportunities that these advances could bring. The areas of particular importance for cancer care included the diagnosis of genetic subtypes of common cancers, the management of common cancers, the stratified use of medicines and pharmacogenomics to target treatment at individuals depending on their genetic makeup and the use of bioinformatics and the role of biobanks. The report highlighted the significance of these scientific developments for healthcare, acknowledged that the existing arrangements, i.e. genetic testing being undertaken within genetics services, would not be sustainable and recommended much greater integration of genomics into mainstream services.

This concept of 'mainstreaming' genetics has been further developed by a report on the integration of genetics into mainstream medicine produced by the Public Health Genomics Foundation (Burton, 2011) at the request of the Joint Committee on Medical Genetics. The report refers specifically to ophthalmology and cardiovascular disease, but the recommendations to integrate genetics into mainstream services apply to all hereditary conditions including cancer. The Joint Committee on Medical Genetics considered the challenges and implications for education, service delivery and commissioning in the Genomics in Medicine Report (Burton et al., 2012), and subsequently the Human Genomics Strategy Group published a report setting out a strategic vision for how healthcare in the UK could benefit from genomic technology and the steps needed to realise this vision (Human Genetics Strategy Group, 2012). Central to implementation is the need to develop a service delivery infrastructure that will enable access to genetic testing and training the workforce in all areas of healthcare to deliver this. Understanding about inheritance, identifying patients who may be at risk, interpreting the results of genetic tests and communicating with patients about inherited diseases is now within the remit of all health professionals.

The implications of genomic medicine for cancer care

Before the 1990s, little was understood about the role of inherited factors in the aetiology of cancer. The study of the genetic predisposition to cancer mainly involved very rare family cancer syndromes, such as familial retinoblastoma. Identification of the genes predisposing to breast and ovarian cancer, *BRCA1* and *BRCA2*, in the mid 1990s raised awareness of the importance of genetic predisposition in the development of common cancers. Until recently, medical geneticists and genetic counsellors used the term 'cancer genetics' to refer to an inherited susceptibility to cancer and the identification of germline mutations to enable an assessment of cancer risk, while cancer specialists used the term to refer to the genetic changes which occur within the cell itself (Plon, 2011).

Public and professional awareness of the role of genes in determining cancer risk grew exponentially in the 10 years following the discovery of *BRCA1* and *BRCA2* such that one UK Regional Genetics Service reported an increase in cancer genetics referrals from <1% (fewer than 20 cases) in all clinical genetics referrals in 1991 to 30% of cases (more than a thousand) in 2000 (Cole and Sleightholme, 2000). The number of referrals continued to rise throughout the 2000s, as seen in data from Guy's Regional Genetics Service showing an increase of 84% between the last quarter of 2002 and the first quarter of 2006 (Izatt, 2006). In-house genetic testing for breast cancer genes increased in the same centre by over 370% between 2005 and 2013 with a 175% increase in the last year of data (Genetics Centre, Guy's Hospital, personal communication).

Genetics has become increasingly important in many aspects of healthcare and is likely to have the greatest impact on our understanding of common chronic diseases, such as cardiac disease, diabetes and cancer. While it is important to acknowledge that 80% of cancer is not due to highly penetrant inherited gene mutations, identifying those affected with or at risk of hereditary cancer is important for healthcare. Advances in genetic technology and the falling cost of genetic testing mean that genetics assessment is far more accessible than it was even 5 years ago. The increase in availability of genetic testing carries with it significant implications for patients and health professionals.

Integrating genomics into cancer care

Throughout the world there has been much discussion about the benefits and challenges of integrating genomics into mainstream healthcare (Collins and Guttmacher, 2001; Halliday et al., 2004; Scheuner et al., 2008). There are published examples of successful implementation of genetic risk assessment by health professionals within cancer care (Grimsey et al., 2010; Harris and Lötter, 2012). Yet health professionals do not always feel confident about assessing risk (Metcalfe et al., 2010), are not always clear whose responsibility it is (Lanceley et al., 2012) and do not always refer patients to genetic counselling, even when a risk assessment has been made (Grover et al., 2004; Meyer et al., 2010).

In a worldwide review of models of genetics in healthcare (Battista et al., 2012), the authors suggested that redefinition and redistribution of roles and responsibilities and sharing of expertise and information between health professionals is required for successful integration of genetics into mainstream healthcare.

Currently genetic testing is only available following genetic counselling which is accessed via genetics services. However, over the next 5 years, as the targeting of cancer treatment through genetic profiling becomes a reality, new genes are discovered, the cost of testing is reduced and the availability and speed of testing is increased, genetic testing is likely to be offered as part of routine cancer management. Research is under way to investigate the clinical and scientific requirements for routine genetic testing to be integrated into cancer care (see <http://mcgprogramme.com>). Whilst these developments promise enormous advances in the diagnosis, treatment and prevention of cancer, the implications for patients, families, health professionals and policy makers will need to be thoroughly investigated and carefully considered (Rahman, 2014).

Summary

Advances in our understanding of the human genome and the clinical application of this knowledge will inevitably lead to major changes in the clinical management of common diseases. It is essential that all health professionals understand the implications of this, accept that managing the genetic aspects of disease is within the remit of their roles and take action to develop the skills and knowledge required to manage the care of their patients in the light of these developments.

References

Battista RN, Blancquaert I, Laberge AM, et al. 2012. Genetics in health care: an overview of current and emerging models. *Publ Health Genom* **15**: 34–45.

Burton H 2011. *Genetics and mainstream medicine*. Cambridge: PHG Foundation.

Burton H, Cole T, Farndon P 2012. *Genomics in medicine*. Cambridge: Joint Committee on Medical Genetics.

Cole TR and Sleightholme HV 2000. ABC of colorectal cancer. The role of clinical genetics in management. *Br Med J* **321**: 943–946.

Collins F and Guttmacher A 2001. Genetics moves into the medical mainstream. *J Am Med Assoc* **286**: 2322–2324.

Department of Health 2003. *Our inheritance, our future: realising the potential of genetics in the NHS*. London: The Stationery Office.

Grimsey E, Howlett D, Allan S, et al. 2010. Implementation and progress review of a nurse-led family history risk assessment clinic. *Eur J Cancer Suppl* **8**: 241.

Grover S, Stoffel EM, Bussone L, et al. 2004. Physician assessment of family cancer history and referral for genetic evaluation in colorectal cancer patients. *Clin Gastroenterol Hepatol* **2**: 813–819.

Halliday JL, Collins VR, Aitken MA, et al. 2004. Genetics and public health—evolution, or revolution? *J Epidemiol Commun Health* **58**: 894–899.

Harris K and Lötter B 2012. Focus on patients with a family history of cancer. *Cancer Nurs Pract* **11**: 14–19.

House of Lords Science and Technology Committee 2009. *Genomic medicine: 2nd report of session 2008–09*. London: The Stationery Office.

Human Genetics Strategy Group 2012. *Building on our inheritance. Genomic technology in healthcare. A report by the Human Genomics Strategy Group*. London: Department of Health.

Izatt L 2006. Re-audit of referral practice to the cancer genetics service at Guy's Hospital—appropriateness and outcome. *J Med Genet* **43** (Suppl): S66.

Lanceley A, Eagle Z, Ogden G, et al. 2012. Family history and women with ovarian cancer: is it asked and does it matter? An observational study. *Int J Gynecol Cancer* **22**: 254–259.

Metcalfe A, Pumphrey R, Clifford C 2010. Hospice nurses and genetics: implications for end-of-life care. *J Clin Nurs* **19**: 192–207.

Meyer LA, Anderson ME, Lacour RA, et al. 2010. Evaluating women with ovarian cancer for *BRCA1* and *BRCA2* mutations: missed opportunities. *Obstet Gynecol* **115**: 945–952.

Plon SE 2011. Unifying cancer genetics. *Genet Med* **13**: 203–204.

Rahman N 2014. Realizing the promise of cancer predisposition genes. *Nature* **505**: 302–308.

Scheuner M, Sieverding P, Shekelle P 2008. Delivery of genomic medicine for common chronic adult diseases: a systematic review. *J Am Med Assoc* **299**: 1320–1334.

World Health Organization 2002. *Genomics and world health: report of the Advisory Committee on Health Research*. Geneva: World Health Organization.

World Health Organization 2004. *Genomics and world health: report of the Advisory Committee on Health Research*. Fifty-Seventh World Health Assembly, A57/16. Geneva: World Health Organization.

Cancer genetics: the basics

Chapter 2

Cancer genetics: the basics. Introduction

Chris Jacobs

Introduction to cancer genetics

In the UK, medical and non-medical health professionals with specialist training and expertise currently provide genetic healthcare via regional genetics centres or services (RGC) which incorporate laboratory and clinical services. Central to the role of the genetics health professional is the provision of genetic counselling. Genetic counselling is defined as 'a communication process which deals with human problems associated with the occurrence, or risk of occurrence, of a genetic disorder in a family' (American Society of Human Genetics, 1975) and which aims to help the individual or family to understand, manage and adapt to hereditary conditions in the way that is most appropriate for them. The central ethos of genetic counselling is non-directiveness (Harper, 2004) and the focus is on the wider family as much as the individual (Parker and Lucassen, 2003), concepts that may be less familiar to non-genetics health professionals. Further discussion of genetic counselling is given in Chapters 31 and 32.

The impact of genetics and genomics on all aspects of healthcare requires new ways of delivering genetic healthcare, which has implications for health professionals in all specialties and settings, not least cancer care. Ensuring adequate levels of knowledge and skills across the workforce is a challenge, and much work has been done in this area to develop competencies, learning outcomes and training packages for health professionals.

This chapter provides an overview of the current situation with regard to the level of knowledge about genetic health in the UK and Europe, outlines the competencies that have been developed for various groups of health professionals and considers the rationale for achieving these competencies. The learning objectives are:

- to be able to describe the competencies and knowledge needed to implement genetics into clinical practice in the UK for non-genetics health professionals;
- to be able to discuss the rationale for achieving these competencies.

Knowledge about genetics/genomics amongst health professionals

People at risk of genetic conditions and parents of children affected by genetic conditions who received genetic information from non-genetics health professionals have identified a need for health professionals to have a greater knowledge and awareness about genetic conditions, greater involvement in patient care and a greater awareness of the impact of genetic information on the wider family (Burke et al., 2007). Amongst physicians, levels of knowledge about genetics that are essential for daily practice have been shown to be low (Baars et al., 2005; Scheuner et al., 2008). A survey of primary-care physicians based in general practice, paediatrics and obstetrics and gynaecology across France, Germany, the Netherlands, Sweden and the UK found that general practitioners (GPs) were the least confident in their ability to carry out defined basic medical genetics tasks. Of those surveyed, 80.4% reported that they had had no training in medical genetics or only undergraduate training. Of the total sample of GPs, only 9% reported feeling confident in their genetics knowledge (Nippert et al., 2011). The picture is similar for nurses. While there are few studies of nurses' actual knowledge of genetics, a systematic review of studies focusing on nurses' competence in genetics found that self-reported knowledge of genetic concepts was generally poor and the amount of genetics education received by nurses was very limited (Godino and Skirton, 2012).

A framework for implementing genetics/genomics into nursing in the UK

Much work has been done to identify the training and educational needs of nurses and the barriers to the integration of genetics into nursing practice. The first genetics education framework was developed for nurses in the UK in 2003 (Kirk et al., 2003). The importance of taking into account genetic and environmental factors was included for the first time in the Nursing and Midwifery Council (NMC) standards for pre-registration nursing education in 2010 (Nursing and Midwifery Council, 2010). However, it seems that nurses do not consistently demonstrate the competencies required for providing healthcare to people with genetic conditions (Skirton et al., 2012).

In a recent report to the Nursing and Midwifery Professional Advisory Board (Genetics in Nursing and Midwifery Task and Finish Group, 2011), barriers to the implementation of genetics in nursing practice were set out. These fall under three main areas: the complexity and uncertainty of genetic healthcare itself and the lack of clarity about what can be achieved; lack of confidence, perceived relevance to practice and interest amongst individual health professionals; and the context and setting for genetic healthcare in terms of competing priorities in nursing education, the limited response of the NMC and the challenges of cross-boundary working. The competence-based framework was revised in 2011 (Kirk et al., 2011) in the context of advances in genetic healthcare, with an additional competency being added to those defined in the 2003 report and up to date guidance being provided for nurse education and training. The additional competency (Statement 8) highlights the importance of providing ongoing nursing care and support to patients and their carers and families with regard to their genetic healthcare needs that may change over time. The revised competencies framework for nurses is shown in Box 2.1. These competencies identify the skills and knowledge required to deliver genetic healthcare by all nurses

Box 2.1 Nursing competencies in genetics/genomics in the UK: revised framework 2011

1. Identify individuals who might benefit from genetic services and/or information through a comprehensive nursing assessment:
   - that recognises the importance of family history in assessing predisposition to disease,
   - recognising the key indicators of a potential genetic condition,
   - taking appropriate and timely action to seek assistance from and refer individuals to genetics specialists, other specialists and peer support resources,
   - based on an understanding of the care pathways that incorporate genetics services and information.

2. Demonstrate the importance of sensitivity in tailoring genetic/genomic information and services to the individual's culture, knowledge, language ability and developmental stage:
   - recognising that ethnicity, culture, religion, ethical perspectives and developmental stage may influence the individual's ability to utilise information and services,
   - demonstrating the use of appropriate communication skills in relation to the individual's level of understanding of genetic/genomic issues.

3. Advocate for the rights of all individuals to informed decision-making and voluntary action:
   - based on an awareness of the potential for misuse of human genetic/genomic information,
   - understanding the importance of delivering genetic/genomic education and counselling fairly, accurately and without coercion or personal bias,
   - recognising that personal values and beliefs of self and individuals may influence the care and support provided during decision-making, and that choices and actions may differ over time.

4. Demonstrate a knowledge and understanding of the role of genetic/genomic and other factors in maintaining health and in the manifestation, modification and prevention of disease expression, to underpin effective practice:
   - which include core genetic/genomic concepts that form a sufficient knowledge base for understanding the implications of specific conditions that may be encountered.

Box 2.1 Nursing competencies in genetics/genomics in the UK: revised framework 2011 *(continued)*

5. Apply knowledge and understanding of the utility and limitations of genetic/genomic information and testing to underpin care and support for individuals and families prior to, during and following decision-making, that:
   - incorporates awareness of the ethical, legal and social issues related to testing, recording, sharing and storage of genetic/genomic information,
   - incorporates awareness of the potential physical, emotional, psychological and social consequences of genetic/genomic information for individuals, family members, and communities.

6. Examine one's own competency of practice on a regular basis:
   - recognising areas where professional development related to genetics/genomics would be beneficial,
   - maintaining awareness of clinical developments in genetics/genomics that are likely to be of most relevance to the client group, seeking further information on a case-by-case basis,
   - based on an understanding of the boundaries of one's professional role in the referral, provision or follow-up to genetics services.

7. Obtain and communicate credible, current information about genetics/genomics, for self, patients, families and colleagues:
   - using information technologies and other information sources effectively to do so, and
   - applying critical appraisal skills to assess the quality of information accessed.

8. Provide ongoing nursing care and support to patients, carers and families with genetic/genomic healthcare needs:
   - being responsive to changing needs through the life-stages and during periods of uncertainty,
   - demonstrating awareness about how an inherited condition, and its implications for family members, might impact on family dynamics,
   - working in partnership with family members and other agencies in the management of conditions,
   - recognising the potential expertise of individuals, family members and carers with genetic/genomic healthcare needs that develops over time and with experience.

Reproduced with permission from Kirk M, Tonkin E and Skirton H, *Fit for practice in the genetics/genomics era: a revised competence based framework with learning outcomes and practice indicators. A guide for nurse education and training*, NHS National Genetics Education and Development Centre, Copyright © 2011.

working with cancer patients, in primary, secondary and tertiary care. Analysis of the process of developing the competencies (Kirk, 2013) highlighted the critical importance of active nurse leadership which is demonstrated by changes to policy, education and practice.

Core learning outcomes in genetics for other non-genetics health professionals in the UK

Following extensive review of the genetics learning needs of GPs (Burke et al., 2005) and non-genetics specialist registrars (Burke et al., 2009), three key areas have been identified in the patient pathway where genetics has an impact on clinical practice: identification of patients, clinical management and communicating genetic information. In addition to the specific learning outcomes for these groups, learning outcomes have been developed generally for clinical practice in the UK, which apply to all clinicians. Table 2.1 summarises these competencies.

The core competencies and learning outcomes have been developed by The NHS National Genetics and Genomics Education Centre in consultation and collaboration with various groups of healthcare professionals and their representative or professional bodies. Full details of the competencies, learning outcomes and practice indicators, together with many educational resources such as patient stories, slides and lesson plans can be found at <http://www.geneticseducation.nhs.uk/for-healthcare-educators/learning-outcome> ('Supporting healthcare educators')

Table 2.1 Summary of the competencies for clinical practice in the UK

Clinical pathway	Core competencies
Identifying patients	Identify where genetics is relevant in your area of practice
	Identify individuals with or at risk of genetic conditions
	Gather multigenerational family history information
	Use multigenerational family history information to draw a pedigree
Clinical management	Recognise a mode of inheritance in a family
	Assess genetic risk
	Refer individuals to specialist sources of assistance in meeting their healthcare needs
	Order a genetic laboratory test
Communicating genetic information	Communicate genetic information to individuals, families and other healthcare staff

Adapted with permission from *I'm in clinical practice*, NHS National Genetics Education and Development Centre, Copyright © 2013, available from: <http://www.geneticseducation.nhs.uk/for-practitioners-62>

Core competencies for health professionals across Europe

Across Europe there is variation in the provision of genetic healthcare. The Education Committee of the European Society of Human Genetics (ESHG) in collaboration with the EuroGentest project agreed to establish a core set of competencies that could apply to all health professionals with the aim of helping individual countries to tailor their education and delivery of genetics services for the future. Three core sets of competencies have been developed: for health professionals working in the general setting, for specialist (non-genetic) health professionals and for specialists in genetics (Skirton et al., 2010). The core competencies can be found on the website for the ESHG and EuroGentest (<http://www.eurogentest.org>).

Summary

Identifying patients who may be at genetic risk, managing genetic aspects of healthcare and communicating genetic/genomic information will become increasingly important for all health professionals working with patients with and at risk of cancer as genetics/genomics becomes more integrated into mainstream medicine. The chapters in this section aim to provide the foundations for health professionals in cancer care to meet the competencies outlined in this introductory chapter.

References

American Society of Human Genetics 1975. Genetic counseling. *Am J Hum Genet* **27**: 240–242.

Baars MJ, Scherpbier AJ, Schuwirth LW, et al. 2005. Deficient knowledge of genetics relevant for daily practice among medical students nearing graduation. *Genet Med* **7**: 295–301.

Burke S, Stone A, Martyn M, Thomas H, Farndon P 2005. *Genetics education for GP registrars.* Birmingham: Centre for Education in Medical Genetics, University of Birmingham.

Burke S, Bedward J, Bennett C, Farndon P 2007. *The experiences and preferences of people receiving genetic information from healthcare professionals.* Birmingham: NHS National Genetics Education and Development Centre.

Burke S, Martyn M, Thomas H and Farndon P 2009. The development of core learning outcomes relevant to clinical practice: identifying priority areas for genetics education for non-genetics specialist registrars. *Clin Med* **9**: 49–52.

Genetics in Nursing and Midwifery Task and Finish Group 2011. *Genetics/genomics in nursing and midwifery: Task and Finish Group report to the Nursing and Midwifery Professional Advisory Board.* London: Department of Health.

Godino L and Skirton H 2012. A systematic review of nurses' knowledge of genetics. *J Nurs Educ Pract* **2**: 173–184.

Harper P 2004. *Practical genetic counselling.* London: Hodder Arnold.

Kirk M, McDonald K, Anstey S, Longley M 2003. *Fit for practice in the genetics era: a competence based education framework for nurses, midwives and health visitors.* Pontypridd: University of Glamorgan.

Kirk KM, Tonkin E, Skirton H 2011. *Fit for practice in the genetics/genomics era: a revised competence based education framework with learning outcomes and practice indicators. A guide for nurse education and training.* Birmingham: NHS National Genetics Education and Development Centre.

Kirk M, Tonkin E, Skirton H. 2014. An iterative consensus-building approach to revising genetics/genomics competency framework for nurse education in the UK. *J Adv Nurs* **70**: 405–420.

Nippert I, Harris HJ, Julian-Reynier C, et al. 2011. Confidence of primary care physicians in their ability to carry out basic medical genetic tasks. A European survey in five countries—Part 1. *J Commun Genet* **2**: 1–11.

Nursing and Midwifery Council 2010. *Standards for pre-registration nursing education*. London: Nursing and Midwifery Council.

Parker M and Lucassen A 2003. Concern for families and individuals in clinical genetics. *J Med Ethics* **29**: 70–73.

Scheuner MT, Sieverding P and Shekelle PG 2008. Delivery of genomic medicine for common chronic adult diseases: a systematic review. *J Am Med Assoc* **299**: 1320–1334.

Skirton H, Lewis C, Kent A and Coviello DA 2010. Genetic education and the challenge of genomic medicine: development of core competences to support preparation of health professionals in Europe. *Eur J Hum Genet* **18**: 972–977.

Skirton H, O'Connor A and Humphreys A 2012. Nurses' competence in genetics: a mixed method systematic review. *J Adv Nurs* **68**: 2387–2398.

Chapter 3

Taking a cancer family history and drawing a family tree

Emma Williams

Introduction to taking a cancer family history and drawing a family tree

This chapter will explain how to approach taking a cancer family history, the type of information required, how to elicit that information, what information is important and why and how to construct and notate a pedigree (family tree). Issues of confidentiality and sensitivity will be addressed as well as suggestions for helping patients to obtain missing information about their family history. The learning objectives for this chapter are:

- to be able to describe the principles of taking an accurate family history and the issues this raises for patients;
- to be able to draw an accurate family tree (pedigree);
- to be able to describe the symbols and notation needed to draw a family tree.

The importance of a cancer family pedigree

When assessing an individual's risk of developing cancer, it is essential to gather information about the family history. Drawing a family tree or pedigree using clear and consistent symbols provides a pictorial representation of the family relationships and those family members affected by cancer that is clearer than a just long written list of relatives (Harper, 2004). From this record of the family history, an accurate risk assessment can be made about whether the family history fits the pattern for a specific inherited cancer syndrome. This assists the health professional in determining the appropriate screening recommendations and deciding whether a referral to cancer genetics services is indicated.

The optimal setting for taking a family history may be in a designated family history clinic. However, with the financial and time pressures exerted on busy NHS clinicians, options may be limited and other settings may need to be explored. For example, it would be appropriate for a GP to enquire about family history when a patient seeks advice about breast screening or is experiencing a change in bowel habits, for a breast care nurse when a patient has investigations into a breast lump or a surgeon or oncologist after a patient has been diagnosed with a cancer. It is important not to assume that another clinician has already explored the family history.

Obtaining family history information in a family history clinic may be a stepwise process. A paper-based family history questionnaire might be sent to patients before the appointment. This is a useful tool as many patients do not know details about their wider family history, and it may encourage them to contact relatives to obtain or confirm information before attending a clinic appointment. Further information may be gathered or consolidated in a clinic setting or during a telephone consultation. It is helpful to set aside sufficient time to obtain or review this information, to explain to the patient that they will be asked a series of questions about their family history and why it is a useful part of their medical care.

A pedigree is a useful way of visualising a cancer family history and helps to build a rapport with the patient. It is important to obtain information about a minimum of three generations on both the maternal and paternal sides of the family, as this helps to demonstrate inheritance patterns. The pedigree can also provide a visual aid for discussing cancer predisposition and inheritance with the patient. The actual process of taking and drawing a family history can be used to elicit the patient's concerns about the family history assessment and give them an idea of their own risk.

There are various computer-based tools available for drawing pedigrees, for example Progeny and Clinical Pedigree. However, it can be just as time-consuming to construct the pedigree in digital form using such tools as it is to draw it by hand, and the computer program is unlikely be available in all clinic settings.

Standard pedigree nomenclature

Standardised symbols and nomenclature have been devised and agreed internationally (Schneider, 2002; Bennett et al., 2008). This ensures that health professionals throughout the world can understand and correctly interpret family history information (Skirton and Patch, 2002). These symbols are illustrated in Fig. 3.1.

When recording a cancer family history it is necessary to denote different types of cancer. Some clinicians use a quadrant system, while others use different types of shading. It is useful to provide a key with the pedigree to show which system is being used. It is also useful to distinguish between cancers that have been confirmed and those that have not, and to indicate any family members who have had a pre-malignant tumour or undergone genetic testing (Schneider, 2002).

How to take and record a family pedigree

Ideally, the following logical approach is used when enquiring about a family history:

1 The first step is to identify the patient whose family history is being documented (the proband) with an arrow (Fig. 3.2). It is important to enquire about the proband's medical history, regardless of whether or not they have a personal history of cancer; to document their date of birth, ethnicity, whether they have any history of benign or malignant tumours and their reproductive history. Other useful information to obtain includes: age at menarche, parity, age at first live birth, age at menopause, history of exogenous hormone use, exposure to carcinogens (e.g. tobacco use and radiation exposure), diet and

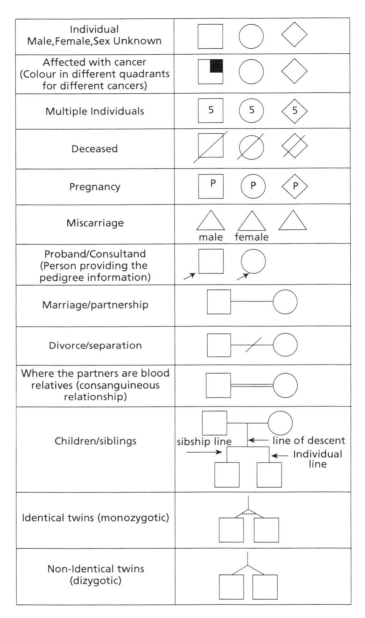

Figure 3.1 Standard pedigree nomenclature.

Adapted from Robin L. Bennett et al., Standardized human pedigree nomenclature: update and assessment of the recommendations of the National Society of Genetic Counselors, *Journal of Genetic Counseling*, Volume 17, Issue 5, pp. 424–433, Copyright © National Society of Genetic Counselors, Inc. 2008 with permission from Springer, Part of Springer Science and Business Media.

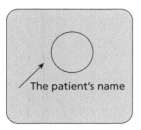

The health professional's name
Date pedigree drawn

Figure 3.2 The proband.

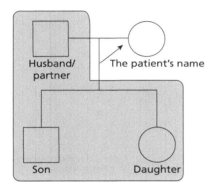

The health professional's name
Date pedigree drawn

Figure 3.3 The proband's immediate family.

lifestyle and surveillance. If the proband has a personal history of cancer, it is important to ask about the primary site of each cancer, age at diagnosis, histological type, ongoing treatment, bilaterality if applicable, previous cancers and past medical history.

2 Next, ask about the proband's partner and children, including how many children they have and whether all the children are with the same partner (Fig. 3.3). If the proband has children with more than one partner, add the second partner on the other side of the proband and draw their children beneath that couple (Fig. 3.4).

3 Step three is to gather information about each relative in turn, starting with the brothers and sisters of the proband, noting their ages and medical history and whether or not they have any children (Fig. 3.5). Continue to move systematically through the family, recording details about both parents. Starting with one parent, ask about their siblings and children. It is also important to ask about the proband's grandparents and their siblings. Many patients are concerned about the risk for their children, so it may also be useful to ask about the family members of their partner (Fig. 3.6). For family members who have been diagnosed with cancer, it is important to ask about the primary site of each cancer and age at diagnosis, where the relative was diagnosed and/or treated and any

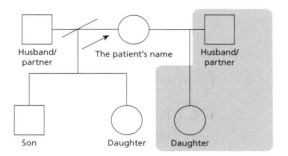

Figure 3.4 Adding different partners of the proband and their children.

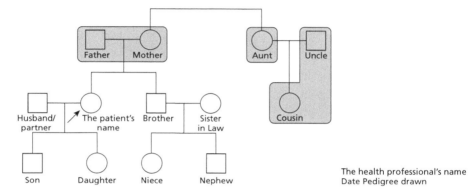

Figure 3.5 The proband's sibling(s) and their family.

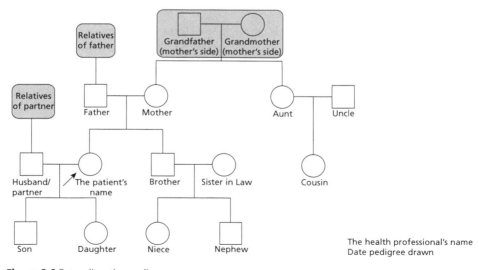

Figure 3.6 Extending the pedigree.

other significant health problems. For family members who have not been diagnosed with cancer, it is helpful to ask about their age and date of birth (if known), or (if deceased) age and cause of death, routine medical history, carcinogen exposure, organ removal/surgery and reproductive history. It is important to document any non-malignant findings that the proband mentions, such as macrocephaly or congenital hypertrophy of the retinal pigment epithelium (CHRPE) as these may be helpful in assessing the family history.

4 Finally, ask about the ethnicity of the grandparents on both sides of the family as this may influence decisions about screening and genetics referral. It is good practice to review the completed pedigree with each patient; they may have additional or revised information to include (Schneider, 2002). It may help to ask, 'Is there anyone else you think we haven't mentioned?' (Skirton and Patch, 2002). It is important to document the name of the proband providing the information, the health professional taking the information and the date the pedigree was drawn.

Confidentiality and family pedigrees

In the UK the Data Protection Act 1998 replaced and broadened the Data Protection Act 1984. The purpose of the Act is to protect the rights and privacy of individuals and to ensure that personal data are processed with the individual's knowledge wherever possible. The Act covers personal data relating to living individuals. Clear guidance is available on issues of consent and confidentiality in relation to genetic testing and sharing genetic information (RCP, 2011).

Under Schedule 3 of the Data Protection Act 1998, information shown on a family pedigree can generally be passed between health professionals without the consent of all those shown on the pedigree if this is necessary for medical purposes (including the purposes of preventative medicine, medical diagnosis, medical research, the provision of care and treatment and the management of healthcare services) (RCP, 2011).

When taking a family history it is important to explain that it may be used to determine the mode of inheritance of a disorder. It is also important to inform patients that the information may be shared with relatives if they seek advice and with other health professionals if necessary for the care of family members. Before information is shared it is good practice to review the information on the pedigree to ensure that only information relevant to the clinical purpose is released. It may be that full names of relatives and other potentially sensitive information do not need to be included (Schneider, 2002).

The Act also contains a requirement that data are processed 'fairly and lawfully'. Some suggest that this wording creates a statutory obligation to comply with the wider requirements of the common law on confidentiality. As yet there are no definite legal judgements resolving this point (RCP, 2011).

Psychosocial aspects of family history taking

The process of taking the family history can provide information about why a patient is seeking cancer risk assessment, reveal beliefs about the causes of cancer in the family and expose feelings and concerns about cancer experiences. Some patients find the construction of a pedigree to be a positive experience, giving them an opportunity to provide information, making them feel listened to and easing anxiety (McCarthy Veach et al., 2003). However, for others, discussing their family history can be emotionally distressing, bringing back memories of births, deaths and illnesses. Some patients find it difficult to discuss cancer and cancer-related illness, which can make the elicitation of information difficult (Schneider, 2002; Evans, 2006).

Challenges of family history taking

Managing sensitive issues that arise during family history taking can be challenging. For example, patients may disclose information about non-paternity, undisclosed adoptions, suicide, mental illness, termination of pregnancy, race/ethnicity and rape/incest. To maintain a constructive relationship with the patient, it is helpful to remain non-judgemental, be guided by the patient's responses and only explore issues further if they are relevant to the purpose of taking the family history. Some questions, such as about consanguinity, are difficult to ask. One way of approaching this would be to ask 'Is it possible that you and your spouse/partner have any relatives in common?'. If non-paternity is suspected, it may be helpful to have a discussion with the mother alone to clarify the situation, and determine whether her partner and other family members know, and if not whether she has thought about ways of informing them. In some cultures, personal or family medical information is viewed as confidential, and may therefore be withheld from healthcare professionals.

Confirming the family history

The patient's ability to recall information, the extent of communication within the family, geographical proximity and the closeness of relationships can affect the accuracy of the reported family history. The patient may have difficulty elucidating information, for example if relatives are deceased, there has been a breakdown in family relationships or because relatives do not talk about cancer diagnoses.

Where family history is uncertain, it may be necessary for the patient to try to confirm diagnoses. This can be time-consuming and emotionally difficult. Health professionals may suggest ways to help the patient obtain this information. For example, it may be easier for a patient to approach an aunt than to discuss a cancer diagnosis with a distant cousin (Schneider, 2002). If cancer was the cause of death it may be possible to obtain a death certificate. For a fee relatives can request this through the General Register Office, provided they have sufficient information to locate it (Schneider, 2002). In the UK, all cancer diagnoses from the 1970s onwards are recorded in cancer registries. If patients are referred to genetics services, cancer diagnoses may be confirmed via the cancer registry. In order to do this information will be required about the deceased relative such as the name, approximate date of birth, date of death and date and location of diagnosis.

Summary

Taking an accurate cancer family history and documenting a clear three-generation pedigree is important to facilitate cancer risk assessment. Taking a family history can raise difficult issues for patients and can be challenging for health professionals and it is important that this is approached with sensitivity and care.

The National Genetics and Genomics Education Centre website (<http:www.geneticseducation.nhs.uk/>) should be helpful for those health professionals whose role involves taking a family history and documenting a pedigree; this website lists specific competencies that could be incorporated into a job description as well as the knowledge and skills framework (KSF) outline. The relevant national occupational standards are: gather multigenerational information, use multigenerational family history information to draw a pedigree and recognise a mode of inheritance in a family.

References

Bennett RL, French KS, Resta RG, Doyle DL 2008. Standardised human pedigree nomenclature: update and assessment of the recommendation of the National Society of Genetic Counselors. *J Genet Counsel* **17**: 424–433.

Evans C 2006. An overview of genetic counselling. *Genetic counselling a psychological approach*, pp. 1–15. Cambridge: Cambridge University Press.

Harper P 2004. Genetic counselling an introduction. *Practical genetic counselling*, 6th edn, pp. 3–20. London: Hodder Arnold.

McCarthy Veach P, Leroy BS, Bartels DM 2003. *Facilitating the genetic counseling process: a practice manual.* New York: Springer.

RCP (Royal College of Physicians, Royal College of Pathologists and British Society for Human Genetics) 2011. *Consent and confidentiality in clinical genetic practice: guidance on genetic testing and sharing genetic information*, 2nd edn. Report of the Joint Committee on Medical Genetics. London: RCP, RCPath.

Schneider K 2002. Collection and interpretation of cancer histories. *Counseling about cancer: strategies for genetic counseling*, 2nd edn, pp. 221–266. New York: Wiley-Liss.

Skirton H and Patch C 2002. The family history. *Genetics for healthcare professionals: a lifestage approach*, pp. 13–30. Oxford: BIOS Scientific.

Chapter 4

Basic cancer genetics

Christine Patch

Introduction to basic cancer genetics

The first draft of the human genome was published in 2001 (International Human Genome Sequencing Consortium, 2001). With the exponential advances in technology and knowledge since then and the increasing importance of genomics in everyday healthcare, health professionals have to have an understanding of both the potential and the limitations of developments in genetics. The use of genetic technology is already moving from the confined area of medical genetics to almost every clinical specialty.

Increasing numbers of genetic factors underpinning the development of cancers are being discovered. The influence of genes on health and disease can be thought of as a continuum, with diseases caused by one major single gene mutation, such as Duchenne muscular dystrophy or Huntington disease, at one end and diseases with a major environmental component, such as infectious diseases, at the other end.

Cancers can be acquired or have an inherited component. In both cases the balance of the cell's machinery controlling growth or cell death is disturbed. This is due to an accumulation of genetic mutations. In this chapter basic aspects of genetics of relevance to cancer will be described and will provide a foundation for the following chapters. The learning objectives for this chapter are:

- to be able to discuss the structure and function of genes;
- to be able to describe the different mechanisms of inheritance of single gene disorders;
- to be able to describe the main modes of inheritance of cancer predisposition genes.

Cells, DNA, chromosomes and genes

Every cell in the body (apart from red blood cells which have no nucleus) carries within its nucleus a copy of the whole human genome. The genome is the total complement of DNA—the genes and all the non-coding sequences in between (Fig. 4.1).

DNA carries in coded form the information that directs the way in which the cell grows, develops and divides and controls the function of the biological systems of the body. It is usually present within the cell as two strands which are organised in the double helix that is now so familiar. The strands are formed from a backbone of sugars and are linked by paired bases. In DNA the bases are thymine (T), adenine (A), cytosine (C) and guanine (G). T and

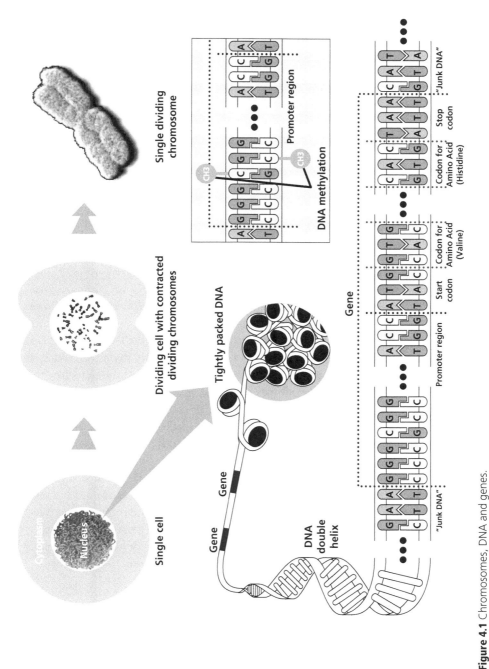

Figure 4.1 Chromosomes, DNA and genes.

A will always pair, as will C and G. This pairing means that the strands of DNA can copy themselves. The specific order of the bases provides the template for sequences of amino acids which are the building blocks of proteins. Each amino acid is coded for by a specific sequence of three bases (a codon).

The genome has portions (the genes) that code for specific amino acid sequences leading to the generation of proteins by the cellular machinery and also large portions of DNA sequence that does not appear to code for genes. There are various estimates as to the number of genes in the human genome, the most recent (from 2012) being about 20 500 protein-coding genes. The function of the remaining 97% of the genome is unclear and is sometimes described as 'junk' DNA. As more is being discovered it is becoming clear that this portion of the genome also has functional effects (The ENCODE Project Consortium, 2012).

Individual genes consist of sequences that provide the code for the amino acids that make up proteins. These coding sequences are called exons; the exons are interspersed with non-coding sequences called introns. There are also regulatory elements which can turn the gene on or off, allowing it to generate the code for the protein or stop it, and other sequences which can make the gene produce more or less protein (Fig. 4.2).

Within the nucleus of the cell, the DNA strand is organised into structures called chromosomes. Chromosomes can be seen by light microscopy in a dividing cell. A picture of the chromosomes is known as a karyotype and the normal human karyotype is 23 pairs of chromosomes—22 autosomes (numbered from 1 to 22) and a pair of sex chromosomes. Women have two identical sex chromosomes known as the X chromosomes and men have an X chromosome and a Y chromosome.

The way in which the DNA is packaged into chromosomes allows the DNA to be copied and passed on during cell division. There are two types of cell division. In mitosis, which is the type of cell division that happens constantly with the human body leading to growth, differentiation and repair, the chromosomes copy themselves before the cell divides and each new daughter cell has a full copy of each pair of chromosomes (i.e. 23 pairs of chromosomes). In meiosis, which is the type of cell division that happens during the formation of eggs and sperm, the chromosomes copy themselves but only one chromosome from each pair goes into the daughter cells, meaning that each sperm or ovum has one copy from each pair of chromosomes (i.e. 23 individual unpaired chromosomes). When fertilisation occurs, the cells of the resulting zygote will thus contain 23 pairs of chromosomes, but one copy of each chromosome will come from the maternal line and one from the paternal. Therefore, a child will inherit half of its genome from its mother and half from its father.

Our genes direct the growth, development and functioning of every bodily system and are the means by which these characteristics are passed from generation to generation.

Gene mutations

A gene mutation is a change in a gene's normal base pair sequence; some mutations are benign and cause no problems while others disrupt the production of the protein. There are different kinds of mutations, for example missense mutations which involve a change in a single base in

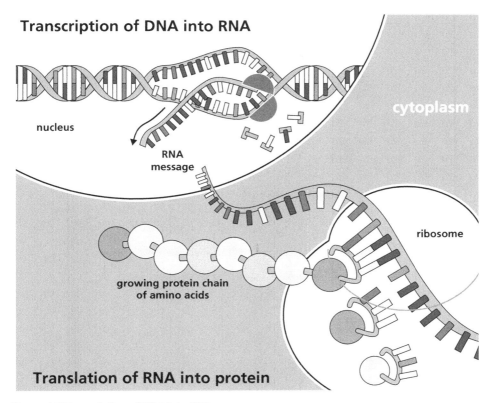

Figure 4.2 Transcription of DNA into RNA.
Reproduced with permission from Marcus Pembrey, *An introduction to the genetics and epigenetics of human disease*, Progress Educational Trust, London, UK, Copyright © 2012, available from <http://www.progress.org.uk/orgfiles/ZORGF000014/geneticsepigenetics.pdf>.

a codon. Missense mutations may be benign, because although there is a change in the codon, and thus the amino acid coded for, if the substituted amino acid is chemically very similar to the original then the properties of the protein may be unchanged. A change in a base may change the protein sequence and disrupt protein function or may introduce a stop codon that stops the protein being made. These changes would probably have functional consequences. An insertion or deletion of a single base may disrupt the reading sequence of the DNA so that it is completely scrambled and no protein is produced; a large insertion or deletion will also disrupt the protein so much that it is not produced. There may also be sequence changes in sequences of DNA that regulate how much or how little of a protein is produced. For more information on different types of mutations see Read and Donnai (2010).

Patterns of inheritance

Gregor Mendel, in his experiments with pea plants in the nineteenth century, is said to have demonstrated that some inherited characteristics are not caused by blending of the

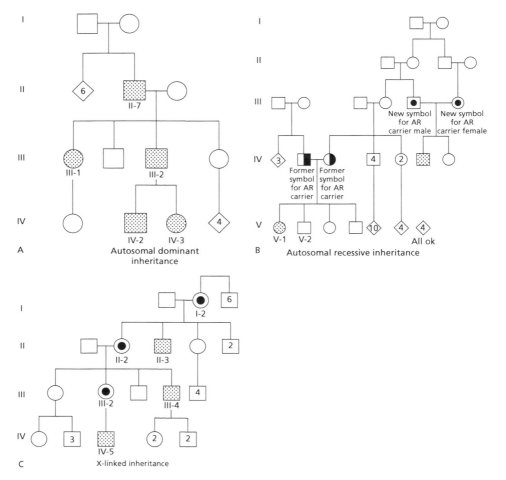

Figure 4.3 Mendelian patterns of inheritance (AR, autosomal recessive).

characteristics of the previous generations as previously thought but by distinct units of heredity—later termed genes (Fairbanks and Rytting, 2001).

The inheritance patterns of diseases in families that are caused by mutations in single genes are called Mendelian. Mendel's experiments demonstrated that genes come in pairs (one on each chromosome) and that if one characteristic is dominant and the other recessive the recessive characteristic will not be expressed unless both members of the gene pair are recessive. In diseases which are caused by mutations in recessive genes, the disease is only manifest when both copies of the gene are mutated. In diseases caused by dominantly inherited genes, only one copy needs to be mutated. The three commonly observed patterns of inheritance are X-linked recessive, autosomal recessive and autosomal dominant (Fig. 4.3).

X-linked recessive inheritance

If a gene is mutated on the X chromosome, the pattern of inheritance that is observed in the family is known as X-linked recessive. Since women have two X chromosomes and men have an X and a Y, a woman will have two copies of all her genes on the X chromosome. Providing only one copy of the gene has a mutation and one copy of the gene is sufficient to produce the protein, she will carry the faulty gene but will herself be unaffected by the condition or only slightly affected. If a man carries the faulty gene, he will develop the condition as he has no corresponding working gene on the Y chromosome. The features of X-linked inheritance that are observed in a family tree are affected males and carrier females, with none of the affected males having affected sons, i.e. there is no male to male transmission.

Autosomal recessive inheritance

The chromosomes other than the sex chromosomes are known as the autosomes. In recessively inherited conditions, in order for the disorder to occur an individual has to inherit two copies of the mutated gene, one from their mother and one from their father. The characteristics of recessive inheritance are that you tend to see the condition in only one generation and males and females are affected equally. As illustrated in Fig. 4.3 the chance of two carrier parents having an affected child is one in four.

Autosomal dominant inheritance

The most common pattern of inheritance in the inherited cancers is autosomal dominant. In autosomal dominantly inherited conditions it is sufficient to inherit one copy of the mutated gene. An individual with the faulty gene will have a high risk of developing the condition, for some diseases it is 100% and for others less. An individual with the faulty gene will have a 50% chance of passing it on to any of their offspring. The features of autosomal dominant inheritance that are observed in a family tree are transmission from generation to generation with males and females affected equally and male to male transmission. As mentioned, some dominantly inherited genetic conditions are not fully penetrant; that is, not all individuals who inherit the mutated gene will develop the condition. This feature of variable penetrance is relatively common in the inherited cancer syndromes. In addition, a mutated gene may have variable expression; that is, one individual may show some features of the condition whereas another with the same mutated gene may show different features. This is also a feature of some inherited cancer syndromes.

Genes and cancer

The following chapters will include more details on specific cancers; however it is important to understand that cancer, as stated in the first paragraph of this chapter, is, in the main, genetic in nature. An accumulation of genetic changes in a cell leads to unrestrained growth and divisions, inhibition of cell differentiation and loss of the normal cell destruction machinery. As the cancerous tumours grow in size they acquire new blood vessels which allow the tumours access to oxygen and nutrients. Eventually tumour cells invade surrounding tissues and spread to other areas of the body. In order for this process to happen there is normally a series of mutations, first in the original cell and then in the subsequent tumour. In families with an inherited cancer susceptibility, one of the mutations may be inherited, which puts the individual a number of steps along the pathway to developing cancer. Other mutations will be acquired by the cells. It takes time to accumulate all the gene mutations that may be necessary for a particular cancer to develop and this contributes towards explaining why the risk of cancer increases with age.

Oncogenes

Mutations in genes that promote cell growth (proto-oncogenes) can lead to uncontrolled cell growth; the mutated gene is known as an oncogene. An analogy that is sometimes used is that the oncogene acts as the accelerator, driving cell growth to occur faster and in a more uncontrolled way. At the cellular level, an oncogene acts in a dominant fashion. Having one copy of an oncogene is sufficient to promote tumour formation or growth. Mutations in proto-oncogenes are usually acquired; however, a rare cancer syndrome, multiple endocrine neoplasia type 2, is caused by inherited mutations in the *RET* proto-oncogene (Frank-Raue and Raue, 2009).

Tumour suppressor genes and the Knudson two-hit hypothesis

Tumour suppressor genes are normally present in our cells, and when they are working properly they control cell growth and the process of cell death (apoptosis). The analogy that is often used is that when working properly they can act as a brake. At the cell level they act in a recessive fashion. Both copies of a tumour suppressor gene have to be mutated for a change in cell growth and tumour development to occur.

Mutations in tumour suppressor genes can be inherited or acquired. This was described by Knudson (1971) in his two-hit hypothesis (Fig. 4.4). Knudson was interested in the genetic mechanism underlying a form of childhood cancer of the eyes called retinoblastoma. It was noted that this tumour could occur in one eye (unilateral) or both eyes (bilateral) and that children of individuals who developed the tumour could also develop the tumour. When he developed his hypothesis it was thought that the tumour could be caused by both inherited (germline) mutations and acquired mutations. Knudson carefully collected data on whether the tumour was bilateral or unilateral and whether it was hereditary or non-hereditary. The hypothesis that emerged was that retinoblastoma is caused when both copies of one specific gene, the retinoblastoma (*RB1*) gene, are mutated. He estimated that many people would acquire a mutation in a *RB1* gene over a lifetime and by chance some people would acquire two mutations. In families with an inherited mutation, all the retinal cells would have one mutated gene—the first hit. Cancer would only develop if the cell also acquired a second mutation in the working copy of the gene—the second hit. People who had an inherited mutation would tend to develop tumours earlier and would tend to develop the tumours in both eyes. However, if the cell never received a second hit then they would not develop a tumour but of course

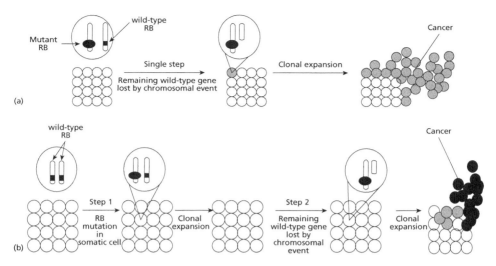

Figure 4.4 Knudson's two-hit hypothesis (RB, retinoblastoma).
Reproduced from Andrew Coop and Matthew J. Ellis, The genetics of inherited cancers, Fig. 1, p. 230, in DA Warrell et al. (ed.), *Oxford Textbook of Medicine,* Fourth Edition, Oxford University Press, Oxford, UK, Copyright © 2003, by permission of Oxford University Press.

could pass the mutated gene to their children who would then be at risk of developing retinoblastoma themselves.

At the cellular level the gene is acting as a recessive gene and the loss of function of the gene caused by both copies of the gene being mutated means that the tumour suppression activity of the gene is no longer in place. The cells can therefore grow and divide uncontrollably leading to the development of cancer. In 1986 the *RB1* gene was discovered and there are many other tumour suppressor genes acting in the same way that have been discovered since then (Knudson, 2001).

DNA repair genes

Every time a cell divides the DNA makes a copy of itself. During this copying process mistakes occur and these mistakes are repaired by proteins produced by genes called mismatch repair genes. If the mismatch repair genes are mutated then mistakes in the sequence of DNA will not be repaired. If these mistakes are in proto-oncogenes, causing them to act as oncogenes, or in tumour suppressor genes, leading to loss of function, then eventually this will lead to uncontrolled cell growth and tumour formation. There are other types of repair genes that repair the damage caused by mutagenic agents, such as large doses of radiation.

Mutations in mismatch repair genes can be acquired over time as a result of ageing or environmental agents but can also be inherited. At the cellular level DNA repair genes need both copies to be mutated and act as recessive genes. In families with an inherited mutation, a single mutation is inherited in a dominant fashion but the individual with the inherited mutation needs to acquire other mutations in order to develop cancer (Peltomäki, 2001).

Cancer is the result of a cascade of genetic changes. These changes may all be acquired but in some families there is an inherited mutation in one of the cancer susceptibility genes. In these families not all individuals will develop cancer since they too have to accumulate additional genetic changes at the cellular level. This is an explanation for the reduced penetrance seen in some families.

Genetic testing in cancer

Genetic testing in cancer may be done at the level of the tumour by analysing the gene mutations to determine treatment. This approach is in the early stages of development but is an active area of interest and research.

Genetic testing may be used in the inherited cancer syndromes to identify those family members who have inherited the susceptibility and may need extra screening or management to help ameliorate the effects of the initial gene mutation.

In genetic testing in families it is important to distinguish between diagnostic testing and predictive or pre-symptomatic testing. Diagnostic testing is performed when the individual with cancer is tested to identify if their cancer is caused by an inherited gene mutation. If the mutation is identified in the individual it is possible to offer at-risk family members without cancer pre-symptomatic or predictive testing. For the majority of the inherited cancer syndromes it is still necessary to identify a disease-causing mutation in the family by testing someone with cancer before a test can be offered to other members of the family. This is because the gene involved may be mutated in many different ways and the result in an unaffected person may be difficult to interpret.

There are a few situations where there are common mutations within a population and testing for those specific 'founder' mutations may give useful information. For example, in the breast/ovarian cancer susceptibility genes *BRCA1* and *BRCA2* there are common mutations in the population of Iceland and the Ashkenazi Jewish population, amongst others. It is thought that these mutations become common in isolated populations by chance. These mutations do not affect the ability to have children, so if by chance a few members of the original small population had the mutation it would spread throughout the population as it grew, providing it remained isolated. In the general population in the UK there has been so much population change over time that there are no founder mutations in these genes that are useful for testing.

References

Fairbanks DJ and Rytting B 2001. Mendelian controversies: a botanical and historical review. *Am J Bot* **88**: 737–752.

Frank-Raue K and Raue F 2009. Multiple endocrine neoplasia type 2 (MEN 2). *Eur J Cancer* **45** (Suppl. 1): 267–273.

International Human Genome Sequencing Consortium 2001. Initial sequencing and analysis of the human genome. *Nature* **409**: 860–921.

Knudson AG 1971. Mutation and cancer: statistical study of retinoblastoma. *Proc Natl Acad Sci USA* **68**: 820–823.

Knudson AG 2001. Two genetic hits (more or less) to cancer. *Nat Rev Cancer* **1**: 157–162.

Peltomäki P 2001. Deficient DNA mismatch repair: a common etiologic factor for colon cancer. *Hum Molec Genet* **10**: 735–740.

Pembrey M 2012. *An introduction to the genetics and epigenetics of human disease*. London: Progress Educational Trust. Available at: <http://www.progress.org.urluk/orgfiles/ZORGF000014/geneticsepigenetics.pdf>

Read AD and Donnai D 2010. *New clinical genetics*, 2nd edn. Oxford: Scion Publishing.

The ENCODE Project Consortium 2012. An integrated encyclopedia of DNA elements in the human genome. *Nature* **489**: 57–74.

Chapter 5

Cancer biology

Audrey Yandle

Introduction to cancer biology

Cancer is a term used for a cluster of diseases that arise from permanently altered cells with different rates of incidence, progression and outcomes but with a number of key biological similarities. Understanding the basic concepts that underpin the biology of cancer is essential for practitioners involved in supporting individuals either with cancer or with a cancer risk as these help to frame clinical approaches, treatment options and prognostic indicators. It can also facilitate communication on cancer-related issues between the practitioner and individuals with cancer or when supporting individuals facing important decisions about cancer screening or cancer treatment. Finally, the exponential growth in the amount of detailed cancer-related information readily available to patients and their families through a variety of sources can sometimes lead to confusion and anxiety and requires the support of healthcare practitioners confident in their own understanding of key cancer-related concepts.

Despite the clear heterogeneity of cancers seen in clinical practice, the cells that populate malignant tumours share some key characteristics; Hanahan and Weinberg (2000) refer to these as the 'hallmarks of cancer'. These characteristics include abnormal and sustained signalling to induce excessive cell proliferation, resistance to or loss of the normal regulators of proliferation, resistance to programmed cell death, the ability to induce angiogenesis, tissue invasion and metastasis and, ultimately, immortality of the cell line. Advances in cancer cell biology have identified that genome instability, cancer-associated inflammation, altered cell metabolism, a supportive and dynamic tumour microenvironment and a complex relationship with the immune system also contribute to the various mechanisms involved in cancer development and progression and to the behaviour of the cancer cell (Hanahan and Weinberg, 2011). Loss of cell differentiation, the process that turns an immature cell into a mature one with specific characteristics and functions, is another essential feature in cancer development and progression (Floor et al., 2012). The archetypal cancer cell exhibits all of these characteristics, but any one individual cancer cell in a tumour may exhibit only some of these 'hallmarks' at any one time and, since malignant tumours are dynamic and evolving entities, the characteristics expressed can alter markedly over time (Floor et al., 2012). Through the use of different strategies, all successful tumours will ultimately achieve uncontrolled growth and a high degree of cellular autonomy.

Although cancer tumours are thought to arise from a single abnormal cell, they eventually consist of a heterogeneous group of cells with mixed growth, survival and metastatic potential. The genetic instability inherent in cancer cells, the changing nature of the environment in and around the tumour, the exposure of cells to noxious substances, inconsistent or restricted access to oxygen and nutrients and the continuous generation of new tumour cells make possible the emergence of new clones with individual characteristics, different capabilities and altered survival advantages. This heterogeneity within the tumour population can limit the success of cancer treatments in the long term and can help to explain the changing behaviour of cancer cells over the life of a tumour.

Cancer-related genetic errors

Cancer arises out of innate and/or acquired genetic errors. Malignant cells are the product of permanent damage to DNA arising from mutations that confer a cluster of key growth and survival advantages alongside the loss of mechanisms that normally protect the genome's integrity, such as the systems that provide genomic stability and the surveillance mechanisms that detect and repair genetic damage. The genetic errors that are seen in cancer are not randomly distributed throughout the genome but are concentrated in the groups of genes that regulate cell growth and division, cell survival, cell death and DNA repair.

The abnormal genes that enhance cancer cell proliferation and survival are known as oncogenes and are generally characterised by increased expression. Mutations in these genes lead to the production of proteins with quantitatively or qualitatively different functions from their normal counterparts or the generation of new, abnormal proteins with novel functions. Multiple copies of oncogenes can often be seen in the cancer genome, resulting in enhanced expression of their gene products. By contrast, tumour suppressor genes are involved in the pathways that help to down-regulate cell proliferation and those that enhance cell death and repair. In cancer, there is a loss of function of tumour suppressor genes due to the loss of genes, the abnormal silencing of genes or through the inactivation of the gene product. Cancer generally develops as a consequence of an accumulation of errors to both oncogenes and tumour suppressor genes.

A number of controls exist to regulate gene expression; one important strategy is termed epigenetic regulation. Epigenetic regulation involves several processes including genomic imprinting, DNA methylation and histone modification (Feinberg and Tycko, 2004). Genomic imprinting refers to the partial or complete silencing of genes on either the maternal or paternal allele in a pre-determined way as part of the normal regulation of gene expression. Loss of appropriate imprinting can lead to over-expression or under-expression of the relevant gene. Methylation is a mechanism that silences genes in normal tissue cells; in cancer it is associated with hypomethylation of oncogenes and hypermethylation of tumour suppressor genes, leading to enhanced oncogene expression and loss of function of tumour suppressor genes. Histones are supporting structures with a number of functions that also participate in the regulation of gene expression and silencing. Alterations in these mechanisms also lead to abnormal expression or silencing (Phillips et al., 2001).

Cancer-associated genetic errors

As part of the chromosomal instability (CIN) of cancer, malignant cells typically contain structural and numerical changes to chromosomes and genes. The first common abnormality is the presence of aneuploidy, a term that refers to an abnormal number of chromosomes. The gain or loss of chromosomes can be commonly seen in cancer. Aneuploidy can occur as a consequence of the mis-segregation of chromosomes during mitosis and is known to occur relatively infrequently during normal cell cycling (Seigel and Amon, 2012). Normal cells that are no longer diploid (that do not have two sets of chromosomes) will generally either undergo apoptosis or be prevented from entering the cell cycle and become senescent. In the context of cancer it is possible that mis-segregation leading to aneuploidy occurs more frequently as a result of the disruption of the pathways that regulate key elements of mitosis, a final step in the cell cycle (Holland and Cleveland, 2012). Aneuploidy may also be an outcome of the stress response of a cancer cell or a short-term adaptation to some selective pressure (Holland and Cleveland, 2012; Seigel and Amon, 2012). Aneuploidy also appears to be associated with loss or inactivation of the p53 tumour suppressor family pathways, enabling the abnormal chromosome number to be tolerated and the cell to re-enter the cell cycle (Aylon and Oren, 2011). Due to its heterogeneity in cancer, it is not currently known if aneuploidy is part of the constellation of abnormal changes that generate cancer, a consequence of other changes that occur during cancer development or both (Hanahan and Weinberg, 2011; Seigel and Amon, 2012). It is thought that aneuploidy may lead to a subsequent increase in mutations, increased oncogene function and decreased tumour suppressor gene function and that it may contribute to the overall genomic instability seen in cancer (Holland and Cleveland, 2012).

Other important cancer-associated somatic mutations include the translocation of genetic information from one chromosome to another, loss of portions of chromosomes, rearrangements of genes within a chromosome and the amplification of genes and proteins through the acquisition of multiple gene copy numbers. Changes in the DNA sequences themselves arise through substitution, deletion or insertion of one or more DNA bases, resulting in changes in the reading frames and the production of proteins with altered function or the inactivation of the gene or protein. Sometimes new DNA material, such as viral DNA, can be incorporated into the genome. In cancer these changes are found in both oncogenes and tumour suppressor genes and can alter a range of pathways including those involved in cell cycling, proliferation-associated cell signalling, programmed cell death, cell survival and the cell's communication with the surrounding microenvironment.

Cell proliferation and the cell cycle

Appropriate cell proliferation enables growth and development, the replacement of damaged, old or dead cells, tissue repair and the maintenance of tissue homeostasis. Cell replication is achieved via the cell cycle, a carefully orchestrated process that leads to the division of one cell into two daughter cells. This involves a tightly regulated series of steps that undertakes the accurate transcribing of the cell's genetic information so as to provide

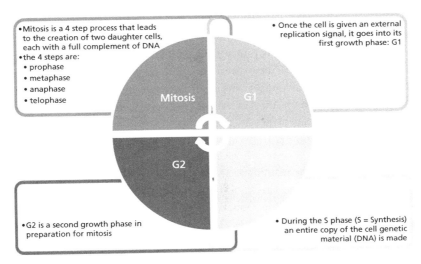

- Mitosis is a 4 step process that leads to the creation of two daughter cells, each with a full complement of DNA
- the 4 steps are:
  - prophase
  - metaphase
  - anaphase
  - telophase

Mitosis

G1

- Once the cell is given an external replication signal, it goes into its first growth phase: G1

G2

- G2 is a second growth phase in preparation for mitosis

- During the S phase (S = Synthesis) an entire copy of the cell genetic material (DNA) is made

Figure 5.1 The cell cycle.

each new cell with a complete set of chromosomes/genes as well as the requisite cellular components for normal cell function. The cell cycle is characterised by a number of distinct steps, shown in Fig. 5.1.

Normal cell replication is initiated when there is a sufficient increase in the concentration of growth factors in the cell's microenvironment followed by their binding to receptors on the cell membrane. Once bound, these factors activate a signalling cascade within the cell, leading to the initiation of the steps that ultimately end in cell division. The signalling cascade progresses through the cell's cytoplasm via molecules referred to as signal transducers, or second messengers, eventually passing into the nucleus via specific nuclear proteins, called transcription factors, involved in gene expression. Transcription factors mediate the access and translation of genetic information contained within DNA.

The cell replication process involves four distinct phases. The first phase is known as Gap_1 or G_1. During this phase the cell grows in size and manufactures proteins, nucleic acids and other necessary cellular building blocks and prepares for DNA replication. The S (synthesis) phase involves the faithful copying of the cell's genetic information. As this process is not without some errors, mechanisms are initiated to identify and undertake any necessary repairs to the genome and its associated structures. Phase G_2 enables final repairs to the DNA and the chromatin condenses into chromosomes. The final phase, mitosis (M), ensures the appropriate segregation of chromosomes to each daughter cell prior to the final separation process (cytokinesis). The cell will then either enter into a non-cycling phase (G_0) or, if required, will start the cycling process once again.

Regulation of the cell cycle

A number of important regulatory proteins are responsible for the cell's progression through the cell cycle; these proteins can either maintain or inhibit the cycling process.

Three main groups of proteins involved in this process are the cyclin-dependent kinases (CDKs), cyclins and cyclin-dependent kinase inhibitors (CDKIs). CDKs permit a cell to progress through the cycle by activating other key proteins and are, as their name suggests, cyclin dependent; that is they require sufficient levels of appropriate cyclins for activation. When cyclin levels drop, the kinases once again become inactive. In order to effectively regulate the process, different cyclin-activated CDKs peak and trough in a coordinated manner through the different stages of the cell cycle. CDKs are responsible for activating a number of proteins, including those involved in DNA replication and mitosis. CDKIs regulate CDKs and cyclins in order to prevent perpetual or inappropriate cycling.

Normally, the cell must go through specific checkpoints in order to complete the replication and division process. These checkpoints provide important safety mechanisms so that cells that are no longer required to replicate or those that have not completed each step correctly can be stopped prior to mitosis. The first restriction point occurs between the G_1 and S phase of the cycle; at this point, if environmental conditions are not suitable for cell division, if the cell is no longer required to divide or if DNA damage is detected, there will be CDKI-mediated cell cycle arrest. Additionally, in order to pass through the checkpoint, the cell must overcome the blocking influence of the tumour suppressor retinoblastoma (*RB*) gene.

In the presence of cellular or DNA damage, CDKIs also prevent progress from G_2 to M (restriction point 2). The identification of DNA damage during the cell cycle can also activate the p53 gene family, key tumour suppressor genes, inducing either DNA repair or cell death. Assessment of DNA damage and repair takes place at various points of the cell cycle and involves a number of strategies that ensure both the fidelity of genetic information between the cell generations and the structural integrity of the genome and its supporting structures, all of which are essential for long-term genetic stability.

Final checkpoints are activated during the spindle-forming and mitosis stages of the cycle, ensuring the appropriate segregation of chromosomes to the daughter cells, promoting the generation of diploid cells and preventing aneuploidy. These checkpoints also involve a number of tumour suppressor genes including *BRCA1* and *BRCA2*, mutated versions of which are associated with breast and ovarian cancers (Deng and Brodie, 2000). Important cell cycle alterations in cancer are the silencing of the *RB* gene, deregulation of CDKs in favour of cycling and over-expression of an important oncogene, *Myc*, a key controller of the cell cycle and proliferation (Evan and Vousden, 2001).

Cell proliferation in cancer

The first fundamental characteristic of cancer is its proliferative potential. Unlike normal cells, which carefully control and restrict proliferation in order to maintain tissue homeostasis, cancer cells develop strategies that enable them to gain control of their proliferative capacity. The loss of key proliferation-associated restrictions both enables the continuous and exponential growth of cell numbers, leading to tumour development, and permits the local invasion of tissue by cancer cells, a process that in normal cell and tissue physiology is prevented by a complex system of locally produced signalling factors and cell to cell interactions (King and Robins, 2006). The loss of processes such as density-dependent inhibition, contact inhibition and anchorage dependence means that cancer cells do not stop proliferation once the tissue reaches a specific density or when cells come into contact with one another. In addition, cancer cells appear to be able to grow and divide without attachment to the supporting structures in the microenvironment.

Important signalling pathways are commonly altered in cancer as a result of oncogene expression. Oncogenes can abnormally code for growth factors such as platelet-derived growth factor (PDGF) and transforming growth factor-α (TGFα). The presence of their cognate receptors on the cancer cell then leads to an autonomous growth loop. Amplification of oncogenes can also lead to over-expression of cell surface growth factor receptors, leading to cell growth in the context of lower concentrations of growth factor. Alternatively, growth factor receptors on the cancer cell surface, such as receptor kinases, can be constitutively activated and therefore do not require the presence of growth factors for signalling. Because they are abnormally activated, these receptors permit the relevant intracellular signalling molecules to be activated, resulting in proliferation signals being sent further down the signalling pathway, ultimately reaching the nucleus.

Cytoplasmic proteins that make up the signalling pathways from the cell surface to the nucleus can themselves be permanently altered into their activated form, leading once again to continuous proliferation signals in the malignant cell. Examples of these pathway signal transducers include the ras, abl and raf proteins. Within the nucleus, transcription factors are fundamental to gene expression as they recognise and bind to specific parts of the gene and recruit RNA polymerase for gene transcription. Deregulation of this part of the pathway will lead to over-expression of oncogenes or reduced expression of tumour suppressor genes.

Cell senescence

Most cells can only undertake a limited number of cell divisions; the term cell senescence refers to the point at which a cell is still able to undertake its normal functions but is no longer able to divide. Cell senescence is important in maintaining the integrity of the cell's genome and is associated with DNA 'tails', referred to as telomeres. Telomeres are repetitions of specific DNA sequences located at the end of chromosomes that serve to indicate where the chromosomes end to prevent them from fusing together during the replication process. Telomeres are also essential for the complete replication of the DNA sequences near the ends of chromosomes, preventing the loss of genetic information. The telomere tails progressively shorten during repeated cell cycling and eventually become too short for safe DNA replication, leading to DNA damage signalling, checkpoint activation and p53-associated cell senescence (Xu et al., 2013). Further replication in the context of short telomeres leads a 'telomere crisis', genomic instability and, generally, cell death (Artandi and DePinho, 2010).

Most differentiated somatic cells are not able to access the necessary instructions to extend shortened telomeres. However, stem cells, cells with self-renewal capacity, are able to produce telomerase, an enzyme that maintains telomere length, enabling the stem cell to divide indefinitely. The ability of normal stem cells to maintain telomere length is important for survival and health; for example, haematopoietic stem cells are the source for production of blood and immune system cells. Telomerase helps to ensure that these stem cells are able to sustain their proliferative capacity so as to meet the requirement for daily production of blood cells throughout the lifespan of the organism. In cancer, continuous proliferation eventually leads to a 'telomere crisis'; however, some malignant cells appear to emerge from this crisis with the capacity to produce telomerase, enabling continued cell proliferation in the context of an unstable genome (Xu et al., 2013).

Cell death

A number of mechanisms can lead to cell death. Necrotic cell death, often an outcome of cellular injury, leads to the disruption of the cell membrane, the breakdown of organelles and the release of cellular debris in the extracellular environment and can activate the inflammatory response. Apoptosis, or programmed cell death, is a controlled, tissue-sparing strategy for the destruction and removal of old, abnormal or injured cells and cells that are no longer required. A number of key apoptotic pathways can be initiated via signals generated either outside the cell or within the cell itself. Cell surface receptors, known as death receptors, are able to detect extracellular death signals and initiate apoptotic pathways within the cell. DNA damage, cell stress and hypoxia can activate the p53 pathway that, in turn, is able to activate an internal apoptotic pathway.

Mitochondria play an important role in apoptosis. They produce pro- and anti-apoptotic proteins such as Bcl-2 and BAX; the balance between cell survival or destruction is, in part, mediated by the balance in the activation of these proteins (King and Robins, 2006). A number of key proteolytic cellular enzymes, known as caspases, are also involved in the apoptotic pathways; these enzymes can be either self-activated or activated by other enzymes. Caspases can inactivate molecules that function to protect the cell from apoptosis, such as members of the Bcl-2 family, prevent DNA replication, disassemble organelles, cut the cell off from neighbouring cells and mark the cell for phagocytosis by immune cells (Phillips et al., 2001). Mitochondria are able to release pro-apoptotic caspase-activating molecules, such as cytochrome c, whereas Bcl-2 prevents its release. The activation of the different apoptotic pathways is, by necessity, a tightly regulated process. Bcl-2 and other related proteins protect the cell from apoptosis and are therefore key regulators of programmed cell death; in cancer, Bcl-2 is often over-expressed (Evan and Vousden, 2001). Additionally, a reduction in death signals or in the number of death receptors or the increased expression of other proteins that inhibit apoptosis confer an important survival advantage to malignant cells (Wong, 2011).

Angiogenesis

A good blood supply is essential for normal cell function, enabling oxygen and nutrients to be delivered to the cell and removing the waste products of cell metabolism. Cancer cells are often metabolically highly active and therefore require a substantive blood supply to meet their needs. Although normally the formation of blood vessels is only instituted in response to a specific need, such as in wound healing, and is a carefully controlled process, in the context of malignancy an 'angiogenic switch' is turned on early in the process of cancer development and subsequently remains active, sprouting new vasculature to feed and support the growing tumour (Baeriswyl and Christofori, 2009). This ongoing angiogenesis is instigated and maintained by the cancer cells themselves, through the manufacture of specific signalling molecules that control the angiogenic process. In particular, vascular endothelial growth factor-A (VEGF-A) and fibroblast growth factor (FGF) are associated with the angiogenesis of cancer (Baeriswyl and Christofori, 2009). In addition, cells of the innate immune system, such as macrophages and mast cells amongst others, also appear to support tumour-associated angiogenesis (Chung and Ferrara, 2011). Cellular hypoxia, inflammatory signals and the action of oncogenes can also act as drivers of the process; however, the resulting blood vessels are often abnormal and distorted (Hanahan and Weinberg, 2011). These abnormal vessels also tend to be friable and leaky and can result in abnormal bleeding, a common cancer-associated sign.

Hypoxia

Oxygenation in tumour environments can fluctuate markedly, and cancer cells can therefore be subjected to hypoxic episodes. Increased oxygen consumption relative to the available oxygen, insufficient or abnormal intra-tumoural vasculature and fluctuations in perfusion may all contribute to cancer cell hypoxia. Hypoxia-inducible factors (HIFs) are transcription factors that assist the cell to adapt to low levels of oxygen by promoting energy production via the glycolytic pathway and through enhanced oncogene (*cMYC*) activity (Shay and Simon, 2012). Hypoxia also induces the presence of tumour-associated macrophages, and HIFs, in turn, may support these immune cells to participate in tumour progression (Shay and Simon, 2012). The cancer cell's hypoxic response also leads to protection from cell death and enhanced signalling for the production of VEGF to increase angiogenesis (Baeriswyl and Christofori, 2009). Hypoxia in the cancer cell can lead to increased gene mutations and to reduced DNA repair, contributing to genetic instability (Bristow and Hill, 2008), and may therefore contribute to the emergence of tumour cells with enhanced metastatic and/or growth and/or survival capabilities.

Invasion and metastasis

An important feature of cancer cells is their ability to invade surrounding tissue and, ultimately, to travel to distant organs to establish new malignant colonies. Only some malignant cells will possess all of the requisite characteristics for migration, immune escape and the ability to seed and home on target organs. Malignant cells appear to achieve this 'cellular freedom' by using key elements of the body's usual mechanisms for cell migration, a normal process during embryonic development and in wound healing (Friedl and Gilmour, 2009). Reduced adhesion to neighbouring cells or to the extracellular matrix, reduced anchorage dependence and contact inhibition all support the cancer cell's capacity for mobility. There is an essential imbalance between the pro-adhesion signals and molecules, which maintain tissue cells in their place and therefore ensure the preservation of normal tissue architecture, and those which encourage cell migration. One such pro-adhesion molecule, E-cadherin, key to normal cell-to-cell adhesion, is, in cancer, often associated with down-regulation or deactivation (Friedl and Gilmour, 2009). Cancer cells also often produce specific factors that can directly facilitate migration and also increase the cell's resistance to apoptosis (Lu et al., 2012).

As both invasion and metastasis are complex processes that pose a number of challenges to the cancer cell, successful expansion or escape can also be achieved through the recruitment of other cells that then either offer general support or directly contribute to the process. For example, the tumour microenvironment is important in that it can either enable or inhibit tumour growth and escape. Stromal cells, those cells that function to support the tumour environment, are in regular communication with the malignant cells and, in response to signals from the cancer cells, can stimulate the malignant cells to invade neighbouring tissue. In contrast, the stroma can also potentially serve to inhibit invasion, depending on the nature of the signals it produces (Sleeman et al., 2012). Cancer cells can also recruit help from immune/inflammatory cells, such as macrophages, that are able to produce enzymes to break down the cellular matrix that constrains the malignant cells, enabling invasion (Pollard, 2004). In addition, immune cells may aid cancer cells to intravasate into the lymphatic or circulatory system, providing an important initial step to ultimate metastatic dissemination (Pollard, 2004).

Tumour immunology

The relationship between cancer and the immune system starts at the inception of cancer. It is hypothesised that abnormal cells are potential targets for destruction by cells of the immune system as part of normal immune surveillance; however, cancer cells appear to evade destruction via a number of possible mechanisms. Immune tolerance of the malignant cell can be a result of naturally low tumour cell immunogenicity and/or the absence of co-stimulatory signal production by the cancer cell (Murphy, 2011). Additionally, a process called immune editing may contribute to cancer's escape from immune regulation through the ongoing destruction of abnormal cells recognised by the immune system and the survival of cancer cells expressing antigens that are poorly recognised by the immune system. Eventually, a critical number of viable cancer cells that do not express antigens capable of inducing a meaningful immune response is reached, enabling the tumour to grow unchecked (Schreiber et al., 2011).

Established tumours commonly contain a range of immune cells; different types of immune cells can be found in distinct parts of the tumour and the surrounding tissue and amongst these are cells that are thought to specifically suppress immune responses in tumours (Murphy, 2011). Cancer cells additionally appear to manipulate their immune environment through the release of pro-inflammatory and other cytokines that ensure continued suppression of immune responses directed at cancer cells. Particular subgroups of immune cells also appear to be influential in ensuring the survival of the cancer cells and the development of metastases (Pollard, 2004). Cancer cells, immune cells and the components of the tumour's extra-cellular matrix engage in interactions that can lead to either tumour suppression or tumour progression. The aberrant behaviour of cancer cells is thought to be, in part, facilitated by the dynamic and complex interactions of the malignant cells with their immediate environment (Bissell and Radiski, 2001; Lu et al., 2012), adding a further dimension to the complex nature of the biology of cancer.

References

Artandi SE and DePinho RA 2010. Telomeres and telomerase in cancer. *Carcinogenesis* **31**: 9–18.

Aylon Y and Oren M 2011. p53: guardian of ploidy. *Mol Oncol* **5**: 315–323.

Baeriswyl V and Christofori G 2009. The angiogenic switch in carcinogenesis. *Semin Cancer Biol* **19**: 329–337.

Bissell MJ and Radiski D 2001. Putting tumours in context. *Nat Rev Cancer* **1**: 46–54.

Bristow RG and Hill RP 2008. Hypoxia, DNA repair and genetic instability. *Nat Rev Cancer* **8**: 180–192.

Carson DA and Lois A 1999. Cancer progression and p53. *Lancet* **346**: 1009–1011.

Chung AS and Ferrara N 2011. Developmental and pathological angiogenesis. *Ann Rev Cell Develop Biol* **27**: 563–584.

Deng C and Brodie SG 2000. Roles of BRCA1 and its interacting proteins. *BioEssays* **22**: 728–737.

Evan GI and Vousden KH 2001. Proliferation, cell cycle and apoptosis in cancer. *Nature* **411**: 342–348.

Feinberg AP and Tycko B 2004. The history of cancer epigenetics. *Nat Rev Cancer* **4**: 143–153.

Finn OJ 2012. Immuno-oncology: understanding the function and dysfunction of the immune system in cancer. *Ann Oncol* **23** (Suppl. 8): viii6–viii9.

Floor S, Dumont JE, Maenhaut C, Raspe E 2012. Hallmarks of cancer: of all cancer cells, all of the time? *Trends Mol Med* **18**: 509–515.

Fridman WH, Pages F, Sautes-Fridman C, Galon J 2012. The immune contexture in human tumours: impact on clinical outcomes. *Nat Rev Cancer* **12**: 298–306.

Friedl P and Gilmour D 2009. Collective cell migration in morphogenesis, regeneration and cancer. *Nat Rev Mol Cell Biol* **10**: 445–457.

Hanahan D and Weinberg RA 2000. Hallmarks of cancer. *Cell* **100**: 57–70.

Hanahan D and Weinberg RA 2011. Hallmarks of cancer: the next generation. *Cell* **144**: 646–672.

Holland AJ and Cleveland DW 2012. Losing balance: the origin and impact of aneuploidy in cancer. *EMBO Rep* **13**: 501–514.

King RJB and Robins MW 2006. *Cancer biology*, 3rd edn. Harlow: Pearson Education.

Lu P, Weaver V, Werb Z 2012. The extra-cellular matrix: a dynamic niche in cancer progression. *J Cell Biol* **196**: 395–406.

Murphy K 2011. *Janeway's immunobiology*, 8th edn. New York: Garland Science.

Phillips J, Murray P, Kirk P 2001. *Biology of disease*, 2nd edn. Oxford: Blackwell Science.

Pollard J 2004. Tumour-educated macrophages promote tumour progression and metastasis. *Nat Rev Cancer* **4**: 71–78.

Schreiber RD, Old LJ, Smyth MJ 2011. Cancer immunoediting: integrating immunity's roles in cancer suppression and promotion. *Science* **331**: 1565–1570.

Seigel JJ and Amon A 2012. New insights into the troubles of aneuploidy. *Ann Rev Cell Develop Biol* **28**: 189–214.

Shay JES and Simon MC 2012. Hypoxia-inducible factors: crosstalk between inflammation and metabolism. *Semin Cell Develop Biol* **23**: 389–394.

Sleeman J, Christofori G, Fodde R, et al. 2012. Concepts of metastasis in flux: the stromal progression model. *Semin Cancer Biol* **22**: 174–186.

Stratton MR 2011. Exploring the genomes of cancer cells: progress and promise. *Science* **331**: 1553–1558.

Weaver BA and Cleveland DW 2006. Does aneuploidy cause cancer? *Curr Opin Cell Biol* **18**: 658–667.

Wong RSY 2011 Apoptosis in cancer: from pathogenesis to treatment. *J Exp Clin Cancer Res* **30**: 2–14.

Xu L, Li S, Stohr BA 2013. The role of telomere biology in cancer. *Ann Rev Pathol: Mech Dis* **8**: 49–78.

Chapter 6

Cancer genetics: the basics. Summary

Lorraine Robinson and Patricia Webb

Introduction to section 2 summary

The chapters in Section 2 introduce the fundamentals of cancer genetics—the important foundations on which understanding and principles of practice are based. It is essential that the knowledge and tenets from this section underpin clinical practice in cancer care and interactions with individuals and their families about cancer family history and genetics.

Chapter 2. Cancer genetics: the basics. Introduction

Chapter 2 offers an overview of the current knowledge required by healthcare professionals and outlines the competencies for practice.

Guided activities for Chapter 2

◆ Non-directiveness is a central ethos of genetic counselling; think about what this means and why it is important in the context of cancer genetics. Reflect on situations in your current practice when you implement this approach and identify how this might apply in your own practice when discussing issues around cancer genetic with patients.

◆ Review the competencies established by the NHS National Genetics and Genomics Education Centre (<http://www.geneticseducation.nhs.uk/for-healthcare-educators/learning-outcome>). Identify your confidence and knowledge in relation to the competencies. It may be helpful to do this with a colleague to establish not only your strengths and areas for development but also those of your service.

◆ One of the key competencies challenging healthcare professionals is identifying individuals with, or at risk of, genetic conditions. Mapping the patient journey is a vital step in accommodating innovation and change in practice as set out by the NHS Institute for Innovation and Improvement in 2012. A useful strategy involves either mapping the journey of your last patient, noting critical points, opportunities that were used or missed to discuss genetics, etc., or mapping the experience of your last 10 patients to identify the main issues, looking particularly for occasions to raise awareness, offer cancer genetics information and identify individuals at risk.

Further resources for Chapter 2

A series of articles in the *Nursing Standard* based around the genetics education framework for nurses. Some articles published to December 2013 are:

Kirk M 2013 Introduction to genetics and genomics: a revised framework for nurses. *Nursing Standard* 28(8): 37–41.
Kirk M, Marshallsay M 2013. Providing nursing care and support to individuals and families with genetic/genomic healthcare needs. *Nursing Standard* 28(16): 39–46.
Tonkin E, Skirton H 2013. The role of genetic/genomic factors in health, illness and care provision. *Nursing Standard* 28(12): 39–46.

See also:

Elwyn G, Gray J, Clarke A 2000. Shared decision making and non-directiveness in genetic counselling. *J Med Genet* 37: 135–138.

Chapter 3. Taking a family history and drawing a family tree

Chapter 3 illustrates the approach, procedures and techniques for taking a family history and drawing a family tree alongside an analysis of issues relating to confidentiality. One of the significant messages of this chapter centres on familiarity and practice in order to develop competence and confidence.

Guided activities for Chapter 3

◆ Access the paper by Bennett et al. (2008) and acquaint yourself with the notation. Fluency and confidence will evolve with practice; regularly drawing and reviewing family trees with colleagues will therefore be helpful.

◆ Read the guidelines of the British Society for Genetic Medicine on consent and confidentiality in genetic testing at <http://www.bsgm.org.uk/media/678746/consent_and_confidentiality_2011.pdf>.

Use the scenarios therein to discuss and identify with colleagues the critical areas within your own setting.

◆ How would you explain to an individual the positive and negative psychosocial aspects of discussing cancer family history?

Further resources for Chapter 3

Jacobs C, Patch C 2013. Identifying individuals who might benefit from genetic services and information. *Nursing Standard* 28(9): 37–42.

Chapter 4. Basic cancer genetics

The key points from Chapter 4 are:

◆ Cancer is a disease caused by the accumulation of genetic mutations in cells.

◆ Mutations may be acquired or inherited.

- Oncogenes promote cell growth.
- Tumour suppressor genes control cell growth and apoptosis.
- Mismatch repair genes repair breaks in DNA.
- Mutations in oncogenes, tumour suppressor genes and mismatch repair genes lead to disruption of the normal mechanisms regulating cell growth, death and differentiation:
- In the inherited cancer syndromes the individual has an increased risk of developing cancer which may occur at a younger age.
- The most common pattern of inheritance in the cancer syndromes is autosomal dominant but further mutations are required before cancer develops in any particular tissue.
- The Knudson two-hit hypothesis explains how both copies of a tumour suppressor gene at the cellular level need to be inactivated before cancer develops and is relevant to many cancers.
- Genetic testing may be used at the level of the tumour to inform treatment decision or in inherited cancer susceptibility syndromes to provide information and tailor screening and prevention strategies.

Guided activities for Chapter 4

- How, for a patient and their family, would you summarise the relationship between cancer and genetics?
- Over the next 2 to 4 weeks take an in-depth look at the coverage about cancer genetics in newspapers, websites, TV and radio programmes, particularly soaps. What message about genetics is being portrayed and what impact might this have on your patients? If there is no coverage why might that be?

Further resources for Chapter 4

National Cancer Institute. *Understanding cancer series*. Available at: <http://www.cancer. gov/cancertopics/understandingcancer>.
Read A and Donnai D 2010. *New clinical genetics*, 2nd edn. Oxford: Scion Publishing.
Skirton H and Patch C 2009. *Genetics for the health sciences*. Oxford: Scion Publishing.
Strachan T and Read A 2010. *Human molecular genetics*, 4th edn. New York: Garland Science.

Chapter 5. Cancer biology

The key points from Chapter 5 are:

- Cancer arises from a range of genetic mutations involved in cell proliferation, survival and death, resulting in a group of cells with distinct advantages over their normal counterparts and with reduced controls over their behaviour.
- Oncogenes enhance proliferation and survival and are amplified in cancer, whereas tumour suppressor genes restrict proliferation and enhance cell death and are silenced or absent in cancer. In cancer, both types of genes are altered.

- Cancer cells arise from a single altered cell but develop new characteristics and behaviours, meaning that tumours contain heterogeneous groups of cells.
- The 'hallmarks of cancer' are the key characteristics of malignancies.
- Tumours have complex and dynamic relationships with their environment and with cells of the immune system—these relationships are integral to cancer development and progression.
- Metastasis is an important step in tumour progression, indicating a high degree of autonomy of cancer cells, and is associated with resistance to treatment and to poorer outcomes.

Guided activities for Chapter 5

- How would you describe the difference between inherited and acquired genetic mutations?
- Consolidate by viewing the videos on the following sites which offer a visual representation of the key issues: <http://www.cancerquest.org/cancer-biology-animations. html> or <http://www.insidecancer.org/>.

Further resources for Chapter 5

Finn OJ 2012. Immuno-oncology: understanding the function and dysfunction of the immune system in cancer. *Ann Oncol* 23 (Suppl. 8): viii6–viii9.

Floor S, Dumont JE, Maenhaut C, Raspe E 2012. Hallmarks of cancer: of all cancer cells, all of the time? *Trends Molec Med* 18: 509–515.

Harrington KJ 2007. The biology of cancer. *Medicine* 36: 1–4.

King RJB and Robins MW 2006. *Cancer biology*, 3rd edn. Harlow: Pearson Education.

Schreiber RD, Ool LJ, Smyth MJ 2011. Cancer immunoediting: integrating immunity's roles in cancer suppression and promotion. *Science* 331: 1565–1570.

References

Bennett RL, French KS, Resta RG, Doyle DL 2008. Standardised human pedigree nomenclature: update and assessment of the recommendation of the National Society of Genetic Counselors. *J Genet Counsel* **17**: 424–433.

Section 3

Genetics of specific cancers

Chapter 7

Genetics of specific cancers. Introduction

Chris Jacobs

Introduction to genetics of specific cancers

The lifetime risk of developing cancer in the UK, Europe, North America and Australasia is one in three; thus many people have at least one relative with cancer. However, most of these cancers are not caused by a high-penetrance gene mutation. Cancer is a multifactorial disease, involving a combination of genetic, lifestyle and environmental factors. This chapter explains the multifactorial nature of the development of cancer and the possible outcomes of the various genetic tests that are currently clinically available within cancer genetics services. The learning objectives for this chapter are:

- to become aware of the contribution of genes, lifestyle and the environment in the development of cancer;
- to understand the different types of genetic test that are clinically available for cancer susceptibility and who can be tested.

The contribution of genes, lifestyle and the environment to the development of cancer

The interaction between genes, the environment and lifestyle is complex and the genetic contribution to cancer varies across cancers, across families and across types of genetic mutation.

In order for cancer to develop, a number of mutations need to occur within an individual cell. Each individual is born with any number of variations in the sequence of their DNA. These individual DNA sequence variations act in combination with environmental and lifestyle factors to contribute a small proportion of the overall risk of disease. Since the mapping of the whole human genome in 2003, genome-wide surveys (genome-wide association studies, GWAS) have explored the relationship between common DNA sequence variations (single nucleotide polymorphisms, SNPs) and predisposition to disease, providing greater insight into the nature and aetiology of many common diseases including cancer. The penetrance (the likelihood that the clinical condition will occur in the presence of the particular genotype) for each SNP varies. Common variants, those present in around 1% or more of the population, generally have a lower level of penetrance,

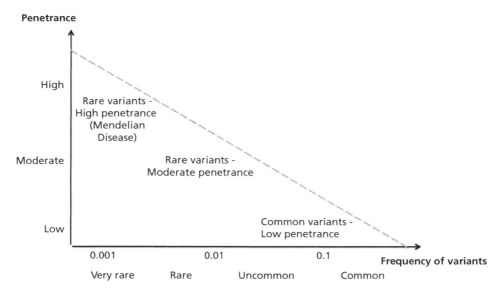

Figure 7.1 Low relative risk tends to be associated with common low-penetrance genetic variants and higher relative risk tends to be associated with rare high-penetrance variants.

Source: data from Mark I. McCarthy et al., Genome-wide association studies for complex traits: consensus, uncertainty and challenges, *Nature Reviews Genetics*, Volume 9, Number 5, pp. 356–369, Copyright © 2008, Rights Managed by Nature Publishing Group.

whereas very rare variants (mutations) occur in around 0.001% of the population and may have a high level of penetrance (McCarthy et al., 2008) (Fig. 7.1).

Cells acquire mutations in their DNA over time (somatic mutations). Most of these somatic mutations are repaired by highly evolved biological mechanisms. As an individual ages these repair mechanisms become less efficient and this can result in the development of cancer. Approximately 80% of cancer is due to a combination of low-penetrance SNPs and acquired somatic mutations that fail to be repaired, resulting in the development of sporadic cancer that appears to occur by chance, often later in life and with no or minimal family history.

Some SNPs are rarer and have a moderate level of penetrance, conferring a greater risk of cancer to the individual. Environmental and lifestyle factors are important in the development of cancer in combination with these moderate-penetrance susceptibility genes that can be passed on in families, although there is no simple pattern of inheritance. The possession of inherited moderate-penetrance susceptibility genes confers a small increased risk on other family members.

The expectation is that genetic profiling looking for multiple individual genetic variants will be possible in the future for personalised therapeutic and public health interventions, such as targeted screening (Pharoah et al., 2008). However, although many SNPs have been detected by GWAS, at present these explain only a small proportion of the heritability of common diseases (Pashayan and Pharoah, 2011).

Just 5–10% of cancer is caused by a mutation in a highly penetrant cancer-predisposing gene. The frequency of these mutations in the general population is low (around 1 in 1000 people). Even in cancers strongly associated with a single gene mutation, the severity and the age of onset of disease vary according to the particular gene mutation, suggesting that penetrance is affected by contributions from modifier genes and the environment (Antoniou et al., 2010; Ramus et al., 2012). The inheritance of these cancer-predisposing mutations is, for the most part, autosomal dominant, and possession of the mutation confers a quantifiable high risk of the disease.

Current practice in genetic testing for highly penetrant cancer-predisposing genes

Currently the only genetic testing that is available within the UK and Europe (Gadziki et al., 2011) involves identifying highly penetrant cancer-predisposing single gene mutations. In the first instance a test is generally offered to a relative with cancer where the family history or tumour histology meet specified criteria based on the likelihood of finding a cancer-predisposing gene mutation. Genetic testing is usually only available to unaffected individuals if a pathogenic mutation has first been identified in an affected relative or the individual has a family history of cancer and is from an ethnic group with a known founder mutation.

In June 2013 the revised National Institute for Health and Care Excellence (NICE) guidelines for familial breast cancer in England and Wales (NICE, 2013) recommended that testing is offered to unaffected individuals with a family history of breast cancer when there is no affected individual available to test if the unaffected individual has a 10% or greater chance of a *BRCA1/2* mutation.

Tumour testing

Sometimes a test may be undertaken on a sample of tumour from a living or deceased individual in order to guide genetic testing and screening in a family. For example, if a family history is suggestive of Lynch syndrome (see Chapter 9), the first steps may be microsatellite instability (MSI) testing and/ or immunohistochemistry (IHC) staining of a tumour sample. Microsatellites are repeats of DNA sequences that are thought to be caused by the failure to correct errors that occur during DNA replication (Baudhuin et al., 2005). The mismatch repair (MMR) system normally recognises and repairs such defects, but where MMR genes are not functioning these errors are not corrected, resulting in genomic instability. A tumour that is microsatellite unstable will trigger germline testing to look for MMR gene defects. Prior to DNA analysis in an individual with MSI, IHC staining may be undertaken to demonstrate expression of the MMR genes. Demonstrating the absence of these gene products (proteins) in a tumour sample helps to target which genes to test for in germline DNA analysis.

Germline testing

Mutation search/diagnostic genetic testing

The first germline genetic test that is undertaken in a family fulfilling the criteria for testing (i.e. when there is a high enough chance of a mutation in the gene being targeted for a genetic test to be offered) is called a mutation search or diagnostic test. In this type of test the targeted gene(s) are systematically searched for using DNA sequencing. There are three possible outcomes of a mutation search test:

1 A pathogenic mutation is identified. This may explain the cause of the cancer in the individual tested or the family (if an unaffected individual is the first person in the family to be tested). When a pathogenic mutation is identified, the risk of further cancer for that individual is usually increased and there are inheritance implications for biological relatives. Most of the common cancer syndromes are passed on by autosomal dominant inheritance. When a mutation is identified at diagnostic testing a predictive genetic test becomes available for family members.

2 No pathogenic mutation is identified. Depending on the gene involved, this outcome reduces the probability that the cancer is due to the gene that has been tested. This result may mean that there is no hereditary cause for the cancer, that current technology is unable to detect the gene fault or that the cancer is due to a mutation in a different gene. In circumstances where an unaffected individual is the first person in the family to be tested because no affected relatives are available for testing, this result requires cautious interpretation and counselling as the gene(s) searched for may not explain the cancers in the family. Other unaffected relatives may also wish to undergo testing if they fulfil the testing criteria. If a mutation is eventually identified in the targeted gene in another family member, then the test can be regarded as a negative predictive test.

3 Variants of uncertain significance (VUS)/unclassified variants (UV) are identified. Sometimes one or more VUS or UV are identified. These are typically missense mutations of unknown functional significance. The outcome of a VUS is the same as for no mutation detected, i.e. predictive genetic testing for the VUS is *not* available for relatives. The cancer risk for the individual and family will be calculated based on the outcome of the testing, the likelihood that other cancer-predisposing genes may be involved and the family history.

Predictive testing

Testing an individual for the presence of a specific cancer-predisposing mutation once a pathogenic mutation has been identified in a biological relative is termed predictive, or sometimes pre-symptomatic, testing. Prior to testing, the probability of finding the mutation will be based on the inheritance pattern and the relationship of the individual undergoing testing to the family member with the mutation. There are two possible outcomes of a predictive test:

1 The familial gene mutation is identified. This is sometimes called a positive predictive test. The associated risk of cancer depends on the penetrance of the mutation. The mutation can be passed on to offspring (depending on the inheritance pattern of the gene).

2 The familial gene mutation is not identified. This is sometimes called a negative predictive test. The individual tested does not carry the familial mutation and does not therefore have the associated risk of cancer. That individual will usually still be at population risk for the cancers in the family. In circumstances where there are some family members with the cancer who do not have the mutation, interpretation of a negative predictive test result requires caution as the mutation may not explain all of the cancers in the family.

Founder mutation testing

Testing may be possible for founder mutations in some populations and for some types of cancer. In this circumstance, affected and unaffected family members may be tested for particular mutations that are known to be more prevalent within particular ethnic groups. The family history criteria for founder mutation testing may be lower than for full mutation search testing because individuals in the ethnic group have a higher pre-test probability of being carriers of the mutation. Interpretation of the results will depend on the ethnicity of the family and the family history.

Developments in genetic testing for cancer susceptibility

Over recent years genetic testing has involved sequencing individual genes in a step-wise manner, taking several weeks to test each gene. The technology for identifying gene mutations is, however, changing rapidly and genetics laboratories are in the very early stages of introducing new methods of clinical sequencing, sometimes called next generation sequencing (NGS). This new technology enables testing of large volumes of genes in a single test with the promise of huge advances in the discovery of cancer-predisposing genes and the prevention, diagnosis and management of the disease (Rahman, 2014).

Careful evaluation of the clinical validity, clinical utility and implications of new tests is essential before such tests are introduced into clinical practice. Many issues surrounding these tests are currently being considered, including managing and storing huge volumes of data, interpreting results, consent for testing, what is tested for and the disclosure of incidental findings (additional findings detected as a result of the testing that may or may not have potential health implications or clinical significance for that individual). The American College of Medical Genetics and Genomics (ACMG) reported in 2013 that laboratories should explicitly seek and report on a minimum list of variants, regardless of the indication for the sequencing, and patients would be required to consent to receiving all of the information before being tested (Green et al., 2013). This position has since been revised (https://www.acmg.net/docs/Release_ACMGUpdatesRecommendations_final.pdf) but the whole debate highlights the challenges surrounding these new approaches to testing for patients, clinicians and laboratories (Burke et al., 2013; Burton and Zimmern, 2013).

Summary

Scientific investigation of the genetic basis of disease has identified many genetic variants of variable penetrance. Testing within the NHS is only available for rare high-penetrance variants (or mutations) which explain only a small proportion of common cancers. There are various types of genetic test available and although these can help some individuals and families to understand their risk, the results need to be interpreted with caution. The introduction of new genetic testing technologies will raise further challenges and require careful implementation.

Chapters 8 and 9 address the risks associated with the particular genes involved in hereditary breast and ovarian cancer and colorectal, gastric cancer and related cancers. Chapter 10 addresses the genetics, screening and management of hereditary prostate cancer. Chapter 11 addresses the genetics and management of rare cancer syndromes.

References

Antoniou AC, Beesley J, McGuffog L, et al. 2010. Common breast cancer susceptibility alleles and the risk of breast cancer for *BRCA1* and *BRCA2* mutation carriers: implications for risk prediction. *Cancer Res* **70**: 9742–9754.

Baudhuin LM, Burgart LJ, Leontovich O, Thibodeau SN 2005. Use of microsatellite instability and immunohistochemistry testing for the identification of individuals at risk for Lynch syndrome. *Fam Cancer* **4**: 255–265.

Burke W, Mathenny Antommaria A, Bennett R, et al. 2013. Recommendations for returning genomic incidental findings? We need to talk! *Genet Med* **15**: 854–859.

Burton H and Zimmern R 2013. *ACMG recommendations on incidental findings: a commentary.* Available at: <http://www.phgfoundation.org/news/13713/> (last accessed 17 February 2014).

Gadzicki D, Evans DG, Harris H, et al. 2011. Genetic testing for familial/hereditary breast cancer-comparison of guidelines and recommendations from the UK, France, the Netherlands and Germany. *J Commun Genet* **2**: 53–69.

Green RC, Berg JS, Grody WW, et al. 2013. ACMG recommendations for reporting of incidental findings in clinical exome and genome sequencing. *Genet. Med.* **15**: 565–574.

McCarthy MI, Abecasis GR, Cardon LR, et al. 2008. Genome-wide association studies for complex traits: consensus, uncertainty and challenges. *Nat Rev Genet* **9**: 356–369.

NICE (National Institute for Health and Care Excellence) 2013. *Familial breast cancer: classification and care of people at risk of familial breast cancer and management of breast cancer and related risks in people with a family history of breast cancer.* NICE Clinical Guideline 164. London: National Institute for Health and Care Excellence.

Pashayan N and Pharoah P 2011. Translating genomics into improved population screening: hype or hope? *Hum Genet* **130**: 19–21.

Pharoah PD, Antoniou AC, Easton DF, Ponder BA 2008. Polygenes, risk prediction, and targeted prevention of breast cancer. *N Engl J Med* **358**: 2796–2803.

Rahman N. 2014. Realizing the promise of cancer predisposition genes. *Nature* **505**: 302–308.

Ramus SJ, Antoniou AC, Kuchenbaecker KB, et al. 2012. Ovarian cancer susceptibility alleles and risk of ovarian cancer in *BRCA1* and *BRCA2* mutation carriers. *Hum Mutat* **33**: 690–702.

Chapter 8

Genetics of breast and ovarian cancer

Deborah Ruddy

Introduction to genetics of breast and ovarian cancer

Breast cancer is a common disease. Worldwide there are over a million new cases diagnosed per year and over 400 000 deaths; there are more than 4.4 million women living with breast cancer (Ferlay et al., 2004). Incidence rates are highest in western Europe and lowest in eastern and central Africa. Incidence in the UK is estimated to be the sixth highest in Europe (Cancer Research UK, 2013) with 80% of breast cancers being diagnosed in women aged 50 and above. In 2010 the lifetime risk of breast cancer in women in the UK was estimated to be 1 in 8 and the lifetime risk for men was estimated to be 1 in 868. In the UK in 2010 there were 11 633 deaths from breast cancer with a female:male ratio of 150:1. Death rates from breast cancer have fallen by 20% in the last 10 years (CRUK, 2013).

Ovarian cancer, which includes cancers of the fallopian tube and primary peritoneal cancer, is less common. In 2008 there were estimated to be 225 000 new cases of ovarian cancer worldwide, with incidence varying considerably between countries (CRUK, 2013). The incidence in more developed countries was almost twice as high as in less developed countries. Ovarian cancer predominantly occurs post-menopausally, with 80% of diagnoses occurring in women over the age of 50. There is a 40% difference between the highest and lowest incidences of ovarian cancer in European countries, with the UK ranking seventh in the European Union. In the UK in 2008 around 6500 women were diagnosed with ovarian cancer. The lifetime risk of ovarian cancer in the UK is 1 in 54. In the UK in 2010 more than 4300 women died from ovarian cancer. However, survival has doubled over the last 30 years with a 5-year survival of around 43% (CRUK, 2013).

The learning objectives for Chapter 8 are:

- to be able to discuss the factors that increase the risk of developing breast and ovarian cancer;
- to be able to describe the hereditary cancer syndromes that are associated with breast and ovarian cancer;
- to understand the rationale behind and criteria for genetic testing for these cancers.

Factors that increase the risk breast or ovarian cancer

Breast cancer

The following factors are known to increase the risk of developing breast cancer:

1 Age: the incidence of breast cancer increases with age, doubling about every 10 years until the menopause, when the rate of increase slows dramatically (Harris et al., 2000).

2 Gender: women are more likely to develop breast cancer than men.

3 Race and geography: for breast cancer, age-adjusted incidence and mortality vary by a factor of up to five between western countries and the Far East, although this difference is diminishing (Ferlay et al., 2004). Studies of migrants from Japan to Hawaii show that the rate of breast cancer in migrants assumes the rate in the host country within one or two generations, indicating that environmental factors are of significant importance (Kolonel et al., 2004).

4 Hormonal factors: women with early menarche or late menopause have an increased risk of developing breast cancer. Women who have a natural menopause after the age of 55 are twice as likely to develop breast cancer as women who experience the menopause before the age of 45.

5 Lifestyle factors: on an individual level, the relationship between fat intake and breast cancer is neither consistent nor strong (Pearce, 2000). Obesity is associated with a twofold increase in the risk of breast cancer in post-menopausal women, whereas amongst pre-menopausal women it is associated with a reduced incidence. Some studies have shown a link between alcohol consumption and the incidence of breast cancer, but the relation is inconsistent and the association may in fact arise due to the confounding effects of dietary or social factors. A clear association between smoking and breast cancer has never been shown.

6 Benign breast disease and breast density: women with severe atypical epithelial hyperplasia have a four to five times higher risk of developing breast cancer than women who do not have any proliferative changes in their breast (Harris et al., 2000). As well as potentially masking the disease from detection by mammography, high breast density is an independent risk factor for breast cancer: those in the upper quartile of breast density are at four- to fivefold increased risk compared with women with a lower breast density (Boyd et al., 2005).

7 Family history: after gender and age, a positive family history is the strongest known predictive risk factor for breast cancer. It has long been recognised that in some families there is hereditary breast cancer which is characterised by an early age of onset, bilaterality and the presence of breast cancer in multiple generations in an apparent autosomal dominant pattern of inheritance (through either the maternal or paternal side of the family), sometimes including tumours of other organs, particularly the ovary and prostate gland (Sellers et al., 1994). It is now known that some of these 'cancer families' can be explained by specific mutations in single 'cancer susceptibility' genes. Although such cancer susceptibility genes are very important, highly penetrant germline mutations are estimated to account for only 5–10% of breast and ovarian cancers overall.

Ovarian cancer

Although reproductive, demographic and lifestyle factors affect the risk of ovarian cancer, the single greatest risk factor for ovarian cancer is a family history of the disease. A meta-analysis of 15 published studies estimated an odds ratio of 3.1 for the risk of ovarian cancer associated with at least one first-degree relative with ovarian cancer (Stratton et al., 1998).

Genetic associations in breast and ovarian cancer

Breast and ovarian cancer are seen in several autosomal dominant cancer syndromes. The syndromes most strongly associated with both cancers are the *BRCA1* and *BRCA2* mutation syndromes. Breast cancer is also a common feature of Li–Fraumeni syndrome (*TP53* mutations) and is seen at an increased frequency in neurofibromatosis type 1 (*NF1* mutations), ataxia telangiectasia (biallelic *ATM* mutations), Cowden syndrome (*PTEN* mutations), Peutz–Jeghers syndrome (*STK11* mutations) and hereditary diffuse gastric cancer syndrome (*CDH1* mutations). In addition, four 'intermediate-penetrance' genes have been identified (*CHEK2, ATM* heterozygotes, *BRIP1* and *PALB2*), and mutations in these genes increase the risk of developing breast cancer. Ovarian cancer is also associated with Lynch syndrome (discussed in Chapter 9).

High-penetrance breast and ovarian cancer predisposition genes

BRCA1 and *BRCA2*: genetics

Mutations in *BRCA1* and *BRCA2* confer a greater than tenfold relative risk of breast cancer. It is estimated that these genes account for 15–20% of familial breast cancer (Turnbull and Rahman, 2008).

BRCA1 is located on chromosome 17q21 and was identified by linkage analysis (Hall et al., 1990) and positional cloning (Miki et al., 1994). Linkage analysis and positional cloning led to the mapping of *BRCA2* in 1994 and its identification in 1995 (Wooster et al., 1994, 1995). *BRCA2* is located on chromosome 13q12.3. *BRCA1* and *BRCA2* are tumour suppressor genes and have important roles in maintaining genomic stability by facilitating the repair of DNA double-strand breaks. *BRCA1* and *BRCA2* are both large genes in which multiple different loss-of-function mutations have been detected. Most recognised disease-associated mutations result in premature protein truncation, and thus loss of protein function, although some missense mutations cause loss of function without truncation. The majority of people who have a *BRCA1* or *BRCA2* mutation have a unique mutation that is specific to them and their family. However, specific recurring mutations have been found in the Ashkenazi Jewish population (and in people from Iceland and Poland). Mutations recur in these groups because of a 'founder' effect (see Chapter 4). In today's Ashkenazi Jewish population three founder mutations (two in *BRCA1* and one in *BRCA2*) account for the majority of the *BRCA* mutations. In the general population, it is estimated that approximately one person in 500 has a mutation in *BRCA1* or *BRCA2*. In contrast, one in 40 Ashkenazi Jewish individuals has one of the recurring mutations. This is clinically relevant, because:

- gene testing (looking specifically for founder mutations in a person of founder ethnicity) can be done generally more quickly and cheaply than 'whole gene' mutation analysis;
- the increased occurrence of *BRCA* founder mutations can have implications for the assessment of the significance of family history in people from particular ethnic groups.

BRCA1 and BRCA2: risks

Estimates of the risk of cancer conferred by mutations in *BRCA1* and *BRCA2* vary according to the ascertainment of the cases studied. It is likely that other genetic factors contribute to the aetiology of some of these cancers. Modifier genes may in the future enable precise figures to be given for risk (Mavaddat et al., 2013). For the time being, however, in clinical practice a range of risks is given to individuals identified as carriers of the *BRCA1/2* gene mutation:

◆ Breast cancer: early studies of large cancer families suggested that the risk of breast cancer by the age of 70 for female carriers may be as high as 87% for *BRCA1* and 84% for *BRCA2*, although these estimates were based on relatively small numbers of families (Easton et al., 1995; Ford et al., 1998). In population-based studies of breast cancer cases (unselected for family history) the risks are lower: 65% for *BRCA1* and 45% for *BRCA2* (Antoniou et al., 2003). Antoniou et al. (2003) observed that the incidence of breast cancer rose to a plateau of 3–4% per year in female carriers of *BRCA1* aged 40–49 (Fig. 8.1), whereas in carriers of *BRCA2* breast cancer incidence rose steeply up to the age 50 and more slowly thereafter (Fig. 8.2).

◆ Contralateral breast cancer (CBC): Metcalfe et al. (2004) estimated the 10-year risk of CBC to be approximately 40% for carriers of *BRCA1/2* who have not had an oophorectomy or taken tamoxifen. In a later study following up women with breast cancer and a *BRCA1/2* mutation for a mean of 11.1 years, women diagnosed with breast cancer before the age of 49 years experienced significantly higher risks of CBC than those diagnosed over the age of 50. The group at highest risk for CBC were women diagnosed with breast cancer before the age of 49 with both ovaries intact and two or

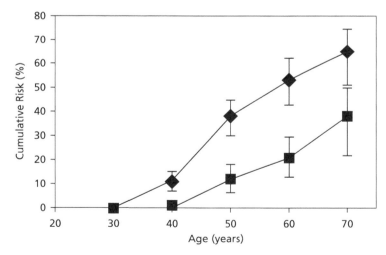

Figure 8.1 Cumulative risk of breast (◆) and ovarian cancer (■) in *BRCA1* mutation carriers.
Reprinted from *The American Journal of Human Genetics*, Volume 75, Issue 2, A. Antoniou, et al., Average risks of breast and ovarian cancer associated with *BRCA1* or *BRCA2* mutations detected in case series unselected for family history: a combined analysis of 22 studies, pp. 1117–1130, Copyright © 2003 The American Society of Human Genetics, with permission from Elsevier, http://www.sciencedirect.com/science/journal/00029297.

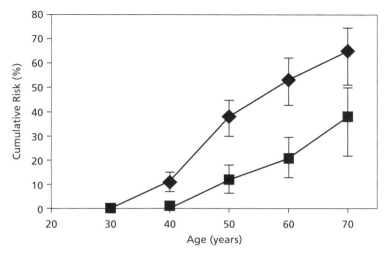

Figure 8.2 Cumulative risk of breast (♦) and ovarian cancer (■) in *BRCA2* mutation carriers.
Reprinted from *The American Journal of Human Genetics*, Volume 75, Issue 2, A. Antoniou, et al., Average risks of breast and ovarian cancer associated with *BRCA1* or *BRCA2* mutations detected in case series unselected for family history: a combined analysis of 22 studies, pp. 1117–1130, Copyright © 2003 The American Society of Human Genetics, with permission from Elsevier, http://www.sciencedirect.com/science/journal/00029297.

more first-degree relatives affected with breast cancer. In these women the 15-year risk of CBC was 68% (Metcalfe et al., 2011).

♦ Ovarian cancer: estimates of the lifetime risk of ovarian cancer range from 22 to 65% for *BRCA1* and from 10 to 35% for *BRCA2* (Mavaddet et al., 2013). Antoniou et al. (2003) found that in carriers of *BRCA1* the risk of ovarian cancer before the age of 40 was low, with the risk rising by 1–2% per annum after the age of 40 (Fig. 8.1). In carriers of *BRCA2* the incidence of ovarian cancer was low before the age of 50 and increased sharply from age 50 to 59 (Fig. 8.2). The prevalence of a pathogenic BRCA1/2 mutation in women with ovarian cancer is estimated to be up to 17% (Trainer et al., 2010).

♦ Breast and ovarian cancer risks associated with Ashkenazi Jewish founder mutations: the risk of breast and ovarian cancer by the age of 70 associated with the three Ashkenazi Jewish founder mutations has been estimated to be 56% and 16%, respectively (Struewing et al., 1997). A meta-analysis by Antoniou et al. (2005) found that up to the age of 70 the two *BRCA1* founder mutations conferred risks of approximately 65% for breast cancer and 14–33% for ovarian cancer, and the *BRCA2* founder mutation conferred risks of 43% for breast cancer and 20% for ovarian cancer.

♦ Male breast cancer: the relative risk of breast cancer is elevated in male carriers of *BRCA2*, with such carriers estimated to have approximately an 8% lifetime risk of breast cancer (Evans et al., 2010a). An elevated risk of prostate cancer has also been demonstrated in *BRCA2* carriers (discussed in detail in Chapter 10).

♦ Other cancer risks associated with *BRCA1/2* mutations: small excesses of a number of other cancers, specifically pancreatic cancer, have been observed in monoallelic (heterozygous) carriers of *BRCA1* and *BRCA2* mutations, but larger studies are required to clarify whether these findings reflect truly elevated risks of these cancers (Thompson and Easton, 2002).

TP53: genetics

Li–Fraumeni syndrome (LFS) is a cancer predisposition syndrome in which there is a high frequency of early onset breast cancer found in association with other young-onset cancers. The associated early mortality and rarity of the condition has impeded collection of sufficient familial samples. P53 was recognised early as a prominent transcription factor central to multiple cellular pathways and is frequently somatically mutated in tumours. These observations led to the proposal of *TP53*, a tumour suppressor gene, as a possible candidate gene for LFS. In 1990 mutational screening of the *TP53* gene revealed causative mutations in the five families studied (Malkin et al., 1990).

TP53: risks

The overall lifetime cancer risk for women with LFS is grossly elevated, predominantly on account of their high risk of breast cancer (Chompret et al., 2000; Birch et al., 2001). Women with a *TP53* mutation are estimated to have 49% risk of developing breast cancer by the age of 50 (Masciari et al., 2012). LFS is rare, and mutations in *TP53* are uncommon in non-Li–Fraumeni breast cancer families (Lalloo et al., 2006). Thus, the familial breast cancer risk attributable to *TP53* mutations is very low.

TP53 mutations are also associated with the development of multiple cancers at a young age. Although most cancer types have been reported to occur in LFS families, the following cancers, particularly when associated with a young age of onset, tend to be specifically associated with LFS (Chompret et al., 2000):

- soft tissue sarcoma
- osteosarcoma
- brain tumour
- pre-menopausal breast cancer
- adrenocortical carcinoma
- leukaemia
- lung cancer.

Intermediate-penetrance breast and/or ovarian cancer predisposition genes

Four intermediate-penetrance breast cancer genes have been identified via mutational screening of candidate genes: *CHEK2*, *ATM*, *BRIP1* and *PALB2*. Mutations in these genes are rare and confer a relative risk of breast cancer of two to four. *RAD50* may also be an intermediate-penetrance breast cancer predisposition gene, but convincing results to date pertain only to a founder mutation detected in the Finnish population; likewise *RAD51C*, although its prominent association seems to be with ovarian cancer (Meindl et al., 2010). The rarity of mutations and modest associated risks are such that the attributable risk of mutations in these genes is low: together *CHEK2*, *ATM*, *BRIP1* and *PALB2* account for approximately 2.3% of excess familial risk (Rahman et al., 2007).

Other genes that can increase breast cancer risk

Five genes associated with syndromic diagnoses are associated with an increased incidence of breast cancer. Cowden syndrome, Peutz–Jeghers syndrome and hereditary diffuse gastric cancer are discussed in Chapters 9 and 11.

Neurofibromatosis type 1 (*NF1* mutations): genetics

Neurofibromatosis type 1 (NF1) is an autosomal dominant disorder, caused by mutations in the *NF1* gene, which has an approximate incidence of 1 in 2500 and a prevalence of 1 in 4000 (Evans et al., 2010b). *NF1* is a tumour suppressor gene, and as such, individuals with *NF1* mutations are at an increased risk of developing cancers, particularly gliomas, malignant peripheral nerve sheath tumours, juvenile chronic myelomonocytic leukaemia, rhabdomyosarcoma and phaeochromocytoma, as well as skin markings, vascular disease, bone deformities and cognitive difficulties (Montani et al., 2011).

NF1: breast cancer risk

Women under the age of 50 with *NF1* mutations have a fivefold increased risk of breast cancer and should be considered for increased breast screening (Sharif et al., 2007).

Ataxia telangiectasia (*ATM* mutations): genetics

Ataxia telangiectasia (A-T) is a rare autosomal recessive neurological disorder, and almost all cases of A-T are caused by homozygous or (more commonly) compound heterozygous mutations in the *ATM* gene (Taylor and Byrd, 2005). A-T is typically diagnosed in early childhood and is characterised by progressive cerebellar degeneration and oculocutaneous telangiectasia. A-T patients with homozygous or compound heterozygote mutations in the *ATM* gene show a predisposition to the development of different types of lymphoid tumours as children or as young adults, and less frequently they may also develop brain and other tumours, associated almost exclusively with absence of ATM kinase activity (Taylor et al., 1996).

ATM: breast cancer risk

Individuals with A-T also show a substantially increased risk of breast cancer at a young age; the estimated risk by the age of 50 years is 45% (Antoniou et al., 2008). Heterozygous female carriers of the *ATM* mutation in A-T families have an increased risk of developing breast cancer without any evidence for an increased risk of lymphoid tumours (Thompson et al., 2005).

Tumour pathology and classification

Breast cancer

Breast tumours may express different proteins, and molecular classification based on the expression of oestrogen receptors (ERs), progesterone receptors (PRs) and human epidermal growth factor receptor (HER2) has proved relevant to prognosis, gene testing and treatment. Triple-negative breast cancer describes a subgroup of tumours that lack ER, PR and HER2 expression (Foulkes et al., 2010). Overall, triple-negative cancers account for approximately 15% of all breast cancers but occur more frequently in younger women and are the predominant subtype in individuals with a germline *BRCA1* mutation (Blows et al., 2010; Foulkes et al., 2010). *BRCA1*-associated tumours are typically high-grade invasive ductal carcinomas in which there is a high incidence of the 'triple-negative phenotype'. No specific distinctive histopathological features have been described in *BRCA2* tumours.

Ovarian and fallopian tube cancer

Ovarian cancer arising in women with *BRCA1* and *BRCA2* mutations is more likely to be invasive serous adenocarcinoma and less likely to be mucinous or borderline. (Lakhani et al., 2004; Liu et al., 2012). Fallopian tube cancer and papillary serous carcinoma of the peritoneum are also part of the spectrum of *BRCA*-associated disease (Crum et al., 2007). Approximately 60% of sporadic ovarian cancers have serous histology. A survey of all published data shows that 94% of *BRCA1*-related ovarian cancers also have serous histology (Berchuck et al., 1998).

Rationale for *BRCA1* and *BRCA2* gene testing

Due to financial and logistical constraints, *BRCA1* and *BRCA2* testing is currently rationed in most countries. Within the UK, *BRCA* testing is typically undertaken if the likelihood of detecting a mutation is 10% or more per gene (Gadziki et al., 2011). Several different methods to determine which cases are eligible for testing are utilised in clinical practice, most of which require specialised knowledge and/or software (Antoniou et al., 2008).

There are no functional tests for *BRCA1* or *BRCA2*; therefore, the classification of mutations that are identified on gene testing relies on imperfect data. The majority of accepted deleterious mutations result in protein truncation and/or loss of functional domains. In 10–15% of all individuals undergoing gene testing with full sequencing of *BRCA1* and *BRCA2* no clearly deleterious mutation will be detected but there will be a variant(s) of uncertain significance (VUS). Identification of a VUS can be challenging for genetic counselling, particularly in terms of estimating cancer risk and risk management. Research is ongoing into the significance of VUS, which are occasionally reclassified as either benign or pathogenic.

Genetic testing criteria for breast and ovarian cancer susceptibility

Mutation testing of *BRCA1/2* and *TP53* may be clinically indicated in women for whom the pathology of the tumour and/or the extent of family history are such that there is a significant likelihood of a mutation being present (typically 10% or more per gene).

Gene testing of the *BRCA1*, *BRCA2* and *TP53* genes is available via regional genetics centres, and if possible gene testing in a family should start with the testing of an affected individual in order to identify a gene mutation. 'Cascade screening' can then be offered to other family members as appropriate, and their risk of developing cancer associated with the particular gene mutation can then be calculated and screening offered as necessary. As technologies change, the criteria used for gene testing will also change. The current UK gene testing guidelines for familial breast cancer are published by the National Institute for Health and Care Excellence (NICE) and were last updated in 2013 (NICE, 2013).

Summary

Breast cancer is a common disease—ovarian cancer is less common. Mutations in the *BRCA1* and *BRCA2* genes account for up to 10% of all cases of breast and ovarian cancer. Mutations in the *BRCA1*, *BRCA2* and *TP53* genes confer high risks of cancer, and genetic testing is offered where there is a 10% or greater chance of a mutation being identified in an individual. Other intermediate-penetrance genes and genes associated with syndromic diagnoses have been identified which contribute to hereditary breast and ovarian cancer.

References

Antoniou A, Pharoah PD, Narod S, et al. 2003. Average risks of breast and ovarian cancer associated with *BRCA1* or *BRCA2* mutations detected in case series unselected for family history: a combined analysis of 22 studies. *Am J Hum Genet* **72**: 1117–1130.

Antoniou A, Pharoah P, Narod S, et al. 2005. Breast and ovarian cancer risks to carriers of the BRCA1 5382insC and 185delAG and 6174delT mutations: a combined analysis of 22 population based studies. *J Med Genet* **42**: 602–603.

Antoniou AC, Cunningham AP, Peto J, et al. 2008. The BOADICEA model of genetic susceptibility to breast and ovarian cancers: updates and extensions. *Br J Cancer* **98**: 1457–1466.

Berchuck A, Heron KA, Carney ME, et al. 1998. Frequency of germline and somatic *BRCA1* mutations in ovarian cancer. *Clin Cancer Res* **4**: 2433–2437.

Birch JM, Alston RD, McNally RJ, et al. 2001. Relative frequency and morphology of cancers in carriers of germline *TP53* mutations. *Oncogene* **20**: 4621–4628.

Blows FM, Driver KE, Schmidt MK, et al. 2010. Subtyping of breast cancer by immunohistochemistry to investigate a relationship between subtype and short and long term survival: a collaborative analysis of data for 10,159 cases from 12 studies. *PLoS Med* **7**(5): e1000279.

Boyd NF, Rommens JM, Vogt K, et al. 2005. Mammographic breast density as an intermediate phenotype for breast cancer. *Lancet Oncol* **6**: 798–808.

Chompret A, Brugieres L, Ronsin M, et al. 2000. P53 germline mutations in childhood cancers and cancer risk for carrier individuals. *Br J Cancer* **82**: 1932–1937.

CRUK (Cancer Research UK 2013). *CancerStats: cancer statistics for the UK.* Available at <http://www.cancerresearchuk.org/cancer-info/cancerstats/> (last accessed 26 December 2013).

Crum CP, Drapkin R, Kindelberger D, et al. 2007. Lessons from BRCA: the tubal fimbria emerges as an origin for pelvic serous cancer. *Clin Med Res* **5**: 35–44.

Easton DF, Ford D, Bishop DT 1995. Breast and ovarian cancer incidence in *BRCA1*-mutation carriers. Breast Cancer Linkage Consortium. *Am J Hum Genet* **56**: 265–271.

Evans DG, Susnerwala I, Dawson J, et al. 2010a. Risk of breast cancer in male *BRCA2* carriers. *J Med Genet* **47**: 710–711.

Evans DG, Howard E, Giblin C, et al. 2010b. Birth incidence and prevalence of tumor-prone syndromes: estimates from a UK family genetic register service. *Am J Med Genet* **152A**: 327–332.

Ferlay J, Bray F, Pisani P, Parkin DM 2004. *GLOBOCAN 2002: cancer incidence, mortality and prevalence worldwide*. IARC CancerBase no. 5, version 2.0. Lyon: IARC Press.

Ford D, Easton DF, Stratton M, et al. 1998. Genetic heterogeneity and penetrance analysis of the *BRCA1* and *BRCA2* genes in breast cancer families. Breast Cancer Linkage Consortium. *Am J Hum Genet* **62**: 676–689.

Foulkes WD, Smith IE, Reis-Filho JS 2010. Triple-negative breast cancer. *N Engl J Med* **363**: 1938–1948.

Gadziki D, Evans DG, Harris H, et al. 2011. Genetic testing for familial/hereditary breast cancer-comparison of guidelines and recommendations from the UK, France, the Netherlands and Germany. *J Commun Genet* **2**(2): 53–69.

Hall JM, Lee MK, Newman B, et al. 1990. Linkage of early onset familial breast cancer to chromosome 17q21. *Science* **250**: 1684–1689.

Harris JR, Lippman ME, Morrow M, Osborne CK 2000. *Disease of the breast*. Philadelphia: Lippincott Williams & Wilkins.

Kolonel LN, Altshuler D, Henderson BE 2004. The multi-ethnic cohort study: exploring genes, lifestyle and cancer risk. *Nat Rev Cancer* **4**: 519–527.

Lakhani SR, Manek S, Penault-Llorca F, et al. 2004. Pathology of ovarian cancers in *BRCA1* and *BRCA2* carriers. *Clin Cancer Res* **10**: 2473–2481.

Lalloo F, Varley J, Moran A, et al. 2006. *BRCA1*, *BRCA2* and *TP53* mutations in very early-onset breast cancer with associated risks to relatives. *Eur J Cancer* **42**: 1143–1150.

Liu J, Cristea MC, Frankel P, et al. 2012. Clinical characteristics and outcomes of *BRCA*-associated ovarian cancer: genotype and survival. *Cancer Genet* **205**: 34–41.

NICE (National Institute for Health and Care Excellence) 2013. *Familial breast cancer: classification and care of people at risk of familial breast cancer and management of breast cancer and related risks in people with a family history of breast cancer*. NICE Clinical Guideline 164. London: National Institute for Health and Care Excellence.

Malkin D, Li FP, Strong LC, et al. 1990. Germ line p53 mutations in a familial syndrome of breast cancer, sarcomas, and other neoplasms. *Science* **250**: 1233–1238.

Masciari S, Dillon DA, Rath M 2012. Breast cancer phenotype in women with *TP53* germline mutations: a Li-Fraumeni syndrome consortium effort. *Breast Cancer Res Treat* **133**: 1125–1130.

Mavaddat N, Peock S, Frost D, et al. 2013. Cancer risks for BRCA1 and BRCA2 mutation carriers: results from prospective analysis of EMBRACE. *J Natl Cancer Inst* **105**: 812–822.

Meindl A, Hellebrand H, Wiek C, et al. 2010. Germline mutations in breast and ovarian cancer pedigrees establish RAD51C as a human cancer susceptibility gene. *Nat Genet* **42**: 410–414.

Metcalfe K, Lynch HT, Ghadirian P, et al. 2004. Contralateral breast cancer in *BRCA1* and *BRCA2* mutation carriers. *J Clin Oncol* **22**: 2328–2335.

Metcalfe K, Gershman S, Lynch HT, et al. 2011. Predictors of contralateral breast cancer in *BRCA1* and *BRCA2* mutation carriers. *Br J Cancer* **104**: 1384–1392.

Miki Y, Swensen J, Shattuck-Eidens D, et al. 1994. A strong candidate for the breast and ovarian cancer susceptibility gene *BRCA1*. *Science* **266**: 66–71.

Montani D, Coulet F, Girerd B, et al. 2011. Pulmonary hypertension in patients with neurofibromatosis type I. *Medicine (Baltimore)* **90**: 201–211.

Pearce N 2000. The ecological fallacy strikes back. *J Epidemiol Commun Health* **54**: 326–327.

Rahman N, Seal S, Thompson D, et al. 2007. *PALB2*, which encodes a BRCA2-interacting protein, is a breast cancer susceptibility gene. *Nat Genet* **39**: 165–167.

Sellers TA, Potter JD, Rich SS, et al. 1994. Familial clustering of breast and prostate cancers and risk of postmenopausal breast cancer. *J Natl Cancer Inst.* **86**: 1860–1865.

Sharif S, Moran A, Huson SM, et al. 2007. Women with neurofibromatosis 1 are at a moderately increased risk of developing breast cancer and should be considered for early screening. *J Med Genet* **44**: 481–484.

Stratton JF, Pharoah P, Smith SK, et al. 1998. A systematic review and meta-analysis of family history and risk of ovarian cancer. *Br J Obstet Gynaecol* **105**: 493–499.

Struewing N, Hartge P, Wacholder S 1997. The risk of cancer associated with specific mutations of *BRCA1* and *BRCA2* among Ashkenazi Jews. *N Engl J Med* **336**: 1401–1408.

Taylor AM, Metcalfe JA, Thick J, Mak YF 1996. Leukemia and lymphoma in ataxia telangiectasia. *Blood* **87**: 423–438.

Taylor AM and Byrd PJ 2005. Molecular pathology of ataxia telangiectasia. *J Clin Pathol* **58**: 1009–1015.

Thompson D, Duedal S, Kirner J, et al. 2005. Cancer risks and mortality in heterozygous *ATM* mutation carriers. *J Natl Cancer Inst* **97**: 813–822.

Thompson D and Easton DF 2002. Cancer incidence in *BRCA1* mutation carriers. *J Natl Cancer Inst* **94**: 1358–1365.

Trainer AJ, Meiser B, Watts K, et al. 2010. Moving towards personalized medicine: treatment-focused genetic testing of women newly diagnosed with ovarian cancer. *International Journal of Gynecological Cancer* **20**(5): 704–716.

Turnbull C and Rahman N 2008. Genetic predisposition to breast cancer: past, present and future. *Ann Rev Genom Hum Genet* **9**: 321–345.

Wooster R, Neuhausen SL, Mangion J, et al. 1994. Localization of a breast cancer susceptibility gene, *BRCA2*, to chromosome 13q12–13. *Science* **265**: 2088–2090.

Wooster R, Bignell G, Lancaster J, et al. 1995. Identification of the breast cancer susceptibility gene *BRCA2*. *Nature* **378**: 789–792.

Chapter 9

Genetics of colorectal, gastric and related gynaecological cancers

Gabriella Pichert

Introduction to genetics of colorectal, gastric and related gynaecological cancers

This chapter focuses on the role and function of genes predisposing to upper and lower gastrointestinal (GI) and related gynaecological cancers. The clinical manifestations of GI cancer syndromes, the cancer risks associated with GI cancer syndromes and the associated tumour pathology are discussed and the most efficient genetic testing strategies are outlined. The clinical manifestations and cancer risks associated with hereditary GI syndromes are summarised in Table 9.1 and diagnostic and germline testing criteria are shown in Table 9.2.

The learning objectives for Chapter 9 are:

- to be able to discuss the influence of cancer genetics in the development of GI cancer syndromes and related gynaecological cancers;

- to be able to describe the implications of these genetic conditions for the client group and healthcare practice.

Colorectal cancer

Between 25 and 30% of all colorectal cancer (CRC) has a familial background and up to 10% of all CRC is due to a single faulty heritable gene. Heritable CRC caused by a faulty gene is in most instances autosomal dominantly inherited. Exceptions are *MUTYH*-associated GI cancers and the rare constitutional mismatch repair-deficiency syndromes which are both autosomal recessive.

Non-polyposis syndromes

Lynch syndrome (LS) or hereditary non-polyposis colon cancer was first described by Lynch et al. (1966) and called 'non-polyposis' to distinguish it from the familial adenomatous polyposis syndrome. LS is responsible for 2–3% of heritable CRC and is caused by heritable mutations in a class of genes called mismatch repair (MMR) genes. These genes repair errors in DNA replication occurring during cell division. Loss of their function leads to an accumulation of replication errors in a variable number of tandem

Table 9.1 Risks of cancer associated with hereditary gastrointestinal syndromes

Syndrome	Clinical manifestations	Cancer risks	Benign pathology	Malignant pathology
Polyposis syndromes				
Classical familial adenomatous polyposis (FAP)	Multiple colonic polyps in adolescence, gastric/small bowel polyps, desmoid tumours, dental abnormalities, osteomas, congenital hypertrophy of retinal epithelium, adrenal masses, thyroid cancer, hepatoblastoma, medulloblastoma (Jasperson and Randall, 1998)	Almost 100% CRC, 0.5% GC, 4–12% small bowel, 2% pancreatic cancer, 1% hepatoblastoma, small but increased risk for bile duct and adrenal gland cancer, 2% thyroid, 1% brain/CNS cancer (Cancer.Net, 2013)	Adenomatous polyps, epidermoid cysts and fibromas	Colonic adenocarcinoma, Small bowel carcinoma, pancreatic adenocarcinoma, medulloblastoma, hepatoblastoma, papillary thyroid cancer, stomach/bile duct adenocarcinoma
Attenuated familial adenomatous polyposis	Variable number of frequently right-sided colonic polyps with later age of onset. Upper GI findings and thyroid cancer risk similar to classical FAP. Other extra-intestinal findings unusual (NCCN, 2013)	70% CRC, 4–12% small bowel, 0.5% GC, 2% pancreatic, 2% thyroid (Cancer.Net, 2013)	Adenomatous polyps	Same as FAP
MUTYH-associated polyposis	Usually > 15 (rarely < 15 or none) colonic polyps, gastric and duodenal polyps, sebaceous gland tumours. 25–36% of patients with CRC have no synchronous polyps (Farrington et al., 2005)	43–100% CRC, 4% duodenal, 38% extra-intestinal malignancies (OC, bladder skin), trend for increased breast cancer risk (Vogt et al., 2009)	Adenomatous, serrated, hyperplastic/mixed hyperplastic and adenomatous polyps, 17% duodenal polyposis	
Peutz–Jeghers syndrome	Gastrointestinal polyps leading to obstruction, intussusception and bleeding. Mucocutaneous hyperpigmentation. Colon, breast, pancreas, stomach, small bowel, ovarian and uterine/cervical cancer (McGarrity et al., 2001).	85% cancer risk at age 70, 33% GI cancer risk at age 60, 31% breast cancer risk at age 60 (Hearle et al., 2006).	Hamartomatous polyps in the GI tract, uterus, bladder, lungs or nasal passage (Schreibman et al., 2005). Mucocutaneous hyperpigmentation, sex cord tumours with annular tubules, Sertoli cell testicular tumours	Adenoma malignum of the cervix

Table 9.1 (continued) Risks of cancer associated with hereditary gastrointestinal syndromes

Syndrome	Clinical manifestations	Cancer risks	Benign pathology	Malignant pathology
Serrated polyposis syndrome	Multiple and/or large serrated polyps of the colon	25–70% of patients have CRC at diagnosis/follow-up (Bujanda, 2012). Median age of diagnosis from 40 to 62 years	Multiple and/or large serrated polyps of the colon	
Non-polyposis syndromes				
Lynch syndrome	CRC, EC, small bowel, ureter and renal pelvis cancer, sebaceous cysts, sebaceous gland adenomas, keratoacanthomas, sebaceous carcinomas, brain tumours (glioblastoma) (Kohlmann and Gruber, 2004)	CRC: 41, 48, 12% for *MLH1*, *MSH2*, *MSH6*, respectively. EC: 54, 21, 16% for *MLH1*, *MSH2*, *MSH6*, respectively. OC: 20, 24, 1% for *MLH1*, *MSH2*, *MSH6*, respectively. All other cancers ≤ 3% (Bonadona et al., 2011)	Sebaceous cysts, sebaceous gland adenomas, keratoacanthomas	CRC with tumour-infiltrating lymphocytes, Crohn-like lymphocytic reaction, mucinous/signet ring differentiation of cancer or medullary growth pattern (Lynch et al., 2009). Transitional cancer of ureter and renal pelvis
Constitutional mismatch repair deficiency syndrome	*Café au lait* patches and other signs of NF1, early CRC, haematological cancers, brain tumours (mostly glioblastomas) and a range of other malignancies (Wimmer and Kratz, 2010)	High risk for LS-associated malignancies, haematological malignancies and brain tumours (NCCN, 2013)	*Café au lait* patches, freckles, Lisch nodules, neurofibromas, tibial pseudarthrosis	
Familial colorectal cancer type X	CRC (Lindor, 2009)	Moderately elevated CRC risk		

Table 9.2 Diagnostic and germline testing criteria for colorectal cancer

Syndrome	Gene and locus	Gene function	Diagnostic criteria	Germline testing criteria
Polyposis syndromes				
Familial adenomatous polyposis	APC, 5q21-q22	Tumour suppression	More than 100 polyps in an individual under 40 years. Fewer than 100 polyps and relative with FAP (Jasperson and Randall, 2011)	Same as diagnostic criteria
Attenuated familial adenomatous polyposis	APC, 5q21-q22	Tumour suppression	Fewer than 100 adenomatous polyps, CRC under 60 years and family history (FH) of multiple adenomatous polyps. Three different diagnostic criteria (NCCN, 2013)	Fewer than 100 adenomatous polyps
MUTYH-associated polyposis	MAP, 1p34.3–32.1	Tumour suppression	15 to a few hundred adenomatous and/or hyperplastic polyps in the absence of APC mutation (Balaguer et al., 2007). FH of recessive inheritance	CRC at age under 50, more than 15 adenomatous polyps
Peutz–Jeghers syndrome (PJS)	STK11/LKB1, 19p13.3	Tumour suppression	Two or more histologically confirmed PJS polyps. Any number of PJS polyps and FH of PJS. Characteristic mucocutaneous pigmentation and FH of PJS. One or more PJS polyps and characteristic mucocutaneous pigmentation (Beggs et al., 2010)	Same as diagnostic criteria
Serrated polyposis syndrome	Unknown	Unknown	Criterion A: 5+ serrated polyps proximal to sigmoid colon, two of which are greater than 10 mm in diameter. Criterion B: any number of serrated polyps occurring proximal to the sigmoid colon in individual with first-degree relative with serrated polyposis. Criterion C: more than 20 serrated polyps any size distributed throughout the colon (Snover et al., 2010)	

Table 9.2 (continued) Diagnostic and germline testing criteria for colorectal cancer

Syndrome	Gene and locus	Gene function	Diagnostic criteria	Germline testing criteria
Non-polyposis syndromes				
Lynch syndrome	*MLH1, MSH2, MSH6, PMS2, EPCAM*	Tumour suppression	Amsterdam II and revised Bethesda criteria	Microsatellite unstable tumour and/or loss of MMR protein expression. Loss of MSH2 expression without *MSH2* germline mutation should prompt testing for deletions in the *EPCAM* gene (Ligtenberg et al., 2009)
Constitutional mismatch repair deficiency syndrome	*MLH1, MSH2, MSH6, PMS2*	Tumour suppression	Patient with malignancy and: *café au lait* patches and/or other NF1 signs, consanguineous parents, FH of Lynch syndrome associated tumours, second malignancy, sibling with childhood cancer	Microsatellite unstable tumour and/or loss of MMR protein expression
Familial colorectal cancer type X	Unknown	Unknown	Amsterdam I positive families with microsatellite stable CRC	

repeats called microsatellites. Approximately 85% of MMR-deficient tumours are due to a germline mutation in MMR genes such as *MSH2*, *MSH6*, *MLH1*, *PMS1* and *PMS2*, leading to a loss of protein expression by the affected gene (Hampel et al., 2005). The main cancers in LS are CRC, endometrial cancer (EC) and ovarian cancer (OC) (Table 9.1). Lifetime risk estimations for rarer cancers in LS vary in the literature. A study by Engel et al. (2012), based on 2118 carriers of MMR gene mutations estimated the cumulative risks at 70 years for the less common cancers in LS for males and females respectively, as follows: gastric 6.7% and 2.6%; small bowel 12% and 3.9%; urinary bladder 5.5% and 3.5%; other urothelium 9.4% and 6%; breast 14% and prostate 9.1%. A similar study estimated that the lifetime risk for any of the rarer cancers did not exceed 3% (Bonadona et al., 2011).

Constitutional mismatch repair-deficiency syndrome (CMMR-D) is another rare non-polyposis colon cancer syndrome in which most patients show *café au lait* patches and other features of neurofibromatosis type 1 (NF1) in addition to haematological malignancies and/or brain tumours and early onset CRC (Table 9.1). As in LS, CRC in CMMR-D shows microsatellite instability (MSI). However, in an overview summarising the findings from 78 CMMR-D patients, five of six brain tumours were microsatellite stable but in three of these five there was loss of expression of MMR proteins (Wimmer and Etzler, 2008).

As testing for germline mutations in MMR genes is time-consuming and expensive, clinical criteria have been developed to select individuals for genetic testing, such as the Amsterdam I criteria (Vasen et al., 1991) followed by the modified Amsterdam II criteria (Vasen et al., 2007) and the much broader and less specific revised Bethesda guidelines (Umar et al., 2004) (Box 9.1). Several risk assessment models have been proposed, based on MSI and immunohistochemistry (IHC) data and/or clinical criteria to predict the likelihood of a germline mutation in one of the MMR genes (Kohlmann and Gruber, 2012).

Funkhauser et al. (2012) in their report for the Association for Molecular Pathology list the different sensitivities of clinical criteria and laboratory tests in detecting LS: the Amsterdam II criteria have a sensitivity of 42–50% with a specificity of 97–98%; the revised Bethesda guidelines have a sensitivity of 95% with a specificity of 14–38%; MSI has a sensitivity of 89% for *MLH1*, 90% for *MSH2* and 76% for *MSH6*; IHC has a sensitivity of 81% for *MLH1*, 88% for *MSH2* and 76% for *MSH6*; and sequencing has a sensitivity of 99.5%. They go on to state that MSI and IHC combined would have detected 100% of LS cases in a set of four CRC series, describing a total of 3369 patients. If the search for the c.1799T>A somatic mutation in the *BRAF* gene was added to MSI and IHC, 100% of MMR-deficient tumours would be identified. Ultimately, the use of clinical selection criteria and laboratory tests will depend on financial considerations and local availability of the different laboratory test methods.

Familial colorectal cancer type X describes families which meet the Amsterdam I criteria (Box 9.1) but have microsatellite stable colorectal cancers. Members of these families have a lower CRC risk than LS families, i.e. a moderately to highly elevated CRC risk, and no increased risks for other cancers.

Box 9.1 The Amsterdam and Bethesda criteria

Definition of Amsterdam I positive families

1. Three or more relatives with CRC in the family.
2. One case is a first-degree relative of the other two.
3. At least two successive generations.
4. One CRC diagnosed under the age of 50.
5. FAP excluded.

Definition of Amsterdam II positive families

1. Three or more relatives with verified LS-related cancers in the family.
2. One case is a first-degree relative of the other two.
3. At least two successive generations.
4. One CRC diagnosed under the age of 50.
5. FAP excluded.

Definition of Bethesda positive individuals/families

1. CRC in a patient under 50 years of age.
2. Presence of synchronous[a], metachronous[b] colorectal or other LS-related tumours[c] regardless of age.
3. CRC with presence of tumour-infiltrating lymphocytes, Crohn's-like lymphocytic reaction, mucinous/signet ring differentiation of cancer or medullary growth pattern in a patient under 60 years of age.
4. CRC in one or more first-degree relatives with a LS-related tumour with one of the cancers being diagnosed before 50.
5. CRC in two or more first- or second-degree relatives with LS-related tumours[c] regardless of age.

[a]Synchronous: diagnosed at the same time.
[b]Metachronous: one cancer diagnosed after the other.
[c]LS-related tumours include CRC, endometrial, stomach, pancreas, biliary tract, small bowel carcinoma, ovarian, transitional cell ureter and renal pelvis, brain (usually glioblastoma) sebaceous gland adenomas and keratoacanthomas.

Adapted by permission from BMJ Publishing Group Limited, *Journal of Medical Genetics*, Guidelines for the clinical management of Lynch syndrome (hereditary non-polyposis cancer), Vasen HFA et al., Volume 44, Issue 6, pp. 353–362, Copyright © 2007, British Medical Journal Publishing Group. Source: data from Umar A et al, Revised Bethesda guidelines for hereditary nonpolyposis colorectal cancer (Lynch syndrome) and microsatellite instability, *Journal of National Cancer Institute*, Volume 96, Issue 4, pp. 261–268, Copyright © Oxford University Press 2004.

Polyposis syndromes

Familial adenomatous polyposis (FAP) was first described by Lockhart-Mummery (1925). FAP is responsible for about 1% of all CRC and causes hundreds to thousands of adenomatous polyps in the bowel, starting in adolescence. Attenuated FAP is characterised by a variable number of polyps which occur later in life and a lower risk of CRC (Table 9.1).

For attenuated FAP there are no universally accepted diagnostic and germline testing criteria and at least three different diagnostic criteria have been proposed (Table 9.2).

Over 1000 unique DNA variants have been reported in the *APC* gene in the Leiden Open Variation Database. The location of the mutation appears to affect the clinical manifestation, which is of interest for the clinical management of these patients (Heinen, 2010). However, further research needs to be done concerning the relationship between the location of mutations and their correlation with disease before the genotype can guide clinical decisions (Laurent-Puig et al., 1998).

MUTYH-**associated polyposis** (MAP) was first described by Al-Tassan et al. (2002) and accounts for less than 1% of all CRC cases (Cleary et al., 2009). MAP is caused by bilalleic mutations in *MUTYH* and therefore shows autosomal recessive inheritance (Table 9.1). Monoallelic *MUTYH* mutations are found in 1–2% of the population (Heinen, 2010). Whether carriers of monoallelic mutations have an increased risk of CRC has not yet been completely clarified, but a recent collaborative meta-analysis showed only a marginally increased risk of CRC in monoallelic carriers (Theodoratou et al., 2010).

Two missense *MUTYH* mutations have been described in the northern European population, c.536A>G in exon 7 and c.1187G>A in exon 13; these are carried by 1–2% of the general population and account for up to 70% of the mutations in northern European individuals suffering from MAP (Nielsen et al., 2009). Common *MUTYH* mutations have also been described in other populations such as Pakistani, Japanese, Korean and Ashkenazi Jewish (Nieuwenhuis and Vasen, 2007). Diagnostic and germline testing criteria for MAP are summarised in Table 9.2. As a specific somatic *KRAS* mutation (G12C, G>T) has been found in 9 of 14 MAP-associated cancers and 13 of 30 adenomas (Lipton et al., 2003), it has been suggested that somatic *KRAS* mutation analysis could be performed to select patients with suspected MAP for germline mutation testing.

The following algorithm for genetic testing for MAP has been suggested (Brand et al., 2012):

1 First search for the two common mutations in northern Europe (van Puijenbroek et al., 2008) or the common mutations found in the patients from other ethnic backgrounds. In heterozygotes, sequence analysis amplification should be performed as well as multiplex ligand probe amplification, although the detection rate for duplications and deletions has so far been reported to be small (Nielsen et al., 2011).

2 If no mutation is detected by targeted mutation analysis, it may still be appropriate to perform sequencing and multiplex ligand probe amplification of the MAP gene if there is a strong clinical suspicion for MAP and the patient does not have a northern European background.

Hamartomatous polyposis syndromes

Peutz–Jeghers syndrome (PJS) was described by Peutz (1921) and Jeghers et al. (1949) and is an autosomal dominantly inherited condition. The hallmarks of PJS are gastrointestinal hamartomas and mucocutaneous pigmentation that may disappear during puberty (Table 9.1). The largest study regarding the incidence of cancers in 419 individuals with PJS ascertained through specialist centres showed that the risk for developing any type of cancer up to the age of 70 was 85% (Hearle et al., 2006). PJS is caused by mutations in the *STK11/LKB1* gene (Table 9.2).

Juvenile polyposis was first described by McColl et al. (1964) and is a heterogeneous disease (Tables 9.1 and 9.2). Mutations in *SMAD4* or *BMPRA1* are found in about 20% of juvenile polyposis patients (Howe et al., 2004). In the largest series published so far, 45% of 102 juvenile polyposis patients had germline mutations and large deletions in the *SMAD4* or *BMPRA1* genes (Calva-Cerqueira et al., 2009). Carriers of *SMAD4* mutations may also have an increased risk of gastric polyps.

Cowden syndrome is another rare hamartomatous syndrome with a wide range of clinical manifestations (discussed further in Chapter 10). In a recent study of 127 patients with *PTEN* germline mutations, 64 of 69 patients who underwent one or more colonoscopies had gastrointestinal polyps and nine of them had CRC before the age of 50; half of the patients had hyperplastic polyps (Heald et al., 2010).

Serrated/hyperplastic polyposis syndrome

Hyperplastic polyposis syndrome was first described by Williams et al. (1980) and was renamed serrated polyposis syndrome by Snover et al. (2010). Serrated polyposis syndrome is a heterogeneous disease and its genetic causes are unknown. The estimates of colon cancer risk vary considerably (Table 9.1) and probably suffer from ascertainment bias.

Gastric cancer

Up to 3% of gastric cancers (GCs) are thought to be due to germline mutations causing a high risk for GC and other cancers. Inherited GC may be of the intestinal or diffuse type and is autosomal dominantly inherited.

Lifestyle factors such as diet and smoking and environmental factors such as *Helicobacter pylori* infection contribute to intestinal-type GC. There are countries with a high incidence of intestinal-type GC (e.g. China and Japan) and countries with a low incidence (e.g. the UK and United States). In countries with a low incidence, the diagnostic criteria for heritable intestinal-type GC are:

1 at least two first- or second-degree relatives with intestinal-type GC or

2 three or more relatives with intestinal-type GC at any age (Chun and Ford, 2012).

However, the genetic basis of heritable intestinal-type GC has not yet been elucidated.

In contrast, 25–30% of families with diffuse-type GC fulfilling the diagnostic criteria listed here carry a germline mutation in the E-cadherin gene (Fitzgerald et al., 2010). The most recent International Gastric Cancer Linkage Consortium criteria (Fitzgerald et al., 2010) for the diagnosis of hereditary diffuse-type GC are:

1 two GCs—one confirmed diffuse-type, one diagnosed at under 50 years of age;

2 three confirmed diffuse GCs in first- or second-degree relatives independent of age of onset;

3 diffuse-type gastric cancer diagnosed below the age of 40 years without a family history;

4 personal or family history (first- or second-degree relatives) of diffuse-type GC and lobular breast cancer, one diagnosed below 50 years of age.

The E-cadherin or *CDH1* gene is a tumour suppressor gene on chromosome 16q22 and was identified in 1998 as a GC-causing gene in a large Maori family (Guilford et al., 1998). Families with diffuse-type GC fulfilling any of the four criteria listed above should be considered for *CDH1* mutation testing. Using the MENDEL program, Pharoah et al. (2001) estimated the cumulative cancer risk by the age 80 in *CDH1* mutation carriers in 11 families to be 67% for men and 83% in women. Females carrying a *CDH1* mutation also have an increased risk for lobular breast cancer which may be as high a 52% throughout their lifetime (Kaurah et al., 2007).

Uterine cancer

Uterine (endometrial) cancer (EC) may occur as part of LS or Cowden syndrome. Depending on the cohort of patients examined, EC is the most common (Bonadona et al., 2011) or the second most common (Stoffel et al., 2009) cancer in women suffering from LS and tends to occur earlier than sporadic EC. Stoffel et al. (2009) analysed 147 *MLH1*, *MSH2* and *MSH6* mutation carriers and 6195 relatives; 155 ECs were observed, with a median age at diagnosis of 47.5 years (range 29–73) (Table 9.1). Patients with EC suspected of having LS may be selected for germline MSI testing and IHC for testing MMR protein expression of their tumour tissue because these tumours are microsatellite unstable in more than 90% of patients (Clarke and Cooper, 2012). The ECs observed in LS comprise a spectrum of tumours very similar to sporadic uterine cancers, including non-endometroid tumours such as uterine papillary serous carcinoma and malignant mixed Mullerian tumours (Broaddus et al., 2006), although in a study including a central pathology review 86% of ECs were of the endometroid type (Bonadona et al., 2011).

EC is also one of the spectrum of cancers seen in Cowden syndrome. The cancer risk may be as high as 28% (Table 9.1) with a tendency to occur earlier than in the general population, even in adolescence (Schmeler et al., 2009).

Ovarian cancer

Ovarian cancer (OC) may occur as part of LS and PJS. In LS, the risk for OC varies according to the gene carrying a mutation (Table 9.1) and may be as low as 1%. The mean age at which OC occurs is considerably lower than in sporadic OC, and in one study the mean age was 42.7 years (Watson et al., 2001) and one-third of women were younger than 40 at the time of diagnosis. A recent retrospective report by Stoffel et al. (2009) showed that over 90% of OCs in LS patients were of epithelial origin and invasive, with the majority being of unspecified epithelial type, serous or endometroid. Women with PJS are at increased risk from two very rare gynaecological tumours: sex cord tumours with annular tubules (ovarian tumours with a histology between a granulosa cell and Sertoli cell tumours) and adenoma malignum (a well-differentiated mucin-producing adenocarcinoma of the cervix with an aggressive behaviour). Sex cord tumours tend to be multifocal, bilateral and benign (Connolly et al., 2000).

Summary

Heritable cancer syndromes are very rare. This means that studies describing cancer risks or clinical features in affected individuals often have an ascertainment bias, are based on small numbers, are retrospective or suffer from a combination of these factors. Therefore, reported cancer risks and frequencies of clinical manifestations are probably overestimated in these syndromes. It is important to keep this in mind when counselling families with an inherited predisposition about their cancer risks and management options.

References

Al-Tassan N, Chmiel NH, Maynard J, et al. 2002. Inherited variants of MYH associated with somatic G:C→T:A mutations in colorectal tumors. *Nat Genet* **30**: 227–232.

Balaguer F, Castellví-Bel S, Castells A, et al. 2007. Identification of MYH mutation carriers in colorectal cancer: a multicenter, case–control, population-based study. *Clin Gastroenterol Hepatol* **5**: 379–387.

Beggs AD, Latchford AR, Vasen HF, et al. 2010. Peutz–Jeghers syndrome: a systematic review and recommendations for management. *Gut* **59**: 975–986.

Bonadona V, Bonaiti B, Olschwang S, et al. 2011. Cancer risks associated with different germline mutations in *MLH1, MSH2, MSH6* genes in Lynch syndrome. *J Am Med Assoc* **305**: 2304–2310.

Brand R, Nielsen M, Lynch H, Infante E 2012. *MUTYH*-associated polyposis. In: *GeneReviews™* [Internet] (ed. RA Pagon, TD Bird, CR Dolan, K Stephens, MP Adam). Seattle: University of Washington, 1993–2013 Available at: <http://www.ncbi.nlm.nih.gov/books/NBK107219/>.

Broaddus RR, Lynch HT, Chen LM, et al. 2006. Pathologic features of endometrial carcinoma associated with HNPCC: a comparison with sporadic endometrial carcinoma. *Cancer* **106**: 87–94.

Bujanda L 2012. Serrated polyposis syndrome: molecular, pathological and clinical aspects. *World J Gastroenterol* **18**: 2452–2461.

Calva-Cerqueira D, Chinnathambi S, Pechman B, et al. 2009. The rate of germline mutations and large deletions of *SMAD4* and *BMPR1A* in juvenile polyposis. *Clin Genet* **75**: 79–85.

Cancer.Net 2013. Familial adenomatous polyposis. Available at: <http://www.cancer.net/cancer-types/familial-adenomatous-polyposis> (last accessed 27 December 2013).

Chun N and Ford JM 2012. Genetic testing by cancer site. Stomach. *Cancer J* **18**: 355–363.

Clarke BA and Cooper K 2012. Identifying Lynch syndrome in patients with endometrial carcinoma: shortcomings of morphologic and clinical schemas. *Adv Anat Pathol* **19**: 231–238.

Cleary SP, Cotterchio M, Jenkins MA, et al. 2009. Germline MutY human homologue mutations and colorectal cancer: a multisite case–control study. *Gastroenterology* **136**: 1251–1260.

Connolly DC, Katabuchi H, Cliby WA 2000. Somatic mutations in the STK11/LKB1 gene are uncommon in rare gynecological tumor types associated with Peutz–Jegher's syndrome. *Am J Pathol* **156**: 339–345.

Engel C, Loeffler M, Schacker H 2012. Risks of less common cancers in proven mutation carriers with Lynch syndrome. *J Clin Oncol* **30**: 4409–4415.

Farrington SM, Tenesa A, Barnetson R, et al. 2005. Germline susceptibility to colorectal cancer due to base-excision repair gene defects. *Am J Hum Genet* **77**: 112–119.

Fitzgerald RC, Hardwick R, Huntsman D, et al. (International Gastric Cancer Linkage Consortium) 2010. Hereditary diffuse gastric cancer: updated consensus guidelines for clinical management and directions for future research. *J Med Genet* **47**: 436–444.

Funkhauser WK Jr, Lubin IM, Monzon FA, et al. 2012. Relevance, pathogenesis, and testing algorithm for mismatch repair-defective colorectal carcinomas. A report of the Association of Molecular Pathology. *J Molec Diagnost* **14**: 91–99.

Guilford P, Hopkins JB, Harraway J, et al. 1998. E-Cadherin germline mutations in familial gastric cancer. *Nature* **392**: 402–405.

Hampel H, Frankel WL, Martin E, et al. 2005. Screening for the Lynch syndrome (hereditary nonpolyposis colorectal cancer). *N Engl J Med* **352**: 1851–1860.

Heald B, Mester J, Rybicki L, et al. 2010. Frequent gastrointestinal polyps and colorectal adenocarcinomas in a prospective series of *PTEN* mutation carriers. *Gastroenterology* **139**: 1927–1933.

Hearle N, Schumacher V, Menko FH, et al. 2006. Frequency and spectrum of cancers in the Peutz–Jeghers syndrome. *Clin Cancer Res* **12**: 3209–3215.

Heinen CD 2010. Genotype to phenotype: analyzing the effects of inherited mutations in colorectal cancer families. *Mutat Res* **693**: 32–45.

Howe J, Sayed M, Ahmed A, et al. 2004. The prevalence of *MADH4* and *BMPR1A* mutations in juvenile polyposis and absence of *BMPR2*, *BMPR1B*, and *ACVR1* mutations. *J Med Genet* **41**: 484–491.

Jasperson KW and Randall WB 1998. APC-associated polyposis conditions [last update 27 October 2011]. In: *GeneReviews*™ [Internet] (ed. RA Pagon, TD Bird, CR Dolan, K Stephens, MP Adam). Seattle: University of Washington, 1993–2013. Available at: <http://www.ncbi.nlm.nih.gov/books/NBK1345/>.

Jeghers H, Mckusick VA, Katz KH 1949. Generalized intestinal polyposis and melanin spots of the oral mucosa, lips and digits. *New Engl J Med* **241**: 993–1005, 1031–1036.

Kaurah P, Macmillan A, Boyd N, et al. 2007. Founder and recurrent *CDH1* mutations in families with hereditary diffuse gastric cancer. *J Am Med Assoc* **297**: 2360–2372.

Kohlmann W and Gruber SB 2004. Lynch syndrome [last update 20 September 2012]. In: *GeneReviews*™ [Internet] (ed. RA Pagon, TD Bird, CR Dolan, K Stephens, MP Adam). Seattle: University of Washington, 1993–2013. Available at: <http://www.ncbi.nlm.nih.gov/books/NBK1211/>.

Laurent-Puig P, Béroud C, Soussi T 1998. *APC* gene: database of germline and somatic mutations in human tumors and cell lines. *Nucleic Acids Res* **26**: 269–270.

Leiden Open Variation Database. Colon cancer gene variant databases: adenomatous polyposis coli. Available at: <http://chromium.liacs.nl/LOVD2/colon_cancer/home.php?select_db=APC> (last accessed 27 December 2013).

Ligtenberg MJ, Kuiper RP, Chan TL, et al. 2009. Heritable somatic methylation and inactivation of *MSH2* in families with Lynch syndrome due to a deletion of the 3' exons of TACSTD1. *Nat Genet* **4**: 122–127.

Lindor NM 2009. Familial colorectal cancer type X: the other half of hereditary non-polyposis colon cancer syndrome. *Surg Oncol Clin N Am* **18**: 637–645.

Lipton L, Halford SE, Johnson V 2003. Carcinogenesis in MYH-associated polyposis follows a distinct genetic pathway. *Cancer Res* **63**: 7595–7599.

Lockhart-Mummery JP 1925. Cancer and heredity. *Lancet* **1**: 427.

Lynch HT, Shaw MW, Magnuson CW, et al. 1966. Hereditary factors in cancer. Study of two large midwestern kindreds. *Arch Intern Med* **117**: 206–212.

Lynch HT, Lynch JF, Attard TA 2009. Diagnosis and management of hereditary colorectal cancer syndromes: Lynch syndrome as a model. *Can Med Assoc J* **181**: 273–280.

McColl I, Busxey HI, Veale AM, Morson BC 1964. Juvenile polyposis coli. *Proc R Soc Med* **57**: 896–897.

McGarrity TJ, Amos CI, Frazier ML, et al. 2001. Peutz–Jeghers syndrome [updated 25 July 2013]. In: *GeneReviews™* [Internet] (ed. RA Pagon, TD Bird, CR Dolan, K Stephens, MP Adam). Seattle: University of Washington, 1993–2013. Available at: <http://www.ncbi.nlm.nih.gov/books/NBK1266/>.

Nielsen M, Joerink-Van De Beld MC, Jones N, et al. 2009. Analysis of *MUTYH* genotypes and colorectal phenotypes in patients with *MUTYH*-associated polyposis. *Gastroenterology* **136**: 471–476.

Nielsen M, Morreau H, Vasen HF, Hes FJ 2011. *MUTYH*-associated polyposis (MAP). *Crit Rev Oncol Hematol* **79**: 1–16.

Nieuwenhuis MH and Vasen HF 2007. Correlations between mutation site in APC and phenotype of familial adenomatous polyposis (FAP): a review of the literature. *Crit Rev Oncol Hematol* **61**: 153–161.

National Comprehensive Cancer Network (NCCN) <http://www.nccn.org/professionals/physician_gls/pdf/colorectal_screening.pdf> (last accessed 2 January 2013).

Peutz JLA 1921. Very remarkable case of familial polyposis of mucous membrane of intestinal tract and nasopharynx accompanied by peculiar pigmentations of skin and mucous membrane. *Nederl Maandschr Geneesk* **10**: 134–146.

Pharoah PD, Guilford P, Caldas C, International Gastric Cancer Linkage Consortium 2001. Incidence of gastric cancer and breast cancer in *CDH1* (E-cadherin) mutation carriers from hereditary diffuse gastric cancer families. *Gastroenterology* **121**: 1348–1353.

Schmeler KM, Daniels MS, Brandt AC, Lu KH 2009. Endometrial cancer in an adolescent: a possible manifestation of Cowden syndrome. *Obstet Gynecol* **114**: 477–479.

Schreibman IR, Baker M, Amos C 2005. The hamartomatous polyposis syndromes: a clinical and molecular review. *Am J Gastroenterol* **100**: 476–490.

Snover DC, Ahnen DJ, Burt RW, et al. 2010. Serrated polyps of the colon and rectum and serrated polyposis. In: *WHO classification of tumours of the digestive system* (ed. FT Bosman, F Carneiro, RH Hruban et al.), pp. 160–165. Lyon: IARC Press.

Stoffel E, Bhramar M, Raymond VM, et al. 2009. Calculation of risk of colorectal and endometrial cancer among patients with Lynch syndrome. *Gastroenterology* **137**: 1621–1627.

Theodoratou E, Campbell H, Tenesa A, et al. 2010. A large-scale meta-analysis to refine colorectal cancer risk estimates associated with MUTYH variants. *Br J Cancer* **103**: 1875–1884.

Umar A, Boland CR, Terdiman JP, et al. 2004. Revised Bethesda guidelines for hereditary non-polyposis colon cancer (Lynch syndrome) and microsatellite instability. *J Natl Cancer Inst* **96**: 261–268.

Van Puijenbroek M, Nielsen M, Tops CM, et al. 2008. Identification of patients with (atypical) *MUTYH*-associated polyposis by KRAS2 c.34G > T prescreening followed by *MUTYH* hotspot analysis in formalin-fixed paraffin-embedded tissue. *Clin Cancer Res* **14**: 139–142.

Vasen HF, Mecklin JP, Khan PM, et al. 1991. The International Collaborative Group on Hereditary Non-polyposis Colorectal Cancer (ICG-HNPCC). *Dis Colon Rectum* **34**: 424–425.

Vasen HFA, Möslein G, Alonso A, et al. 2007. Guidelines for the clinical management of Lynch syndrome (hereditary non-polyposis cancer). *J Med Genet* **44**: 353–362.

Vogt S, Jones N, Christian D, et al. 2009. Expanded extracolonic tumor spectrum in MUTYH-associated polyposis. *Gastroenterology* **137**: 1976–1985.

Watson P, Bützow R, Lynch HT, et al. 2001. The clinical features of ovarian cancer in hereditary nonpolyposis colorectal cancer. *Gynecol Oncol* **82**: 223–228.

Williams GT, Arthur JF, Bussey HJ, Morson BC 1980. Metaplastic polyps and polyposis of the colorectum. *Histopathology* **4**: 155–170.

Wimmer K and Etzler J 2008. Constitutional mismatch repair-deficiency syndrome: Have we so far seen only the tip of the iceberg? *Hum Genet* **124**: 105–122.

Wimmer K and Kratz CP 2010. Constitutional mismatch repair-deficiency syndrome. *Haematologica* 95: 699–701.

Chapter 10

Genetics of prostate cancer

Elizabeth Bancroft, Audrey Ardern-Jones,
and Rosalind Eeles

Introduction to genetics of prostate cancer

Prostate cancer is now the commonest cancer in men in the western world. In the UK there are over 40 000 new cases per year and a lifetime risk of prostate cancer of 1 in 9. The fact that there is a large difference in the incidence of prostate cancer worldwide indicates that lifestyle risk factors are important, though as yet no definite risk factors have been identified. These differences may be due to the interplay of genetic, environmental and social influences (such as access to healthcare), which may affect the development and progression of the disease. The estimated number of men with latent prostate cancer (i.e. cancer that is present in the prostate gland but never detected or diagnosed during the patient's life) is greater than the number of men with clinically detected disease who present with symptoms. A better understanding is needed of the genetic and biological mechanisms that determine why some prostate cancers remain clinically silent while others cause serious, even life-threatening, illness. This chapter outlines the genetic risk for men with and without a family history of developing the disease and the latest research. The learning objectives for this chapter are:

- to understand prostate cancer;
- to be able to examine the genetic factors that contribute to the development of prostate cancer;
- to understand genetic research and the implications for screening and management in prostate cancer;
- to be able to discuss the influence of cancer genetics in the development of prostate cancer;
- to be able to describe the implications for the client group and healthcare practice.

Prostate cancer

Prostate cancer is mainly a disease of older men, the median age at diagnosis being 72 years. Around 20% of cases occur in men under the age of 65. Over the past 10 to 15 years there have been many advances in the management of prostate cancer, but there is a great deal of controversy about the best management for patients with early, non-metastatic disease.

The rate of tumour growth varies from very slow to moderately rapid, and some patients may have prolonged survival even after the cancer has spread to distant sites, such as bone. The approach to treatment is influenced by age and coexisting medical problems. It is well known that many men, especially those with localised tumours, die of another illness without ever having had any problems with their prostate cancer diagnosis.

Screening for prostate cancer

Currently the best biomarker test available is measurement of the level of serum prostate-specific antigen (PSA). This test can lead to the diagnosis of localised prostate cancer for which potentially curative treatment can be offered. However, PSA screening has only moderate accuracy, with a low level of specificity and sensitivity; it misses disease in some and gives false-positive results in others. The routine use of PSA screening remains a contentious issue as there is currently no evidence that the benefits of a programme of PSA-based screening of the general population would outweigh the harms. There is international variation in screening recommendations. Some physicians will carry out a digital rectal examination (DRE) in conjunction with a PSA test, but this is not recommended as a screening test in asymptomatic men (Burford et al., 2010). The screening of men with a significant family history is more widely supported, and there is evidence that it can have potential psychological benefits (Bratt et al., 2002).

Many prostate cancers are diagnosed as a result of routine screening, especially in the United States where PSA testing is widespread. When detected through screening, the patient is usually asymptomatic with early stage localised disease. However, in other parts of the world where screening is less common, men may present with symptoms of urinary obstruction such as decreased urinary stream, urgency, hesitancy, nocturia or incomplete bladder emptying—though such symptoms may well have benign causes. Some patients present with bone pain or pathological fractures that are the result of widespread disease.

Risk factors for prostate cancer

The three most important risk factors are age, race and having a family history of prostate cancer. Many other risk factors, including lifestyle, diet and hormonal factors, are being investigated in ongoing epidemiological research projects. As with breast and colon cancer families, clustering of cases of men with prostate cancer has been reported frequently. However, at least some familial aggregation is due to increased prostate cancer screening in families thought to be at high risk.

Genetic risk factors for prostate cancer

One of the most important and well-researched risk factors for prostate cancer is family history. Having a first-degree relative (e.g. a brother or father) with prostate cancer increases the risk of prostate cancer to approximately twice that for men in the general population (Edwards and Eeles, 2004). The risk is inversely related to the age of the affected relative. Therefore the younger a man is diagnosed, the greater the risk to his relatives, with the risk being increased fourfold for cases diagnosed before the age of 60. An analysis of a Swedish database reported that the cumulative (absolute) risks of prostate cancer amongst men in families with two or more affected relatives were 5, 15 and 30% by the ages of 60, 70 and 80, respectively, compared with 0.45, 3 and 10% at the same ages in the general population. The risks were higher still if the affected father was diagnosed before the age of 70. Furthermore, there is a higher risk in black men, who have a 2.87–3.19-fold increased risk compared with white men in the UK (Ben-Shlomo et al., 2008). Interestingly, Lichtenstein et al. (2000) found that there is an increased risk in monozygotic rather than in dizygotic twins, supporting the hypothesis that genetic factors play an important role in the development of prostate cancer. Furthermore, aggressive disease is also known to have a heritable component (Hemminki et al., 2008).

Genetic research in prostate cancer

Until very recently little progress had been made in identifying genes predisposing to an increased risk of prostate cancer. Early work involved genetic linkage studies; such studies examine the co-inheritance of two genetic loci that lie close together on a chromosome in order to identify disease-causing genes. However, this approach has been mainly limited to genes with rare, highly penetrant alleles because it lacks the statistical power to detect genes conferring a moderate risk of cancer. Genetic linkage studies have been successful in identifying high-risk genes associated with other common cancers such as breast cancer, ovarian cancer and colorectal cancer. Linkage studies and molecular analyses which assess the co-segregation of the disease with genetic markers have indicated several regions that may be involved in the development of prostate cancer. However, replicating these findings has proved to be difficult, suggesting that prostate cancer is genetically complex and involves many genes (Goh et al., 2012).

Studies of candidate genes (i.e. genes considered as possible disease-causing genes) have detected a number of possible associations with prostate cancer risk, but replicating the results has proved challenging. Mutations in *BRCA2* and possibly *BRCA1* have been identified by several groups as conferring an increased risk of prostate cancer, and these will be discussed in more detail later.

More recently attention has focused on genome-wide association studies (GWAS), which involve the testing of genetic variants in large series of cases (people with the disease) versus controls (people without the disease or with a low probability of having it). GWAS provide a powerful means of identifying lower-risk genetic variants that cannot be detected by linkage studies.

GWAS have led to the identification of 77 genetic variants (single nucleotide polymorphisms, SNPs) associated with prostate cancer risk (Eeles et al., 2013). Indeed, current research shows that approximately 30% of the familial risk of prostate cancer can be explained by these SNPs. SNPs associated with prostate cancer have been found in the *KLK2* (kallikrein-related peptidase 2, hK2) and *KLK3* (PSA) regions on chromosome 19. Kallikreins are a subgroup of enzymes called serine proteases. PSA is one such serine protease; it is secreted by the prostate gland, and as already mentioned is used as a biomarker for prostate cancer. SNPs in this region have been shown to affect PSA levels.

MacInnis et al. (2011) published a risk prediction algorithm that could potentially be used in the clinic to predict the probability of developing prostate cancer based on both SNP profiles and family history information. The ability to test someone for risk-associated SNPs has the potential to be useful in targeting screening and prevention strategies at those men who are at the highest genetic risk. The combined effect of several of these SNPs in one person could be quite significant. It is estimated that men in the top 1% of the risk distribution could have a 4.7-fold increased risk compared with the population average (Eeles et al., 2013). Given the controversy about the general use of PSA screening, it is possible that SNP profiling will be of particular use in helping to identify which individuals to screen, reducing unnecessary screening tests and improving economic viability (Pash-ayan et al., 2011). Therefore knowledge about these SNPs and their biological role has implications for counselling individuals regarding their risk of prostate cancer.

BRCA1, *BRCA2* and *HOXB13* genes and prostate cancer

Rare variants predisposing to prostate cancer

Mutations in *BRCA1* and *BRCA2* have been identified as conferring an increased risk of prostate cancer. These dominantly inherited, highly penetrant gene mutations were discovered in the mid to late 1990s to increase the risk of breast and ovarian cancer, as described Chapter 8. Their role in the development of prostate cancer was established later.

BRCA2 is an example of a rare variant where clear evidence exists that mutations in the gene result in an increased risk of prostate cancer. This was demonstrated in publications by the Breast Cancer Linkage Consortium (BCLC) which analysed men in breast–ovarian cancer families. Their data estimated that men with germline *BRCA2* mutations have an approximately fivefold increased relative risk of prostate cancer. This increases to over a sevenfold increase in families with young-onset cases (under 65 years). It has been estimated that between 1.2 and 2% of early onset prostate cancer cases (diagnosed under 65 years) may be attributable to *BRCA2* mutations (Kote-Jarai et al., 2011).

The relative risk of prostate cancer in young *BRCA1* mutation carriers has been contentious, but a recent study by Leongamornlert et al. (2012) has corroborated the previous BCLC data showing that *BRCA1* mutation carriers also have an increased risk of prostate cancer (about 3.8-fold) up to the age 65.

In addition rare variants in *HOXB13* have been identified in the research setting. A rare recurrent mutation (G84E) has been reported to be associated with prostate cancer risk (Xu et al., 2013). Further confirmation and characterisation is necessary before translat-ing this information into clinical testing programmes. However, it is known that *HOXB13* plays a role in development of the prostate and binds to the androgen receptor. Indeed, this is the first gene shown to account for a small percentage of inherited prostate cancer, especially early onset disease. Current research suggests that this variant is present in 5% of prostate cancer families, mainly of European descent.

Furthermore, the *NBS1* founder mutation 657del5 plays a role in the development of prostate cancer, and research suggests that heterozygous carriers of the *NBS1* founder mutation exhibit increased risk of prostate cancer (Cybulski et al., 2004a). Germline mutations in the Chek2 kinase gene (*CHEK2*) have been associated with a range of cancer types. In Poland, on average, men who carry a mutation have a 1.8-fold increased risk of prostate cancer, and it is estimated that mutations in *CHEK2* are responsible for about 7% of all prostate cancer cases in Poland (Cybulski et al., 2004b). As yet, no genetic testing is being done in the clinical setting, but this may change in the near future.

BRCA-associated prostate cancer in diagnosed men

Different groups around the world have also published data showing that *BRCA2* mutation carriers have more aggressive prostate cancers with a worse prognosis (Gallagher et al., 2010; Castro et al., 2013). These mutation carriers will have been tested in a genetics clinic and will be aware of the risks of breast and ovarian cancer for their female relatives. The fact that a man is a mutation carrier has important clinical implications, because carriers diagnosed with prostate cancer could be targeted for more aggressive treatment strategies.

Increasingly, targeted drugs such as poly(ADP-ribose) polymerase (PARP) inhibitors have been tested in other tumour sites in patients harbouring germline *BRCA* mutations, with promising response rates (Fong et al., 2010). This could potentially provide a further therapeutic option for prostate cancer in *BRCA* mutation carriers. If the efficacy of targeted agents such as these is proven, it may lead to more prostate cancer patients undergoing *BRCA2* mutation testing. As mentioned before, the data for *BRCA1* mutation carriers remain less clear and further analysis is needed to ascertain the association with clinical/treatment parameters and prognosis, although there is the suggestion that the disease may be more aggressive with a poorer prognosis in these carriers too (Castro et al., 2013).

Prostate screening for BRCA carriers and their relatives

There is an ongoing international study evaluating the efficacy of screening in *BRCA* mutation carriers (the IMPACT study, <http://www.impact-study.co.uk>), and until this study is completed there can be no definite guidelines for the management of *BRCA1/2* mutation carriers, although PSA screening could be considered from the age of 40 (or 10 years younger than the youngest case in the family).

Screening for men with a family history of prostate cancer

Studies evaluating the optimal methods for prostate cancer screening are ongoing. The PROFILE study (Eeles et al., personal communication), a pilot study using primary prostate biopsy (10-core trans-rectal ultrasound biopsy irrespective of PSA in men aged 40–69 years) in a cohort of 100 men with a family history of prostate cancer, has recently been completed. The study detected a higher number of clinically significant prostate cancers (as defined by UK National Institute for Health and Care Excellence treatment guidelines, which determine which tumours need radical treatment rather than active surveillance) compared with population-based PSA screening from the European Randomised Screening for Prostate Cancer (ERSPC) trial (Schroder et al., 2012).

The Targeted PSA Screening (TAPS) study looked at the feasibility of targeting screening at high-risk groups (Melia et al., 2006) and identified a number of key issues. The study aims were to investigate the rate of uptake of screening using PSA testing and the referral rate in male relatives of men already diagnosed with prostate cancer below the age of 65 years. Relatives of men with prostate cancer aged between 45 and 69 years were recruited, eligible men being contacted via their affected relatives. It was found that discussing the study in person with prostate cancer patients yielded a higher recruitment rate than postal invitations. It was also found that there was a high level of previous PSA screening within this cohort. Interestingly, men were far more likely to opt for screening within the study if they were married/cohabiting rather than single. The results of the TAPS study have important implications for the design of targeted screening programmes in higher-risk groups and highlight that further research is needed into the management of these groups.

There are preliminary data on PSA thresholds and PSA screening without DRE in high-risk populations based on genetic analyses or family history (Mitra et al., 2011). There have been a limited number of studies evaluating the role of PSA screening in men with first-degree relatives with prostate cancer. These have shown an increased risk of prostate cancer for men with a family history, and Valeri et al (2002) found an association between early onset disease and increased risk of prostate in first-degree relatives. A study of men with at least one first- or second-degree relative with prostate cancer who underwent prostate biopsy showed that 25.3% had prostate cancer (Canby-Hagino, 2007).

Genetic testing in men at risk of prostate cancer

Several studies have looked at opinions about genetic testing amongst men with a family history of prostate cancer and have found a very high level of interest, with studies reporting that 90–98% of men would be interested in being tested if a test were to become available (Bratt et al., 2000; Cormier et al., 2002; Cowan et al., 2008). Weinrich et al. (2002) and Myers et al. (2000) reported a very high level of interest (86–87%) in genetic testing amongst African-American men without a family history of prostate cancer. This suggests that there could be a high demand from the target population for genetic testing in the future.

The association of genetic variants with treatment variables

Currently there are multiple options for the treatment of prostate cancer, even for those men with metastases. There is a variable response to each of the treatments, but this variability is not yet understood. However, genetic variants could be an explanation for the differing responses to treatment. Researchers investigating the causes of the variation in radiation toxicity initially targeted known candidate genes, for example the DNA repair pathway genes, but the results have been conflicting (Barnett et al., 2009). More recently, the results of GWAS studies associated with radiation toxicity are emerging. Kerns et al. (2010) have so far published three separate papers detailing GWAS in radiotherapy cohorts. Collaborations as part of the Radiogenomics Consortium are currently under way to increase patient numbers so as to better evaluate the effect of genetic variants on radiation toxicity. Thus, the most important aim of this research would be tailor treatment according to risk.

Genetic variants have also been reported to be associated with outcomes from other treatment modalities. In patients who underwent radical prostatectomies, genes reported to be related to the aggressiveness and progression of disease have been identified in various studies, including androgen pathway genes (Strom et al., 2004). This research was done on patients with somatic prostate cancer not germline prostate cancer. Perez et al (2010) identified a SNP with a protective effect in the EGFR (epidermal growth factor receptor) gene. This somatic polymorphism has been associated with decreased biochemical relapse rates in men following prostatectomy. However, further replication studies are still required to validate these findings.

In those undergoing androgen deprivation therapies for prostate cancer, several candidate gene loci have been implicated to be associated with resistance to hormonal therapy. Again, a more complete understanding of such complexities could in the future help doctors to tailor the hormone therapy.

There have been fewer reports concerning the association of genetic variants with the response chemotherapy or the toxicity of chemotherapy. SNPs relating to drug metabolism are thought to predict for adverse reactions (Narita et al., 2012); however, SNPs implicated in this pathway have also been reported to be associated with a poorer prognosis (Sissung et al., 2008).

Summary

In conclusion, as increasing numbers of genetic variants are identified as being involved in the development and progression of prostate cancer ongoing research is needed to understand the biological role of these variants. It is likely that in the future men will be tested for these genetic variants to identify those at increased risk as well as to determine which treatments will be the most effective for an individual. Correlating genetic profiles with tailored treatment plans according to an individual's risk profile could reduce toxicity and benefit the patient. This would also have economic benefits for the health service. Furthermore, increased understanding of the role of the variants may potentially identify new prognostic markers and develop new targets for future therapy.

References

Barnett GC, West CM, Dunning AM, et al. 2009. Normal tissue reactions to radiotherapy: towards tailoring treatment dose by genotype. *Nat Rev Cancer* **9**: 134–142.

Ben-Shlomo Y, Evans S, Ibrahim F, et al. 2008. The risk of prostate cancer amongst black men in the United Kingdom: the PROCESS cohort study. *Eur Urol* **53**: 99–105.

Bratt O 2002. Hereditary prostate cancer: clinical aspects. *J Urol* **168**: 906–913.

Bratt O, Damber JE, Emanuelsson M, et al. 2000. Risk perception, screening practice and interest in genetic testing among unaffected men in families with hereditary prostate cancer. *Eur J Cancer* **36**: 235–241.

Burford DC, Kirby M, Austoker J 2010. Prostate cancer risk management programme information for primary care; PSA testing in asymptomatic men. Evidence document. NHS Cancer Screening Programmes. Available at: <http://www.cancerscreening.nhs.uk/prostate/pcrmp02.pdf> (last accessed 15 April 2014).

Canby-Hagino E, Hernandez J, Brand TC et al. 2007. Prostate cancer risk with positive family history, normal prostate examination findings, and PSA less than 4.0 ng/mL. *Urology* **70**: 748–752.

Castro E, Goh C, Olmos D, et al. 2013. Germline *BRCA* mutations are associated with higher risk of nodal involvement, distant metastasis and poor survival outcomes in prostate cancer. *J Clin Oncol* **31**: 1748–1757.

Cormier L, Valeri A, Azzouzi R, et al. 2002. Worry and attitude of men in at–risk families for prostate cancer about genetic susceptibility and genetic testing. *Prostate* **51**: 276–285.

Cowan R, Meiser B, Giles GG, et al. 2008. The beliefs, and reported and intended behaviors of unaffected men in response to their family history of prostate cancer. *Genet Med* **10**: 430–438.

Cybulski L, Gorski B, Debniak T, et al. 2004a. *NBS1* is a prostate cancer susceptibility gene. *Cancer Res* **64**: 1215–1219.

Cybulski L, Gorski B, Huzarski T, et al. 2004b. A novel founder *CHEK2* mutation is associated with increased prostate cancer risk. *Cancer Res* **64**: 2677–2679.

Edwards SM and Eeles RA 2004. Unravelling the genetics of prostate cancer. *Am J Med Genet C: Semin Med Genet* **129C**: 65–73.

Eeles RA, Olama AA, Benlloch S, et al. 2013. Identification of 23 new prostate cancer susceptibility loci using the iCOGS custom genotyping array. *Nat Genet* **45**: 385–391.

Fong PC, Yap TA, Boss DS, et al. 2010. Poly(ADP)-ribose polymerase inhibition: frequent durable responses in *BRCA* carrier ovarian cancer correlating with platinum-free interval. *J Clin Oncol* **28**: 2512–2519.

Gallagher DJ, Gaudet MM, Pal P, et al. 2010. Germline *BRCA* mutations denote a clinicopathologic subset of prostate cancer. *Clin Cancer Res* **16**: 2115–2121.

Goh CL, Schumacher FR, Easton D, et al. 2012. Genetic variants associated with predisposition to prostate cancer and potential clinical implications. *J Intern Med* **271**: 353–365.

Hemminki K, Ji J, Forsti A, et al. 2008. Concordance of survival in family members with prostate cancer. *J Clin Oncol* **26**: 1705–1709.

Kerns SL, Ostrer H, Stock R, et al. 2010. Genome-wide association study to identify single nucleotide polymorphisms (SNPs) associated with the development of erectile dysfunction in African-American men after radiotherapy for prostate cancer. *Int J Radiat Oncol Biol Phys* **78**: 1292–1300.

Kote-Jarai Z, Leongamornlert D, Saunders E 2011. *BRCA2* is a moderate penetrance gene contributing to young-onset prostate cancer: implications for genetic testing in prostate cancer patients. *Br J Cancer* **105**: 1230–1234.

Leongamornlert D, Mahmud N, Tymrakiewicz M, et al. 2012. Germline *BRCA1* mutations increase prostate cancer risk. *Br J Cancer* **106**: 1697–1701.

Lichtenstein P, Holm NV, Verkasalo PK et al. 2000. Environmental and heritable factors in the causation of cancer-analyses of cohorts of twins from Sweden, Denmark and Finland. *N Engl J Med* **343**: 78–85.

MacInnis RJ, Antoniou AC, Eeles RA, et al. 2011. A risk prediction algorithm based on family history and common genetic variants: application to prostate cancer with potential clinical impact. *Genet Epidemiol* **35**: 549–556.

Melia J, Dearnaley D, Moss S, et al. 2006. The feasibility and results of a population-based approach to evaluating prostate-specific antigen screening for prostate cancer in men with a raised familial risk. *Br J Cancer* **94**: 499–506.

Mitra AV, Bancroft EK, Barbachano Y, et al. 2011. Targeted prostate cancer screening in men with mutations in *BRCA1* and *BRCA2* detects aggressive prostate cancer: preliminary analysis of the results of the IMPACT study. *Br J Urol Int* **107**: 28–39.

Myers RE, Hyslop T, Jennings-Dozier K, et al. 2000. Intention to be tested for prostate cancer risk among African-American men. *Cancer Epidemiol, Biomarkers Prevent* **9**: 1323–1328.

Narita S, Tsuchiya N, Yuasa T, et al. 2012. Outcome, clinical prognostic factors and genetic predictors of adverse reactions of intermittent combination chemotherapy with docetaxel, estramustine phosphate and carboplatin for castration-resistant prostate cancer. *Int J Clin Oncol* **17**: 204–211.

Pashayan N, Duffy SW, Chowdhury S, et al. 2011. Polygenic susceptibility to prostate and breast cancer: implications for personalised screening. *Br J Cancer* **104**: 1656–1663.

Perez CA, Chen H, Shyr Y, et al. 2010. The EGFR polymorphism rs884419 is associated with freedom from recurrence in patients with resected prostate cancer. *J Urol* **183**: 2062–2069.

Schroder FH, Hugosson J, Roobol MJ, et al. 2012. Prostate-cancer mortality at 11 years of follow-up. *N Engl J Med* **366**: 981–990.

Sissung TM, Danesi R, Price DK, et al. 2008. Association of the CYP1B1*3 allele with survival in patients with prostate cancer receiving docetaxel. *Mol Cancer Ther* **7**: 19–26.

Strom SS, Gu Y, Zhang H, et al. 2004. Androgen receptor polymorphisms and risk of biochemical failure among prostatectomy patients. *Prostate* **60**: 343–351.

Valeri A, Cormier L, Moineau MP, et al. 2002. Targeted screening for prostate cancer in high risk families: early onset is a significant risk factor for disease in first degree relatives. *J Urol* **168**: 483–487.

Weinrich S, Royal C, Pettaway CA, et al. 2002. Interest in genetic prostate cancer susceptibility testing among African American men. *Cancer Nurs* **25**: 28–34.

Xu J, Lange E, Lu L, et al. 2013. HOXB13 is a susceptibility gene for prostate cancer: results from the International Consortium for Prostate Cancer Genetics (ICPCG). *Hum Genet* **132**: 5–14.

Chapter 11

Genetics of rare cancer syndromes

Adam Shaw

Introduction to genetics of rare cancer syndromes

This chapter focuses on the rare cancer predisposition syndromes that may occasionally be encountered in clinical practice. Although each one has a unique combination of associated tumours and other clinical features, they are linked by the underlying molecular function of their associated genes and the need for a holistic and multidisciplinary approach to their management. The syndromes covered in this chapter are listed in Table 11.1.

The learning objectives for this chapter are:

- to be able to discuss the influence of cancer genetics in the development of rare cancer syndromes;
- to be able to describe the implications for the client group and healthcare practice.

Birt–Hogg–Dubé syndrome (BHDS)

BHDS is a very rare entity, and with only around 200 cases reported in the medical literature prevalence is likely to be low, although it may be under-recognised. The condition is caused by loss of function mutations in the *FLCN* gene on chromosome 17p11.2. *FLCN* operates as a tumour suppressor gene in the kidney but has different roles in other tissues. For example mutations in *FLCN* result in the development of emphysema-like bullae in the lungs (Menko et al., 2009).

BHDS is associated with a predisposition to renal tumours, most commonly chromophobe tumours and oncocytoma which are often multifocal and bilateral. The risk of developing renal tumours is reported in various studies to be between 6 and 34%, but is most likely to be at the lower end of this range. Tumours are typically slow growing and benign, and present from around 30 years of age. Other classical features of BHDS include benign papular lesions of the skin occurring in adulthood and multiple lung cysts presenting as spontaneous, and possibly recurrent, pneumothorax. The skin lesions can be subtle, and are small hamartoma, histologically described as fibrofolliculoma, trichodiscoma or angiofibroma.

On computed tomography (CT) imaging, 90% of patients will have visible pulmonary cysts but most individuals remain asymptomatic, with only a third reporting dyspnoea, chest pain or other symptoms suggestive of pneumothorax.

Genetic testing for the *FLCN* gene may help clarify the diagnosis in those patients with few features. A molecular diagnosis may help define prognosis and risk to relatives. A mutation

Table 11.1 Syndromes covered in this chapter

Syndrome name (abbreviation)	Gene(s)	Predominant tumour types
Birt–Hogg–Dubé syndrome (BHDS)	FLCN	Renal oncocytoma/chromophobe
Carney complex (CNC)	PRKAR1A	Adrenal hyperplasia, thyroid carcinoma, pancreatic carcinoma
Cowden syndrome (CS)/PTEN hamartoma syndrome	PTEN	Breast carcinoma, thyroid carcinoma, endometrial carcinoma
Familial atypical mole and melanoma (FAMM)	CDKN2A, CDK4	Melanoma
Gorlin syndrome/basal cell naevus syndrome (BCNS)	PTCH	Basal cell carcinoma, medulloblastoma
Hereditary leiomyomatosis and renal cell cancer (HLRCC)	FH	Cutaneous and uterine leiomyoma, renal carcinoma
Hereditary paraganglioma/phaeochromocytoma (PGL/PCC)	SDHA, SDHB, SDHC, SDHD, SDHAF2, TMEM127, MAX, VHL, RET	Paraganglioma, phaeochromocytoma
Muir–Torre syndrome (MTS)	MLH1, MSH2, MSH6	Sebaceous carcinoma, colorectal adenocarcinoma, endometrial carcinoma, ovarian adenocarcinoma
Multiple endocrine neoplasia type 1 (MEN1)	MEN1	Prolactinoma, gastrinoma, insulinoma
Multiple endocrine neoplasia type 2 (MEN2)	RET	Medullary thyroid cancer, phaeochromocytoma, parathyroid hyperplasia
Peutz–Jehgers syndrome (PJS)	STK11	Gastrointestinal (GI) hamartoma, GI adenocarcinoma, breast carcinoma
Von Hippel–Lindau disease (VHL)	VHL	Hemangioblastoma, renal cell carcinoma, phaeochromocytoma

is identifiable in around 90% of clinically diagnosed cases, and around half have a mutation at a known mutation hotspot in exon 11 (Khoo et al., 2002; Toro et al., 2008).

Renal tumour screening should be offered, but given the benign course of tumour growth, intervention is rarely warranted for tumours that are less than 3 cm in size. Most units offer screening by either ultrasound or magnetic resonance imaging (MRI) from 20 years of age with an interval of 12–18 months. To reduce the risk of pulmonary complications, patients would be advised to avoid smoking and SCUBA diving. BHDS is an autosomal dominant condition with variable expressivity, and first-degree relatives of an affected individual may be at risk.

Carney complex

Carney complex is an extremely rare syndrome caused by loss-of-function mutations in the *PRKAR1A* tumour suppressor gene on chromosome 17q24 (Groussin et al., 2006).

Table 11.2 Tumours occurring in Carney complex

Tumour	Benign/malignant	Prevalence
Primary pigmented nodular adrenocortical disease	Benign	25%
Thyroid adenoma	Benign	Up to 75%
Thyroid carcinoma	Malignant	Rare
Growth hormone-secreting adenoma	Benign	10% symptomatic, up to 75% asymptomatic
Testicular Sertoli cell	Mostly benign	Up to 100% of men
Psammomatous melanotic schwannoma	Benign with risk of malignant transformation	10%
Cardiac myxoma	Benign	Mostly childhood
Breast myxoma	Benign	About 50% of women
Cutaneous myxoma	Benign	About 90%
Pancreatic	Malignant	Unknown

Affected individuals develop skin and mucosal lentigines (flat areas of increased pigment) as well as a propensity to a variety of tumours (Table 11.2). The most common of these include endocrine tumours such as primary pigmented nodular adrenocortical disease (PPNAD), growth hormone-secreting adenoma, thyroid carcinoma and myxoma, which can affect many organs.

PPNAD is associated with adrenocorticotropic hormone (ACTH)-independent overproduction of cortisol (hypercortisolism), and thus presents with the Cushing syndrome of central obesity, reduced muscle bulk and skin thinning (Bertherat et al., 2009).

Cowden syndrome/*PTEN* hamartoma syndrome

Cowden syndrome is one of a group of conditions, collectively termed the *PTEN* hamartoma syndromes. They are all very rare with a combined incidence of around 1 in 200 000. *PTEN* is a tumour suppressor gene located on chromosome 10q23.3 which has important functions in controlling the cell replication cycle and regulating apoptosis. Constitutional loss-of-function mutations in *PTEN* may cause Cowden syndrome, Bannayan–Riley–Ruvalcaba syndrome (BRRS) or Lhermitte–Duclos disease (dysplastic gangliocytoma of the cerebellum), which are now believed to be different clinical presentations of the same condition (Blumenthal and Dennis, 2008). Somatic mutations of *PTEN* are commonly seen in sporadic tumours.

Cowden syndrome conveys an increased risk of breast, endometrial and thyroid cancer. The lifetime risk of breast cancer in affected women is estimated to be up to 77%. Women also have up to a 10% lifetime risk of endometrial cancer. Men and women have around a 10–38% lifetime risk of non-medullary thyroid cancer, which is most commonly of follicular histology (Tan et al., 2012; Bubien et al., 2013).

Other features include hamartoma of the gastrointestinal (GI) tract and multiple cutaneous lesions such as facial trichilemmoma, papillomatous papules, acral keratoses, lipoma and fibroma. Affected individuals may also have an increased head circumference (macrocephaly). In the UK, women are offered annual mammograms from 40 to 59 followed by 3 yearly mammograms within the NHS Breast Screening Programme (NICE, 2013). Annual examination and ultrasound of the thyroid should be considered.

Genetic testing of *PTEN* is available and is frequently required to confirm the diagnosis as the clinical presentation can be non-specific or mild. *PTEN*-related conditions are inherited as autosomal dominant traits, but the clinical presentation can vary within families both in terms of severity and presentation, with some relatives presenting as Cowden syndrome and others as BRRS.

Familial atypical mole and melanoma (FAMM)

FAMM is caused by mutations in the *CDKN2A* gene on chromosome 9p21.3 or the *CDK4* gene on 12q14. *CDKN2A* is a complex gene, in that the gene sequence is read in different ways to create two separate proteins called p16 and p14. Both p16 and p14 have tumour suppressor function. Specific mutations in *CDK4* make its protein product resistant to inhibition by p16, suggesting that *CDK4* operates as an oncogene (Puntervoll et al., 2013).

Mutations in *CDKN2A* and *CDK4* are principally associated with an increased risk of melanoma. The risk of melanoma in the general population varies significantly with geography, with a low incidence in northern Europe (about 8 in 100 000) and a high incidence in Australia (about 37 in 100 000). Melanoma risk in individuals with *CDKN2A* and *CDK4* mutations also shows some variation, with a 45–60% risk to age 80 in Europe and a 52–90% risk in Australia (Goldstein et al., 2007; Cust et al., 2011). Mutations in *CDKN2A* are also believed to be associated with an increased risk of pancreatic cancer (up to 17% lifetime risk).

Testing for *CDKN2A* and *CDK4* mutations is available, and may help clarify risk to individuals and allow relatives to benefit from predictive genetic testing. Testing may be considered in individuals with multiple (three or more) melanomata or with an isolated melanoma but with a family history of melanoma and/or pancreatic cancer. Mutation carriers should exercise extreme caution in the sun, wear long-sleeved clothing, hats, high-factor sun screen and avoid the mid-day sun and sun-beds. Regular surveillance by a dermatologist is recommended, and photographic mole-mapping techniques can be useful. No screening of asymptomatic individuals for pancreatic cancer is known to be effective, but patients should be aware of the symptoms.

Gorlin syndrome/basal cell naevus syndrome

Gorlin syndrome affects around 1 in 50 000 individuals and is caused by loss-of-function mutations or deletions of the *PTCH* gene on chromosome 9q22.3. *PTCH* acts as a regulator of the sonic hedgehog (SHH) signalling pathway, which is important in cell growth and regulation. The hallmark of Gorlin syndrome is the development of multiple basal cell carcinoma (BCC) and basal cell naevi from the teenage years. The other principal cancer risk is medulloblastoma which occurs in early childhood in around 3% of patients (Kimonis et al., 1997; Lo Muzio, 2008).

Non-cancer features are common and are frequently used to make the diagnosis. Odontogenic keratocysts (often noted by dentists, and visible on orthopantogram, OPG) occur from mid childhood, and are present in 90% of patients by 40 years. Other skeletal features include bifid, fused, splayed or missing ribs, and fused vertebrae (noted on chest X-ray). Craniofacial features include macrocephaly with a prominent forehead, cleft lip/palate in some and calcification of the falx cerebri which can be seen on skull X-ray. An examination of the skin of the hands and feet can reveal palmar/plantar pits, which are of no consequence but can aid in the diagnosis.

The diagnosis of Gorlin syndrome is usually made clinically on the presence of multiple BCC with other typical features. Genetic testing of the *PTCH* gene is available and may aid management in patients where the clinical diagnosis is unclear or clarify the risk to relatives. Gorlin syndrome is inherited as an autosomal dominant condition, but with variable expressivity between family members. Up to 50% of cases are *de novo* mutations, with no family history.

Individuals with Gorlin syndrome are advised to have an annual dermatological assessment for BCC from the age of 12, use high-factor sun block and avoid exposure to the sun. Treatment for the BCC is standard, with wide local excision; radiotherapy should be avoided due to the propagation of further BCC within the radiation field. A recent study found the SHH pathway inhibitor vismodegib was effective in treating and preventing BCC in Gorlin syndrome, but with frequent side effects (Tang et al., 2012). Patients should alert their dentist to the diagnosis, due to the high prevalence of jaw cysts.

Hereditary leiomyomatosis and renal cell cancer (HLRCC)

HLRCC was only described in 2001 and its incidence is unknown, although it is likely to be rare. It is caused by loss-of-function mutations in the *FH* gene on chromosome 1q43 (Launonen et al., 2001). The most common features are cutaneous and uterine leiomyoma, which are benign tumours of smooth muscle fibres. Cutaneous leiomyoma typically occur from mid childhood, and can be tender and painful in cold weather. Uterine leiomyoma are more commonly known as fibroids and are common in the general population. However, in patients with HLRCC the fibroids are often larger and multiple, with a younger age of onset, and transformation to uterine leiomyosarcoma is reported. Ten to 16% of reported cases of HLRCC have developed renal cell carcinoma. Pathologically, these have been type 2 papillary, tubulo-papillary or collecting duct tumours. Aggressive tumour progression has been reported, with many tumours having metastasised at presentation (Wei et al., 2006).

FH is a gene that encodes a protein known as fumarate hydratase, which is an important enzyme is cellular biochemistry as part of the Krebs cycle. Heterozygous loss-of-function mutations throughout the gene have been reported in HLRCC. Of note is that bi-allelic mutations in *FH* cause the autosomal recessive disorder fumarate hydratase deficiency.

Surveillance for renal cancer is advised and the most appropriate modality and screening interval will be dependent on the patient's age and risk. The earliest reported case of renal cancer is 11 years, although most patients have been in their 30s or 40s. Annual MRI or CT are likely to be the most sensitive modalities, but the risk of general anaesthesia in children and the cumulative radiation dosage of CT must also be considered. Ultrasound performed at 6-monthly intervals may therefore have a role in childhood screening from 10 years, switching to MRI when tolerated (van Spaendonck-Zwarts et al., 2012). HLRCC is an autosomal dominant disorder and relatives at risk should be clinically assessed and offered genetic testing if available.

Hereditary paraganglioma/phaeochromocytoma

Paraganglioma (PGL) is a tumour of the chain of neuroendocrine cells that run each side of the length of the spine. Phaeochromocytoma (PCC) is essentially a PGL that occurs in the adrenal medulla and typically secretes catecholamines. Benign PGL/PCC cause symptoms through their size (mass effect) and/or the effects of catecholamine hypersecretion, such as hypertension, palpitations, sweating, headache and anxiety.

These rare tumours usually occur sporadically, but a number of genes have been shown to be associated with a predisposition to PGL/PCC, and they are summarised in Table 11.3. Four of these (*SDHA*, *SDHB*, *SDHC* and *SDHD*) encode parts of the succinate dehydrogenase (SDH) enzyme, which is important for mitochondrial function, while *SDHAF2* is involved in stabilising the SDH enzyme. Multiple tumours, tumours occurring at a young age or malignant/metastatic tumours are more suggestive of an underlying genetic susceptibility (Fishbein and Nathanson, 2012).

SDHD and *SDHAF2* exhibit a parent-of-origin effect, known as imprinting. Although humans have two copies of these genes (one on each chromosome) only the copy that has been inherited from the father is expressed (used). This means that if an individual inherits a *SDHD* or *SDHAF2* mutation from their father they are at risk

Table 11.3 Genes associated with PGL/PCC

Gene	Locus	Comment
SDHD	11q23.1	Imprinted
SDHB	1p36.13	
SDHC	1q23.3	
SDHA	5p15.33	
SDHAF2	19q13.12	Imprinted
MAX	14q23.3	
VHL	3p25	See von Hippel–Lindau disease
RET	10q11	See Multiple endocrine neoplasia type 2
TMEM127	2q11.2	

of PGL/PCC, but if they inherit it from their mother the mutation is silenced and the risk is reduced.

Around a third of the carriers of a gene mutation will develop either PGL or PCC by the age of 30, and around 80% by the age of 50 years. Most PGL/PCC tumours are benign with a low risk of malignant transformation, but tumours associated with mutation in *SDHB* and *MAX* have a higher risk of malignancy (Jafri and Maher, 2012).

Molecular genetic testing for disease-causing variants in *SDHA*, *SDHB*, *SDHC*, *SDHD*, *SDHAF2*, *MAX*, *TMEM127*, *VHL* and *RET* is clinically available. The majority of families have mutations in either *SDHD* or *SDHB*. Relatives known to be at risk of PGL/PCC should be offered annual screening for plasma metanephrines from the age of 10.

Muir–Torre syndrome (MTS)

MTS is an infrequently described subtype of Lynch syndrome (LS) with co-occurrence of both sebaceous tumours (sebaceous adenoma, epithelioma, carcinoma) and colorectal cancer or other LS-related malignancy.

MTS has now been shown to be due to mutations in the mismatch repair genes *MLH1*, *MSH2* and *MSH6* and is therefore described as allelic to Lynch syndrome. Identical mutations have been described in both MTS and LS, raising the possibility that they are not distinct entities. Indeed it is likely that sebaceous tumours are a less common manifestation of LS than the core triad of colorectal, ovarian and endometrial tumours. Nonetheless, certain families appear to exhibit a high prevalence of sebaceous tumours, and in these families a diagnosis of MTS is justified.

Cutaneous sebaceous tumours are relatively uncommon in the general population, and so when they do occur consideration should be given to the diagnosis of MTS. A family history or previous personal history of LS-related cancers or sebaceous tumours, or a young age of onset (under 50 years), warrants discussion with clinical genetics services. Further investigation with tumour studies (microsatellite instability, immunohistochemistry for MLH1, MSH2, MSH6 protein expression) and/or constitutional DNA analysis may be appropriate (Ko, 2010).

Management and surveillance is as for LS, with affected individuals offered colorectal cancer screening by colonoscopy at 2-yearly intervals from the age of 25 to 75 years. Prophylactic oophrectomy may be offered to women from the age of 40, and advice on symptom awareness for other tumours should be given. MTS is an autosomal dominant susceptibility syndrome, and relatives should be offered appropriate advice, genetic testing and surveillance.

Multiple endocrine neoplasia type 1 (MEN1)

MEN1 is a very rare entity, probably affecting around 1 in 100 000 people. It is caused by loss-of-function mutations in the *MEN1* tumour suppressor gene on chromosome 11q13. *MEN1* encodes a nuclear protein that is involved in DNA repair mechanisms (Pilarski and Nagy, 2012).

Around 30–80% of patients will develop a hormone-secreting pancreatic adenoma, such as a gastrinoma or insulinoma. Pituitary tumours, most commonly a prolactinoma, occur in 15–50%. Other almost universal non-cancer features are facial angiofibroma and parathyroid hyperplasia. Angiofibroma are small, red, papular lesions that are present in 90% of patients. Hyperparathyroidism may present with a variety of non-specific symptoms including malaise, fatigue, abdominal pain and bone/joint pains. It can also cause kidney stones and osteoporosis. MEN1 accounts for around 10% of patients who present with primary hyperparathyroidism (Thakker et al., 2012).

Genetic testing for *MEN1* mutations should be considered in any patient with co-occurrence of two or more of the above features, or with young age of onset of any of these features. Affected individuals (or at-risk relatives) should have annual screening for hypercalcaemia (serum calcium measurement) and prolactin. *MEN1* is an autosomal dominant condition, with the offspring of an affected parent being at a 50% risk.

Multiple endocrine neoplasia type 2 (MEN2)

MEN2 is a term used to describe conditions associated with an increased risk of medullary thyroid cancer (MTC) with or without other features, which include phaeochromocytoma, mucosal neuromas and physical changes to body habitus. They are all caused by activating mutations in the *RET* proto-oncogene on chromosome 10q11, which encodes a cell surface receptor that is present in tissues derived from the neural crest. While mutations that cause over-activity of this gene cause tumour susceptibility (MEN2), loss-of-function mutations cause abnormal development of the nerve ganglia in the colon (Hirschsprung disease) (Machens et al., 2009).

MEN2 conditions affect around 1 in 30 000 people, and account for up to 20% of cases of medullary thyroid cancer. The subtypes of MEN2 are:

- non-syndromic familial medullary thyroid cancer (FMTC)
- MEN2a—MTC, phaeochromocytoma, and parathyroid hyperplasia
- MEN2b—MTC, phaeochromocytoma, mucosal neuroma, enlarged lips, abnormal (long-limbed) body habitus.

MEN2a is the most common subtype accounting for 60% of cases and is typically associated with MTC in early adulthood. MEN2b is associated with early childhood MTC, abnormal body habitus with long limbs, enlarged lips and mucosal neuroma (Pilarski and Nagy, 2012).

The lifetime risk of MTC in MEN2 approaches 100% in some subtypes. It may present with a lump in the neck or with diarrhoea secondary to hypercalcitonaemia, and tumours metastasise early. Histologically, MTC affects the calcitonin-producing cells (C-cells) of the thyroid, with invasion into the follicles. Screening for MTC is recommended every 6 months by clinical examination and serum calcitonin, calcium and parathyroid hormone levels. Screening is commenced at 6 months of age in MEN2b and 5 years in MEN2a, and prophylactic thyroidectomy is indicated. Phaeochromocytoma screening is indicated in MEN2a and MEN2b.

Genetic analysis of the *RET* gene should be considered in any patient with MTC or with two or more other features of MEN2. For a mutation to increase the activity of a protein it must usually affect a specific part of the protein, and so many families will have the same or a similar mutation.

Peutz–Jehgers syndrome (PJS)

PJS is a rare autosomal dominant disorder, classically characterised by the development of histologically distinct Peutz–Jehgers polyps and hyperpigmented macules, most commonly in the peri-oral and peri-anal regions. Estimates of prevalence vary greatly, but it is rare and likely to affect in the region of 1 in 100 000 individuals. It is caused by mutations in the *STK11* gene on chromosome 19p13.3 (Resta et al., 2013).

Peutz–Jeghers polyps are benign hamartomatous tumours which can falsely appear invasive due the interleaving of smooth muscle and mucosal cells that extend into the muscularis propria. They develop most commonly in the GI tract, in particular in the small intestine where they can cause intussusception (causing abdominal pain, intestinal obstruction and/or rectal bleeding). The pigmentation abnormalities are most notable in early to mid childhood, and can fade with age.

It is important to diagnose PJS as it is also associated with an increased risk of malignancy, especially GI and breast cancers. Around 20% of patients develop cancer by 40 years of age, and around 60% by 60 years. Adenoma occur throughout the GI tract, and colorectal and gastric cancers are common. The lifetime risk of pancreatic cancer is around 17%, and around 30% of women develop breast cancer by 60 years (Hearle et al., 2006; Mehenni et al., 2006; Resta et al., 2013).

Surveillance for GI tumours is recommended by endoscopy, capsule endoscopy and colonoscopy. Women should be offered annual mammography from 40 to 59 years, before entering the national breast screening programme with mammography every 3 years (NICE, 2013). Although the diagnosis is often made on the basis of clinical and histological features, genetic testing of *STK11* can be useful in patients presenting with equivocal features or for predictive testing in known families.

Von Hippel–Lindau disease (VHL)

VHL is a rare multisystem disorder affecting around 1 in 36 000 people. The condition is caused by loss-of-function mutations in the tumour suppressor gene *VHL* on chromosome 3p25.

Clinically, the condition is characterised by hemangioblastoma of the brain, spinal cord and retina. Other common features are renal cysts and renal cell carcinomas, PCC and PGL. Less frequent, but nonetheless suggestive, are cystic lesions of other organs, including the pancreas, the epididymis in males and the broad ligament in females, and endolymphatic sac tumours of the inner ear causing variable hearing loss and/or balance problems. Hemangioblastoma, although a benign tumour, is a major cause of morbidity in VHL, affecting 60–80% of patients and presenting throughout life. Renal tumours occur in around 70% of patients by the age of 60, are typically of clear cell histology and may be multifocal or bilateral (Barontini and Dahia, 2010).

As a complex multisystem disease, VHL is often managed in a multidisciplinary setting. Those at risk should have blood pressure and ophthalmological monitoring from 5 years of age. Phaeochromocytoma screening by way of annual plasma metanephrine analysis should commence at 11 years. Although most hemangioblastoma would not be treated surgically unless symptomatic, brain MRI is performed 3-yearly from 15 years. Annual renal imaging for cysts and renal carcinoma is advised from 16 years (Maher et al., 2011).

VHL accounts for around a third of sporadic cerebellar hemangioblastoma, and molecular analysis of the *VHL* gene should be considered in such cases. *VHL* is also included on gene panel tests for renal carcinoma and PCC.

Summary

The syndromes described in this chapter are all individually rare, but are associated with significant morbidity. They often present with unusual or multiple tumours, and the occurrence of a rare tumour or multiple tumours in any patient should prompt consideration of an underlying genetic diagnosis. Knowledge of the natural history of these conditions allows appropriate surveillance and management, and patients will often require input from several medical/surgical specialties.

References

Barontini M, Dahia PL 2010. VHL disease. *Best Pract Res Clin Endocrinol Metab* **24**: 401–413.

Bertherat J, Horvath A, Groussin L, et al. 2009. Mutations in regulatory subunit type 1A of cyclic adenosine 5'-monophosphate-dependent protein kinase (PRKAR1A): phenotype analysis in 353 patients and 80 different genotypes. *J Clin Endocrinol Metab* **94**: 2085–2091.

Blumenthal GM, Dennis PA 2008. PTEN hamartoma tumor syndromes. *Eur J Hum Genet* **16**: 1289–1300.

Bubien V, Bonnet F, Brouste V, et al. 2013. High cumulative risks of cancer in patients with *PTEN* hamartoma tumour syndrome. *J Med Genet* **50**: 255–263.

Cust AE, Harland M, Makalic E, et al. 2011. Melanoma risk for *CDKN2A* mutation carriers who are relatives of population-based case carriers in Australia and the UK. *J Med Genet* **48**: 266–272.

Fishbein L and Nathanson KL 2012. Pheochromocytoma and paraganglioma: understanding the complexities of the genetic background. *Cancer Genet* **205**: 1–11.

Goldstein AM, Chan M, Harland M, et al. 2007. Features associated with germline *CDKN2A* mutations: a GenoMEL study of melanoma-prone families from three continents. *J Med Genet* **44**: 99–106.

Groussin L, Horvath A, Jullian E, et al. 2006. A *PRKAR1A* mutation associated with primary pigmented nodular adrenocortical disease in 12 kindreds. *J Clin Endocrinol Metab* **91**: 1943–1949.

Hearle N, Schumacher V, Menko FH, et al. 2006. Frequency and spectrum of cancers in the Peutz–Jeghers syndrome. *Clin Cancer Res* **12**: 3209–3215.

Jafri M and Maher ER 2012. The genetics of phaeochromocytoma: using clinical features to guide genetic testing. *Eur J Endocrinol* **166**: 151–158.

Khoo SK, Giraud S, Kahnoski K, et al. 2002. Clinical and genetic studies of Birt–Hogg–Dubé syndrome. *J Med Genet* **39**: 906–912 [erratum in *J Med Genet* **40**: 150].

Kimonis VE, Goldstein AM, Pastakia B, et al. 1997. Clinical manifestations in 105 persons with nevoid basal cell carcinoma syndrome. *Am J Med Genet* **69**: 299–308.

Ko CJ 2010. Muir–Torre syndrome: facts and controversies. *Clin Dermatol* **28**: 324–329.

Launonen V, Vierimaa O, Kiuru M, et al. 2001. Inherited susceptibility to uterine leiomyomas and renal cell cancer. *Proc Natl Acad Sci USA* **98**: 3387–3392.

Lo Muzio L 2008. Nevoid basal cell carcinoma syndrome (Gorlin syndrome). *Orphanet J Rare Dis* **3**: 32.

Machens A, Lorenz K, Dralle H 2009. Constitutive RET tyrosine kinase activation in hereditary medullary thyroid cancer: clinical opportunities. *J Intern Med* **266**: 114–125.

Maher ER, Neumann HP, Richard S 2011. Von Hippel–Lindau disease: a clinical and scientific review. *Eur J Hum Genet* **19**: 617–623.

Mehenni H, Resta N, Park JG, et al. 2006. Cancer risks in *LKB1* germline mutation carriers. *Gut* **55**: 984–990.

Menko FH, Van Steensel MA, Giraud S, et al. 2009. [European BHD Consortium] Birt–Hogg–Dubé syndrome: diagnosis and management. *Lancet Oncol* **10**: 1199–1206.

NICE (National Institute for Health and Care Excellence) 2013. *Familial breast cancer: classification and care of people at risk of familial breast cancer and management of breast cancer and related risks in people with a family history of breast cancer.* Clinical Guidelines 164. London: National Institute for Health and Care Excellence.

Pilarski R and Nagy R 2012. Genetic testing by cancer site: endocrine system. *Cancer J* **18**: 364–371.

Puntervoll HE, Yang XR, Vetti HH, et al. 2013. Melanoma prone families with *CDK4* germline mutation: phenotypic profile and associations with MC1R variants. *J Med Genet* **50**: 264–270.

Resta N, Pierannunzio D, Lenato GM, et al. 2013. Cancer risk associated with *STK11/LKB1* germline mutations in Peutz–Jeghers syndrome patients: results of an Italian multicenter study. *Dig Liver Dis* **45**: 606–611.

Tan MH, Mester JL, Ngeow J, et al. 2012. Lifetime cancer risks in individuals with germline PTEN mutations. *Clin Cancer Res* **18**: 400–407.

Tang JY, Mackay-Wiggan JM, Aszterbaum M, et al. 2012. Inhibiting the hedgehog pathway in patients with the basal-cell nevus syndrome. *N Engl J Med* **366**: 2180–2188.

Thakker RV, Newey PJ, Walls GV, et al. 2012. Clinical practice guidelines for multiple endocrine neoplasia type 1 (MEN1). *J Clin Endocrinol Metab* **97**: 2990–3011.

Toro JR, Wei MH, Glenn GM, et al. 2008. *BHD* mutations, clinical and molecular genetic investigations of Birt–Hogg–Dubé syndrome: a new series of 50 families and a review of published reports. *J Med Genet* **45**: 321–331.

Van Spaendonck-Zwarts KY, Badeloe S, Oosting SF, et al. 2012. Hereditary leiomyomatosis and renal cell cancer presenting as metastatic kidney cancer at 18 years of age: implications for surveillance. *Fam Cancer* **11**: 123–129.

Wei MH, Toure O, Glenn GM, et al. 2006. Novel mutations in *FH* and expansion of the spectrum of phenotypes expressed in families with hereditary leiomyomatosis and renal cell cancer. *J Med Genet* **43**: 18–27.

Chapter 12

Genetics of specific cancers. Summary

Patricia Webb and Lorraine Robinson

Introduction to section 3 summary

The chapters in Section 3 concentrate on the genetics of cancer, detailing the genes involved in specific hereditary cancers and the risks associated with cancer-predisposing mutations in those genes.

Chapter 7. Genetics of specific cancers. Introduction

Chapter 7 provides a firm base for beginning to think about the genetic influences in cancer. Cancer develops from a *combination* of many factors, of which genetic mutations may be one. Cancers are a complex group of diseases. The author establishes two significant statistics that need to be remembered when considering cancer genetics: first, across the UK, the United States and Australia the lifetime risk of developing cancer is one in three; second, just 5–10% of cancer is caused by a mutation in a high-risk cancer-predisposing gene. The relevance of these statistics is that low relative risk tends to be associated with common low-penetrance variants and higher relative risk with rare high-penetrance variants. In the UK genetic testing within the NHS is currently only available for rare high-penetrance variants (mutations) that explain only a small proportion of common cancers.

Guided activity for Chapter 7

- ◆ From your own experience reflect on genetic testing that has been undertaken in patients in your care. What type of genetic test did the patient have? Would genetic testing have been available for other relatives as a result of this testing?

Further reading for Chapter 7

Bush WS, Moore JH 2012. Chapter 11: Genome-wide association studies. *PLoS Comput Biol* 8(12): e1002822.

Chung CC, Wagner CSM, Jesus G-B, Chanock SJ 2010. Genome-wide association studies in cancer—current and future directions. *Carcinogenesis* 31: 111–120.

Chapters 8–11. Genetics of specific cancers and rare syndromes

Each of these chapters focuses on a particular type of cancer or cancer syndrome—identifying the genes involved for specific hereditary cancer syndromes, the family history that would suggest a genetic mutation and the risks associated with these genes.

Guided activities for Chapters 8–10

◆ With a colleague consider and discuss the influence of cancer genetics in the development of the cancers mentioned in Chapters 8–10 and the cancer syndromes associated with the genes involved.

Guided activities for Chapter 8

◆ Identify the criteria for genetic testing from the National Institute for Health and Care excellence (NICE) Clinical Guideline 164 for familial breast cancer (<http://www.nice.org.uk/CG164>).

◆ Consider the breast cancer family histories in Figs. 12.1 and 12.2:

 • For Fig. 12.1 explain why *BRCA1/2* genetic testing is possible in this family. Which family member would be the best person to refer to genetic services in the first instance? What type of genetic testing might they be offered?

 • For Fig. 12.2 consider how you might explain to the patient (indicated with an arrow) that this family is not eligible for genetic testing.

Further resources for Chapter 8

Antoniou AC, Beesley J, McGuffog L, et al. 2010. Common breast cancer susceptibility alleles and the risk of breast cancer for *BRCA1* and *BRCA2* mutation carriers: implications for risk prediction. *Cancer Res* 70: 9742–9754.

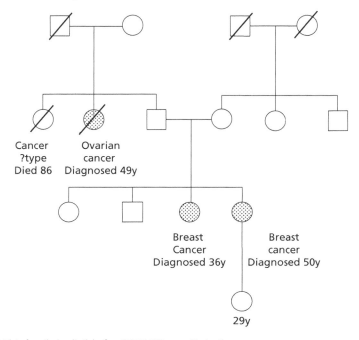

Figure 12.1 This family is eligible for *BRCA1/2* genetic testing.

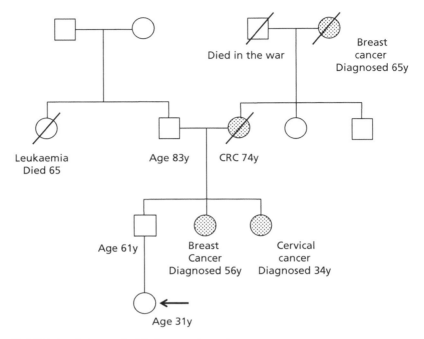

Figure 12.2 This family is not eligible for genetic testing.

Guided activities for Chapter 9

- ◆ Consider the colorectal cancer family histories in Figs. 12.3–12.5:
  - For Fig. 12.3 explain why this family history does not meet the Bethesda or Amsterdam criteria. How might you explain to the patient (marked with an arrow) that genetic testing is not indicated?
  - For Fig. 12.4 explain why this family history meets the Bethesda criteria. It may be possible to test a tumour sample from the patient (marked with an arrow) for

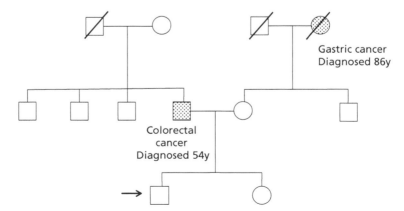

Figure 12.3 This colorectal cancer family history does not meet the Bethesda or Amsterdam criteria.

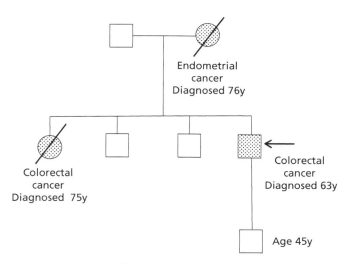

Figure 12.4 This colorectal cancer family history meets the Bethesda criteria.

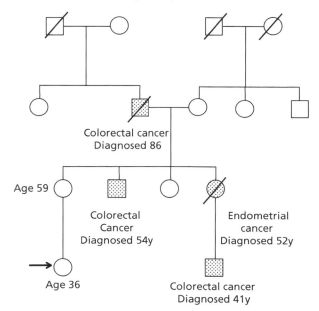

IHC staining showed loss of expression of MLH1 protein
MLH1 mutation identified at diagnostic testing

Figure 12.5 This family history meets the Amsterdam criteria.

microsatellite instability. Consider what the outcomes of this testing might be and how you might explain tumour testing to the patient.

- For Fig. 12.5 explain why this family history meets the Amsterdam criteria. Predictive genetic testing is available in this family. What is the chance that the patient (marked with an arrow) carries the familial *MLH1* mutation? Which family member would you refer first for predictive testing (the patient or her mother) and why?

Further resources for Chapter 9

Lynch HT, Lynch JF, Attard TA 2009. Diagnosis and management of hereditary colorectal cancer syndromes: Lynch syndrome as a model. *Can Med Assoc J* 181: 273–280.

Guided activities for Chapter 10

♦ Consider how an increased understanding of the genetic basis of prostate cancer may impact on prostate cancer treatment.

♦ Look at the website for the IMPACT study (<http://www.impact-study.co.uk>) to understand more about ongoing research into hereditary prostate cancer.

Guided activities for Chapter 11

♦ Consider which rare cancer syndromes could possibly arise in your specialty. Make a note of the genes involved and the clinical features.

Section 4

Cancer risk assessment and communicating risk

Chapter 13

Cancer risk assessment and communicating risk. Introduction

Chris Jacobs

Introduction to cancer risk assessment and communicating risk

It is important that cancer risk is assessed as accurately as possible in order to assist the patient and the clinician with making informed risk management decisions. The way in which risk is communicated may impact on patients' understanding and decision-making.

This chapter explains the principles of risk assessment—identifying the key questions to address when assessing risk in the cancer care setting, briefly discussing the types of risk assessment tool available, considering the factors that can impact on risk perception and presenting some strategies for risk communication. The learning objectives for this chapter are:

- to be able to understand the underlying principles critical to the assessment of a cancer family history;
- to become aware of the types of risk assessment tool available;
- to understand the factors that can have an impact on risk perception;
- to consider risk communication strategies.

Risk in the context of cancer family history

The concept of risk is complex and poorly understood by the general public and health professionals (Gigerenzer and Edwards, 2003). In the context of cancer family history, risk refers to the probability that an individual might carry a specific cancer-predisposing gene mutation or be affected with a specific genetic cancer disorder. Assessment of cancer risk is based on the information that is available at a particular point in time and should be regarded as an 'ongoing process of analysis of estimates' (Baptista, 2005).

Cancer risk factors

Cancer risk factors may be inherited or acquired. All individuals have an inherited level of cancer risk associated with their individual baseline set of genetic variants, ranging from highly penetrant mutations to low-penetrance variants. Individuals at increased risk because of inherited mutations with high penetrance can sometimes, but not always, be identified because they have a strong family history of cancer.

Risk of cancer is not, however, fixed at birth and is affected by acquired, and often modifiable, lifestyle choices and events such as diet, weight, smoking, alcohol consumption and reproductive choices. Cancer risk is also altered by broader influences, such as social, economic, occupational and environmental factors. Modifiable risk factors ultimately influence risk by causing acquired (somatic) genetic changes or alterations in gene expression, which either increase or decrease cancer risk. Ageing is of course a non-modifiable risk factor because it increases exposure to life and environmental events, which in turn increase the likelihood of acquired genetic changes, thus increasing cancer risk.

Assessing cancer family history

In order to assess cancer risk from family history there are some key general questions that need to be asked (Table 13.1) in addition to the specific questions related to the type of cancer in the family that are addressed in Chapters 14 and 15.

Categorising and calculating cancer risk from the family history

In a genetics service where full information is generally gathered about the family history, including verification of diagnoses and clinical and histological features of various cancers and/or genetic testing, a specific individualised risk assessment may be possible. However, even when a cancer-predisposing gene mutation is identified it is not possible to give definite answers about whether someone will develop cancer or not. Instead it is necessary to make an estimation of that individual's cancer risk. It is important to be mindful of the dynamic nature of family history, ensuring that patients are aware that if the family history changes the cancer risk assessment may also change.

There are several validated risk assessment models available to estimate the probability of carrying a cancer-predisposing single gene mutation, such as those described in this section. Genome-wide association studies (GWAS) are likely to generate new and more comprehensive risk prediction models.

The models used in familial breast cancer calculate the probability of a *BRCA1/2* mutation; some take into account risk factors related to family history, such as the Gail model (Gail et al., 1989) and the Manchester model (Evans et al., 2004, 2009), and some are based on the genetic risks (i.e. penetrance, mode of inheritance or mutation frequencies), such as BRCAPRO (Berry et al., 2002) or BOADICEA (Antoniou et al., 2004). There are limitations to all of these models, both in terms of the practicality of using them and the accuracy of risk assessment (Amir et al., 2010).

The empirically based Amsterdam and Bethesda criteria (see Box 9.1) provide a guide to risk assessment in families with colorectal and Lynch syndrome-related cancers. Genetic risk prediction models have been developed to identify the probability of carrying a mismatch repair gene mutation (PREMM(1,2,6), MMRPro and MMRPredict) associated with Lynch syndrome. Although it is reported that these models are superior at predicting risk than clinical criteria alone (Kastrinos et al., 2013) they have yet to be independently validated in large studies.

Table 13.1 Indicators of hereditary cancer risk, key general questions to ask of the family history in order to elicit the information and rationale for the questions

Indicators of hereditary cancer risk	Key questions to ask of the family history in order to identify the indicators of risk	Rationale
A known genetic mutation in the family	Has anyone in the family been found to carry a cancer-predisposing gene mutation/fault?	If a gene mutation has been identified, genetic testing may be possible and a more specific risk assessment can be made. Sometimes it is reported within families that a relative has a gene mutation when in fact they have an unclassified variant. It is always best to ask for confirmation, such as a letter from a genetics department or a laboratory report
Multiple cancers in the family	How many relatives are affected with cancer? Have any relatives developed more than one primary cancer?	Establishing the number of cancers in the family and whether individuals have had more than one primary cancer helps with understanding the likelihood of a genetic predisposition to cancer
Similar types or clustering of cancers in the family	What type of cancer did each relative have?	It is important to be aware of the types of cancers that may be relevant to a particular genetic syndrome, such as breast, ovarian and prostate cancer or colorectal, gastric and endometrial cancer. Ideally, abdominal and pelvic cancers should be verified as these are not always accurately reported. This may need to be undertaken by the genetics service and so it is useful to gather details of the name, date of birth and treatment
Cancers on the same side of the family	Which side of the family are the affected relatives on?	If there are cancers on both sides of the family, they will need to be assessed separately as there may be a risk from both the maternal and paternal family history
Young ages at diagnosis	What are the ages at diagnosis of relatives with cancer?	Gathering this information is important for identifying early onset cancer which is more likely to be due to a cancer-predisposing gene mutation
Close relationship between the individuals with cancer and between the individuals with cancer and the person seeking risk assessment (i.e. the proband)	What is the relationship of the affected relatives to each other and to the proband? What is the current age or age at death of each relative (with and without cancer)?	Most cancer syndromes are dominantly inherited but it is important to remember that recessive inheritance can occur with some cancer syndromes. Finding out the current age or age at death of intervening unaffected relatives helps with calculating risk in a dominantly inherited cancer syndrome
Clinical or histological features that are relevant to a cancer syndrome	Are there any clinical or histological signs of hereditary cancer?	In some hereditary cancer syndromes there are particular clinical or histological features. This information may need to be obtained by the genetics service. If details of histology are available in secondary care it is helpful to provide these with a genetics referral
Ethnicity that may increase the risk of a founder mutation	What is the ethnic background of the family?	In some ethnic groups there is a greater prevalence of particular founder mutations

Various tools and charts are available for categorising family history risk or identifying patients suitable for genetics referral based on the number of affected relatives, the ages at diagnosis and the cancer type. It is important to ensure that the tools being used are up to date. Health professionals in cancer care are advised to discuss the use of particular tools with their genetics centre and to refer to national guidelines where available.

Risk perception

Much work has been undertaken in the area of risk perception, mostly in families at risk of hereditary breast and ovarian cancer. Women from breast and ovarian cancer families often perceive their risk of developing breast cancer to be high. Perception of high risk is associated with worry, distress and in some cases symptoms of depression (Brain et al., 1999). Consequently, many women are motivated to request an appointment to discuss their family history in order to find out the risk for themselves and other family members, reduce worry and seek genetic testing and preventative measures (Van Asperen et al., 2002). A systematic review of cancer genetic risk assessment for individuals at risk of familial breast cancer found that following genetic counselling, risk perception was more accurate and breast cancer-related distress was reduced (Hilgart et al., 2012).

There are fewer studies examining risk perception for other cancers. A study of 65 adult women at 50% risk of a cancer-predisposing mutation found that perceived risk for colon cancer was significantly higher than for extracolonic cancers and that risk perception was significantly more accurate following genetic counselling (Hadley et al., 2008). Men with a family history of prostate cancer are more likely to overestimate their risk when compared with men without a family history (Miller et al., 2001).

Communicating risk

Risk communication is a large component of genetic counselling and much work has been done in the field of cancer genetics to examine how genetics health professionals communicate risk (Lobb et al., 2004; Michie et al., 2005) and what patients understand from the risk communication process (Phelps et al., 2008). There is some evidence that risk communication in genetic counselling benefits patients' knowledge and risk perception but there is less evidence of benefit to anxiety, satisfaction and behaviour (Edwards et al., 2008). Several studies have shown that the context and format in which risks are conveyed can affect people's risk perception, coping, adjustment and decisions (Croyle and Lerman, 1999; Timmermans et al., 2008). Risk information and the way it is communicated is one aspect of a whole range of factors that influence decision-making, highlighting the importance of tailoring risk communication to the individual. There are a number of strategies for communicating risk:

♦ Absolute versus relative risk. There are many ways of presenting risk. Presenting the absolute risk over a specified period of time (i.e. the individual's actual risk) is preferable to presenting the relative risk (i.e. the comparative risk between two or more groups) (O'Doherty and Suthers, 2007). For example, 'You have a one in three chance of developing cancer in your lifetime' (absolute risk) is less confusing than 'Women with a strong family history of breast cancer are at three times the population risk' (relative risk).

◆ Explaining risk in numbers and words. Much work has been done examining the use of verbal expression to substitute numerical risk formats. It has been suggested that patients do not understand risk in numbers (Hallowell et al., 1997), although other studies have concluded that presenting risk in numbers is effective (Marteau et al., 2000). Using words to describe risk can be problematic, due to the variance in the range of numerical probabilities relating to a verbal expression and the individual interpretation of quantifying words. For example, a 'high risk' of cancer may mean to the health professional that the patient's risk is high enough to meet the screening criteria, while for the patient it may mean that cancer is inevitable. For some individuals risk is perceived as a binary outcome (I will get it or I won't) no matter how it is presented (Parsons and Atkinson, 1992).

◆ Consistency of risk formats. Throughout the risk communication process it is important to be consistent in framing the risk. For example, it is confusing to say 'You have one in three lifetime chance of developing breast cancer, a 10% chance of developing ovarian cancer and a high chance of a genetic mutation.'

◆ Visualising risk. There is limited evidence of understanding being improved by presenting risk in visual formats (O'Doherty and Suthers, 2007). It can be helpful to work through the pedigree and risk assessment tool with a patient to show them how the risk assessment has been reached.

◆ Loss versus gain framing. The way in which risk information is framed influences risk perception (Julian-Reynier et al., 2003). Framing risk in a positive as well as a negative way is therefore important: for example, 'You have one chance in three that you will develop cancer in your lifetime. That means there is a two out of three chance that you will never develop cancer.'

◆ Putting the risk in context for the individual. However risk is presented, cancer risk perception is largely based on emotional responses and previous cancer experience, which ultimately drive how the patient behaves in terms of cancer screening, genetic counselling and genetic testing (Zikmund-Fisher et al., 2010). Making risk relevant and in context for the individual helps to give it meaning.

There is no overall consensus on the effectiveness of the many strategies for communicating risk. However, there does appear to be agreement on using a multistep process to communicate risk (Julian-Reynier et al., 2003). In this approach the health professional:

1 assesses the patient's beliefs about the causes of cancer, prior perception of risk, preferences for risk communication style, knowledge, expectations, level of anxiety and coping style;

2 uses this assessment to tailor the risk communication to the individual, putting the information in context for the individual and their family;

3 checks understanding and provides feedback, for example in the form of a letter or leaflet.

Summary

There are several models available for cancer risk assessment, but at present these generally focus on the probability of identifying a high-penetrance cancer-predisposing single gene mutation. Assessing risk based on cancer family history is helpful in identifying patients who may benefit from genetic counselling/testing and/or enhanced screening. It is important when communicating risk to assess the patient's prior perception of their risk, tailor the communication to the individual and check understanding. Chapters 14 and 15 explain the specific risk factors, risk categories and risk assessment tools for breast and ovarian and colorectal and related cancers.

References

Amir E, Freedman OC, Seruga B, Evans DG 2010. Assessing women at high risk of breast cancer: a review of risk assessment models. *J Natl Cancer Inst* **102**: 680–691.

Antoniou AC, Pharoah PP, Smith P, Easton DF 2004. The BOADICEA model of genetic susceptibility to breast and ovarian cancer. *Br J Cancer* **91**: 1580–1590.

Baptista PV 2005. Principles in genetic risk assessment. *Ther Clin Risk Manag* **1**: 15–20.

Berry DA, Iversen ES Jr, Gudbjartsson DF, et al. 2002. BRCAPRO validation, sensitivity of genetic testing of *BRCA1/BRCA2*, and prevalence of other breast cancer susceptibility genes. *J Clin Oncol* **20**: 2701–2712.

Brain K, Norman P, Gray J, Mansel R 1999. Anxiety and adherence to breast self-examination in women with a family history of breast cancer. *Psychosom Med* **61**: 181–187.

Croyle RT and Lerman C 1999. Risk communication in genetic testing for cancer susceptibility. *J Natl Cancer Inst Monogr* **1999**(25): 59–66.

Edwards A, Gray J, Clarke A, et al. 2008. Interventions to improve risk communication in clinical genetics: systematic review. *Patient Educ Counsel* **71**: 4–25.

Evans DG, Eccles DM, Rahman N, et al. 2004. A new scoring system for the chances of identifying a *BRCA1/2* mutation outperforms existing models including BRCAPRO. *J Med Genet* **41**: 474–480.

Evans DG, Lalloo F, Cramer A, et al. 2009. Addition of pathology and biomarker information significantly improves the performance of the Manchester scoring system for *BRCA1* and *BRCA2* testing. *J Med Genet* **46**: 811–817.

Gail MH, Brinton LA, Byar DP, et al. 1989. Projecting individualized probabilities of developing breast cancer for white females who are being examined annually. *J Natl Cancer Inst* **81**: 1879–1886.

Gigerenzer G and Edwards A 2003. Simple tools for understanding risks: from innumeracy to insight. *Br Med J* **327**: 741–744.

Hadley DW, Jenkins JF, Steinberg SM, et al. 2008. Perceptions of cancer risks and predictors of colon and endometrial cancer screening in women undergoing genetic testing for Lynch syndrome. *J Clin Oncol* **26**: 948–954.

Hallowell N, Statham H, Murton F, et al. 1997. 'Talking about chance': the presentation of risk information during genetic counseling for breast and ovarian cancer. *J Genet Counsel* **6**: 269–286.

Hilgart JS, Coles B, Iredale R 2012. Cancer genetic risk assessment for individuals at risk of familial breast cancer. *Cochrane Database Syst Rev* **2**: CD003721.

Julian-Reynier C, Welkenhuysen M, Hagoel L, et al. 2003. Risk communication strategies: state of the art and effectiveness in the context of cancer genetic services. *Eur J Hum Genet* **11**: 725–736.

Kastrinos F, Balmana J, Syngal S 2013. Prediction models in Lynch syndrome. *Fam Cancer* **12**: 217–228.

Lobb EA, Butow PN, Barratt A, et al. 2004. Communication and information-giving in high-risk breast cancer consultations: influence on patient outcomes. *Br J Cancer* **90**: 321–327.

Marteau TM, Saidi G, Goodburn S, et al. 2000. Numbers or words? A randomized controlled trial of presenting screen negative results to pregnant women. *Prenat Diagn* **20**: 714–718.

Michie S, Lester K, Pinto J, Marteau TM 2005. Communicating risk information in genetic counseling: an observational study. *Health Educ Behav* **32**: 589–598.

Miller SM, Diefenbach MA, Kruus LK, et al. 2001. Psychological and screening profiles of first-degree relatives of prostate cancer patients. *J Behav Med* **24**: 247–258.

O'Doherty K and Suthers GK 2007. Risky communication: pitfalls in counseling about risk, and how to avoid them. *J Genet Couns* **16**: 409–417.

Parsons E and Atkinson P 1992. Lay constructions of genetic risk. *Sociol Health Illness* **14**: 437–455.

Phelps C, Bennett P, Brain K 2008. Understanding emotional responses to breast/ovarian cancer genetic risk assessment: an applied test of a cognitive theory of emotion. *Psychol Health Med* **13**: 545–558.

Timmermans DR, Ockhuysen-Vermey CF, Henneman L 2008. Presenting health risk information in different formats: the effect on participants' cognitive and emotional evaluation and decisions. *Patient Educ Counsel* **73**: 443–447.

Van Asperen CJ, Van Dijk S, Zoeteweij MW, et al. 2002. What do women really want to know? Motives for attending familial breast cancer clinics. *J Med Genet* **39**: 410–414.

Zikmund-Fisher BJ, Fagerlin A, Ubel PA 2010. Risky feelings: why a 6% risk of cancer does not always feel like 6%. *Patient Educ Counsel* **81** (Suppl.): S87–S93.

Chapter 14

Risk assessment in breast and ovarian cancer

Vishakha Tripathi and Charlotte Eddy

Introduction to risk assessment in breast and ovarian cancer

Breast and ovarian cancer are common malignancies affecting women in the general population. In the UK, prevalence figures for breast and ovarian cancer in the population setting are 1 in 8 and 1 in 54, respectively (CRUK, 2010). Approximately 10% of families affected by breast and ovarian cancer may have a hereditary component causing their specific family history. When assessing cancer-related family histories distinct patterns can be identified with the aid of some key factors and concepts. This chapter will focus on the specific characteristics which help in assessing and categorising cancer risk in breast and ovarian cancer families. The learning objectives for this chapter are:

- to be able to discuss the relationship between increased risk and family history for breast and ovarian cancer;
- to be able to explain near population, moderate-risk and high-risk categories of breast and ovarian cancer.

Family history and cancer risk

Breast and ovarian cancer are relatively common. It is therefore important to distinguish between cancers arising due to single gene mutations leading to hereditary breast and ovarian cancer (HBOC) and those that occur sporadically as a result of non-hereditary factors. Recent developments in genetic testing methods have shed further light on the presence of genes that confer lower cancer risks as well as numerous single nucleotide polymorphisms which are likely to contribute to breast and ovarian cancer risk in families that do not display a cancer pattern consistent with single gene mutations. Therefore, cancer risk can be thought of as occurring on a continuum along which defined thresholds are set that determine the risk management options available. This highlights the importance of accurate risk assessment when faced with a family history of breast and ovarian cancer, which in turn allows appropriate screening and preventative interventions to be accessed by the proband and their relatives.

Familial risk in breast and ovarian cancer

The first observations linking breast cancer occurrence and familial risk were made in the 1940s by Penrose (Penrose et al., 1948), and this work has now been validated through numerous studies in twins, families with breast and ovarian cancer and population-based studies. Breast and ovarian cancer can be inherited together (i.e. HBOC) and also individually as part of other autosomal dominant cancer syndromes. Before assessing and quantifying the familial risk and likelihood of a single gene mutation in a family with HBOC, it is important to learn about the typical features of the HBOC spectrum which can be used in conjunction with other less specific family history clues described in this chapter. The presence in the family history of the findings described in the following subsections would raise suspicion of HBOC caused by a single gene mutation.

Breast cancer

A positive personal (affected proband) and/or family history of young-onset breast cancer remains the strongest epidemiological factor in high-risk families. Breast and/or ovarian cancers occurring in multiple members on the same side of a family over more than one generation are suggestive of an autosomal dominant pattern. Cross-sectional studies have demonstrated that between 10 and 20% of individuals diagnosed with breast cancer have a close relative with the condition (Hoskins, 1995).

Multiple breast primaries are a strong indicator of inherited risk. Contralateral breast cancer risks have now been well established in families with known *BRCA* mutations and support the presence of an underlying inherited susceptibility as the cause of multiple primaries (Robson et al., 1998; Dong and Hemminki, 2001). In contrast, rates of bilateral disease are much lower in the near population risk group (Reding et al., 2010).

Triple-negative breast cancer

Studies have shown the presence of *BRCA* mutations in approximately 11% of triple-negative breast tumours (see Chapter 8) diagnosed under the age of 50, despite the absence of a dominant family history (Balmana et al., 2011). The receptor status of a tumour can usually be verified through a histopathology report or by documentation from the proband's oncologist or breast surgeon. This information should be actively probed, particularly if the proband developed young-onset breast cancer in the absence of other significant family history, as it could potentially alter their genetic testing and management options.

Male breast cancer is a known risk factor for inherited susceptibility. Although the incidence of breast cancer in men is lower than in women (approximately 1%), having a *BRCA2* mutation increases a man's risk of breast cancer (Evans et al., 2010). Therefore the diagnosis of breast cancer in a man should alert a clinician to the possibility of HBOC, particularly if there are female relatives with HBOC-related cancers. Other known non-hereditary risk factors like gynaecomastia and Klinefelter syndrome, which are risk factors for male breast cancer, should be queried in the absence of a significant cancer family history.

Ovarian cancer

Having a first-degree relative with ovarian cancer remains the strongest risk factor for the development of the disease in family members (Piver, 1996). The occurrence of breast and ovarian cancer in families with *BRCA* mutations is now well known. Both types of cancer may occur in the same individual or within the same family. Having more relatives with ovarian cancer increases the likelihood of HBOC from the population risk figure of 1 in 54 (or 2%) to 1 in 5–10 in families with two affected relatives aged under 60 or over 60, respectively (Lalloo et al., 2005). The risk of ovarian cancer increases in tandem with the probability of there being an inherited cause, which is represented in the Manchester scoring system (Table 14.1).

Young-onset high-grade serous ovarian cancer

Ovarian cancers associated with *BRCA* mutations are more likely to be invasive serous adenocarcinomas and less likely to be of mucinous or borderline pathology (Piek et al., 2003). Ovarian cancer is less accurately reported and understood by lay people; therefore, patient reports of ovarian cancers in relatives should be verified. Ovarian cancers are far less common than breast cancers, and 10–15% of all ovarian cancers diagnosed are caused by *BRCA* mutations (Risch et al., 2001).

Table 14.1 Manchester score

Age	*BRCA1*	*BRCA2*
FBC < 30	6	5
FBC 30–39	4	4
FBC 40–49	3	3
FBC 50–59	2	2
FBC > 59	1	1
MBC < 60	5 (if *BRCA2* tested)	8
MBC > 59	5 (if *BRCA2* tested)	5
Ovarian cancer < 60	8	5 (if *BRCA1* tested)
Ovarian cancer > 59	5	5 (if *BRCA1* tested)
Pancreatic cancer	0	1
Prostate cancer < 60	0	2
Prostate cancer > 59	0	1

FBC, female breast cancer; MBC, male breast cancer. Age is in years.

Scores are added for each cancer in a direct lineage.

Fallopian tube cancer

Recent studies have shown that cancers originating in the fallopian tubes are also part of the HBOC and *BRCA* spectrum; this can include cancer in the adenexa and the distal or fimbrial end of the fallopian tube (Medeiros et al., 2006; Domchek et al., 2010).

Primary peritoneal cancer

Cells forming the peritoneum are known to have the same embryological origin as those forming the ovaries. For this reason, although it is much rarer, women with primary peritoneal cancer (not metastatic) would fit the HBOC spectrum.

Ovarian cancer only families

Recent research has identified mutations in the genes *RAD51C* and *RAD51D* that also predispose to ovarian cancer (Loveday et al., 2011; Pelttari et al., 2011), and the families in which these novel genes were identified showed a paucity of breast cancer only family histories. Health professionals should therefore query the possibility of HBOC in such families.

Prostate cancer

Prostate cancer is the second most common malignancy to affect men, with the vast majority of diagnoses occurring in men aged 50 or over. The presence of a family history remains a strong risk factor, with approximately 42% of risk being derived from heritable factors (Carter et al., 1992; Lichtenstein et al., 2000). Therefore, young-onset prostate cancer in a family with breast and ovarian cancer is likely to be significant and suggestive of HBOC.

Pancreatic cancer

While there are many environmental risk factors that contribute to pancreatic cancer risk, a well-known association in the inherited context is that between *BRCA2* mutations and pancreatic adenocarcinoma, with carriers having a 3.5-fold increase in risk in comparison with the general population (Murphy et al., 2002). Pancreatic cancer is the tenth most common malignancy in the UK and affects approximately 1 in 77 men and 1 in 79 women in the population (CRUK, 2011). In those with a family history of the disease, 17% will harbour a *BRCA2* mutation (Iqbal et al., 2012). In families with breast and ovarian cancer any pancreatic cancer diagnosis should be probed, particularly as it may change the family's eligibility for genetic testing if this information is missed and the threshold of detecting a mutation (10% or more) is not met based on initial family history collection.

Rare *BRCA2* related cancers

Ocular melanoma has been reported in *BRCA2* families in some studies (Liede et al., 2004). Gall bladder and bile duct carcinoma (Breast Cancer Linkage Consortium, 1999) are also known to occur in *BRCA2* families but are rare.

Risk categorisation: near population, moderate-risk and high-risk groups of breast and ovarian cancer

As already mentioned, familial risk of breast and ovarian cancer can be seen to occur along a continuum. The greater the number of affected relatives who are closely related to the proband, and the younger they are at the time of diagnosis, the higher the level of inherited risk. For the purpose of genetic assessment, family histories are placed into one of three risk categories which are 'near population risk', 'moderate risk' and 'high risk'. This concept of a cancer risk continuum is illustrated in Fig. 14.1 through the use of the risk categories and a risk assessment model called the Manchester score (Table 14.1). With a progressive increase in the strength of family history, the risk category also increases, as does the likelihood of there being a single gene mutation.

The National Institute for Health and Care Excellence (NICE) guidance (NICE, 2013) suggests using either a manual model such as the Manchester scoring system or a computer-based model like BOADICEA (Breast and Ovarian Analysis of Disease Incidence and Carrier Estimation Algorithm) (Antoniou et al., 2004, 2008) to assess the inherited risk of breast cancer.

The Manchester score was devised by Evans et al. in 2004 to provide a robust, easy to use and quick method of calculating the probability of detecting a *BRCA1/2* mutation in a family with a cancer family history. It does not, however, estimate an individual's probability of being a carrier. In 2009 it was updated with histopathological information to reflect advances in the understanding of *BRCA*-related tumour characteristics such as tumour type and hormone receptor status (Evans et al., 2009). Scores are assigned based on the tumour type and age of the affected individual. A score of 15 equates to a 10% likelihood of detecting a *BRCA* mutation and is the current threshold for offering genetic testing according to NICE guidelines (NICE, 2013). It does not take into account rare *BRCA*-related cancers or special cases where *BRCA* founder mutations may be prevalent in specific populations. Application of the Manchester score is illustrated by the use of adapted family histories (see Figs 14.3 and 14.4).

BOADICEA also estimates the likelihood of carrying a *BRCA1/2* mutation but in an individual, and is therefore dependent on the sensitivity of the testing method used. It requires access to a computer and can be time-consuming to perform during a clinical consultation. In contrast to the Manchester score, it does incorporate information regarding Ashkenazi Jewish ancestry as well as the results of any *BRCA1/2* testing that has already been performed in the family. Non-genetic factors, however, are currently not taken into account in the BOADICEA model. A paper validating the performance of both these models and others reported that BOADICEA is well calibrated and has a superior discriminatory power to most other models for detecting families likely to harbour *BRCA* mutations (Antoniou et al., 2008).

Secondary-care providers can use methods that calculate carrier probability, such as BOADICEA or the Manchester scoring system, to help determine eligibility for referral to specialist genetic services and genetic testing thresholds (NICE, 2013).

Key

yrs, years
Br Ca, breast cancer
Ov Ca, ovarian cancer
FDR, first-degree relative
SDR, second-degree relative
< less than
> greater than
* Refer to Manchester Score in Table 14.1 for values

• Breast cancer refers to a diagnosis in a female, unless otherwise stated as being male.

• Cancers can be in the same person, meaning a women could have breast and ovarian cancer under 60 years, but they must be primary cancers and not secondary or recurrences.

• Cancers can be on the paternal or maternal side of the family, but you must assess each lineage as two separate entities. If affected relative is SDR through a male FDR, then the female moves up one place to a FDR.

Risk category	Lifetime risk of breast cancer	Equivalent family histories									
		Minimum corresponding Manchester scores*									
Near population risk	< 17% or 1 in 6 to 1 in 8	FDR with Br Ca >40 yrs	1 Ov Ca >60 yrs								
		2–6	10								
Moderate risk	17% to 30% or 1 in 6 to 1 in 4	FDR with Br Ca <40 yrs	2 FDR or SDR relatives with Br Ca at an average of >50 yrs	3 FDR or SDR diagnosed with Br Ca at an average age of >60 yrs	1 Ov Ca <60 yrs FDR						
		12+	12+	8+	12+						
High risk	>30% or 1 in 3	2 FDR or SDR with Br Ca at average age of <50 years	3 FDR or SDR relatives diagnosed with Br Ca at an average age of <60 years	4 relatives diagnosed with Br Ca at any age (at least one a FDR)	1 FDR with bilateral Br Ca both diagnoses < 50 yrs	Bilateral Br Ca in 1 FDR <55 yrs or SDR & 1 Br Ca in FDR or SDR at average age < 60 yrs	Male Br Ca & Br Ca in FDR or SDR <50 yrs	Male Br Ca & 2Br Ca in FDR or SDR <60 yrs	1 Ov Ca any age & 1 Br Ca < 50 yrs (one person must be a FDR)	1 Ov Ca & 2 Br Ca at average < 60 yrs (can be FDR or SDR)	2 Ov Ca any age
		12+	4–8	6	13	10+	16+	18+	16+	18 +	20+
Gene carrier BRCA1 BRCA2 TP53	Specific to each gene but > 30% or 1 in 3										

Elevated Inherited Risk →

Increasing Family History →

Figure 14.1 Continuum of breast and ovarian cancer risk.

Near population, moderate- and high-risk categories

The types of family history for each of these risk groups are shown in Fig. 14.1, Figure 14.2.

◆ Near population risk: individuals at near population risk are managed in primary care as there is no evidence to support a hereditary basis for occurrences of cancer in the family. This group faces lifetime risks of breast cancer of less than 17% and referral to a genetics service is not appropriate.

◆ Moderate risk: individuals at moderate risk have a lifetime risk of breast cancer of between 17 and 30%. In such cases the possibility of inherited factors confers a slight increase in risk, warranting early screening (NICE, 2013), but the chance of a *BRCA1/2* mutation is not high enough to warrant genetic testing.

◆ High risk: this category of risk indicates that the individual has a 30% or greater chance of developing HBOC in their lifetime. High-risk families usually have evidence of a dominant cancer pattern with family members developing breast, ovarian and related cancers at relatively young ages (less than 50 years). It is recommended that these families are referred to clinical genetics for a formal assessment.

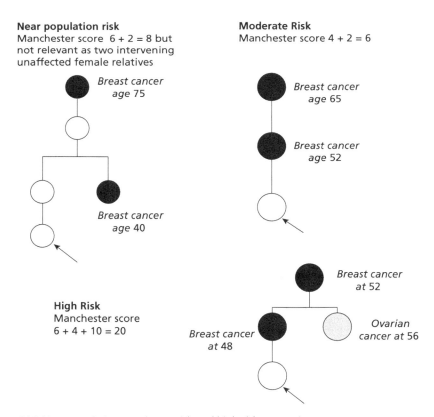

Figure 14.2 Near population, moderate-risk and high-risk categories.

Advances in understanding of cancer genetics, the interpretation of genetic test results and the emergence of new genetic testing methods has allowed informative testing of individuals from high-risk families that do not have a cancer diagnosis themselves where the individual has 10% or greater chance of a BRCA1/2 mutation. Testing of these unaffected relatives has now been incorporated into NICE guidance (NICE, 2013) and referral teams will need to alter previous principles to effectively identify these eligible individuals.

Changing family histories and risk

Reported family history can change, both during and after an assessment (Glanz et al., 1999). This is highlighted in the following example:

> Susan was concerned about her risk of breast cancer. During the discussion it became apparent that her father had thought his maternal aunt had 'female cancer', most likely endometrial cancer, but he was uncertain about the exact diagnosis.
>
> Based on this family history Susan was assessed to be at moderate risk of breast cancer (Fig. 14.3).
>
> With a Manchester score of 8 she was not eligible for genetic testing within the NHS. Susan was asked to try to verify her paternal great aunt's cancer diagnosis. The death certificate confirmed that she had ovarian cancer and that her grandmother had actually had breast cancer twice (Fig. 14.4). Two occurrences of breast cancer 5 or more years apart on either side should be considered as bilateral breast disease.
>
> This new information put Susan into the high-risk category and confirmed that the family history was consistent with HBOC. The Manchester score was now 29 which meant that a genetics referral for Susan's paternal grandmother was indicated to discuss genetic testing.

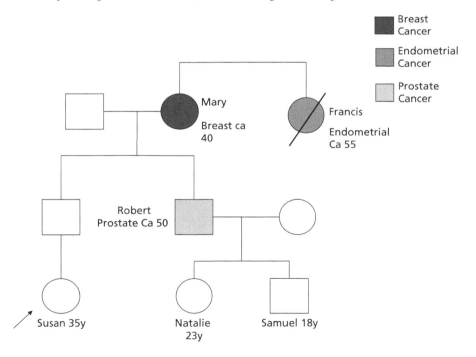

Manchester score: (Prostate Ca <59) 2 + (Breast Ca 40–49) 6 = 8

Figure 14.3 Risk assessment prior to confirmation of family history.

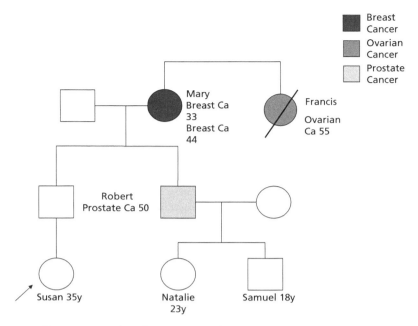

Manchester score: (Prostate Ca <59) 2 + (Breast Ca 30–39) 8 + Breast
Ca 40–49) 6 + (Ovarian Ca <59) 13 = 29

Figure 14.4 Change of family history upon confirmation of cancer (ca, cancer).

Due to time constraints, it is not always possible to obtain confirmation of all cancer diagnoses in a family. For this reason, using a logical approach and choosing to confirm only those cancers which could change the management options for the proband and the family is justified. As this example demonstrates, cancer confirmations may alter a family's risk assessment and eligibility for genetics referral.

Summary

This chapter shows that HBOC is identifiable from distinct patterns in cancer family histories. An increasing number of affected relatives in direct lineage on either side of the family increases the risk of breast or ovarian cancer for individuals in those families and is the basis for triage into the categories of near population, moderate and high risk of breast and ovarian cancer.

References

Antoniou AC, Pharoah PPD, Smith P, Easton DF 2004. The BOADICEA model of genetic
susceptibility to breast and ovarian cancer. *Br J Cancer* **91**: 1580–1590.

Antoniou AC, Hardy R, Walker L, et al. 2008. Predicting the likelihood of carrying a *BRCA1* or *BRCA2*
mutation: validation of BOADICEA, BRCAPRO, IBIS, Myriad and the Manchester scoring system
using data from UK genetics clinics. *J Med Genet* **45**: 425–431.

Balmana J, Díez O, Rubio IT, Cardoso F 2011. *BRCA* in breast cancer: ESMO clinical practice guidelines. *Ann Oncol* **22**: vi31–vi34.

Breast Cancer Linkage Consortium 1999. Cancer risks in *BRCA2* mutation carriers. The Breast Cancer Linkage Consortium. *J Natl Cancer Inst* **91**: 1310–1316.

Carter BS, Beaty TH, Steinberg GD, et al. 1992. Mendelian inheritance of familial prostate cancer. *Proc Natl Acad Sci USA* **89**: 3367–3371.

CRUK (Cancer Research UK) 2010. *Ovarian cancer incidence statistics*. Available at: <http://www.cancerresearchuk.org/cancer-info/cancerstats/types/ovary/incidence/> (last accessed 19 November 2012).

CRUK (Cancer Research UK) 2011. *Pancreatic cancer incidence*. Available at: <http://www.cancerresearchuk.org/cancer-info/cancerstats/types/pancreas/incidence/> (last accessed 24 July 2013).

Domchek SM, Friebel TM, Garber JE, et al. 2010. Occult ovarian cancers identified at risk-reducing salpingo-oophorectomy in a prospective cohort of *BRCA1/2* mutation carriers. *Breast Cancer Res Treat* **124**: 195–203.

Dong C and Hemminki K 2001. Multiple primary cancers of the colon, breast, and skin (melanoma) as models for polygenic cancers. *Int J Cancer* **92**: 883–887.

Evans DGR, Eccles DM, Rahman N, et al. 2004. Medical genetics in practice: A new scoring system for the chances of identifying a *BRCA1/2* mutation outperforms existing models including BRCAPRO. *J Med Genet* **41**(6): 474–480.

Evans DGR, Susnerwala I, Murton F, et al. 2010. Risk of breast cancer in male *BRCA2* carriers. *J Med Genet* **47**: 710–711.

Glanz K, Grove J, Le Marchand L, Gotay C 1999. Underreporting of family history of colon cancer: correlates and implications. *Cancer Epidemiol Biomarkers Prevent* **8**: 635–639.

Hoskins KF, Stopfer JE, Calzone KA, et al. 1995. Assessment and counseling for women with a family history of breast cancer. A guide for clinicians. *J Am Med Assoc* **273**: 577–585.

Iqbal J, Ragone A, Lubinski J, et al. (Hereditary Breast Cancer Study Group) 2012. The incidence of pancreatic cancer in *BRCA1* and *BRCA2* mutation carriers. *Br J Cancer* **107**: 2005–2009.

Lalloo F, Kerr B, Friedman J, Evans G 2005. *Risk assessment and management in cancer genetics*. Oxford: Oxford University Press.

Lichtenstein P, Holm NV, Verkasalo PK, et al. 2000. Environmental and heritable factors in the causation of cancer—analyses of cohorts of twins from Sweden, Denmark, and Finland. *New Engl J Med* **343**: 78–85.

Liede A, Karlan BY, Narod SA 2004. Cancer risks for male carriers of germline mutations in *BRCA1* or *BRCA2*: a review of the literature. *J Clin Oncol* **22**: 735–742.

Loveday C, Turnbull C, Ramsay E, et al. 2011. Germline mutations in *RAD51D* confer susceptibility to ovarian cancer. *Nat Genet* **7**: 879–882.

Medeiros F, Muto MG, Lee Y, Elvin JA, et al. 2006. The tubal fimbria is a preferred site for early adenocarcinoma in women with familial ovarian cancer syndrome. *Am J Surg Pathol* **30**: 230–236.

Murphy KM, Brune KA, Griffin C, et al. 2002. Evaluation of candidate genes *MAP2K4*, *MADH4*, *ACVR1B*, and *BRCA2* in familial pancreatic cancer: deleterious *BRCA2* mutations in 17%. *Cancer Res* **62**: 3789–3793.

NICE (National Institute for Health and Care Excellence) 2013. *Familial breast cancer: classification and care of people at risk of familial breast cancer and management of breast cancer and related risks in people with a family history of breast cancer*. Clinical Guidance 164. London: National Institute for Health and Care Excellence.

Pelttari LM, Heikkinen T, Thompson D, et al. 2011. *RAD51C* is a susceptibility gene for ovarian cancer. *Hum Molec Genet* **20**: 3278–3288.

Penrose LS, Mackenzie HJ, Karn MN 1948. A genetic study of human mammary cancer. *Ann Eugenics* **14**: 234–266.

Piek K, Torrenga B, Hermsen B, Verheijen RH, et al. 2003. Histopathological characteristics of *BRCA1* and *BRCA2* associated intraperitoneal cancer: a clinic-based study. *Fam Cancer* **2**: 73–78.

Piver MS 1996. Prophylactic oopherectomy: reducing the U.S. death rate from epithelial ovarian cancer. A continuing debate. *Oncologist* **1**: 326–330.

Reding KW, Bernstein JL, Langholz BM, et al. 2010. Adjuvant systemic therapy for breast cancer in *BRCA1/BRCA2* mutation carriers in a population-based study. *Breast Cancer Res Treat* **123**: 491–498.

Risch HA, McLaughlin JR, Cole DE, et al. 2001. Prevalence and penetrance of germline *BRCA1* and *BRCA2* mutations in a population series of 649 women with ovarian cancer. *Am J Hum Genet* **68**: 700–710.

Robson M, Gilewski T, Haas B, et al. 1998. *BRCA* associated breast cancer in young women. *J Clin Oncol* **16**: 1642–1649.

Chapter 15

Risk assessment in colorectal, gastric and related gynaecological cancers

Sarah Rose and Vicki Kiesel

Introduction to risk assessment in colorectal, gastric and related gynaecological cancers

Colorectal (bowel) cancer is the fourth most common cancer in the UK, affecting 1 in 19 women and 1 in 14 men (CRUK, 2013). In 2010, there were 40 695 new cases of colorectal cancer (CRC) in the UK: 22 834 (56%) in men and 17 861 (44%) in women (CRUK, 2013). The incidence of CRC is strongly associated with increasing age. Gastric (stomach) cancer (GC) is less common, affecting 1 in 64 men and 1 in 120 women (CRUK, 2013). Gynaecological cancers that can be genetically linked to CRC and GC include ovarian and endometrial/uterine (womb) cancers. Ovarian cancer affects 1 in 51 women and endometrial cancer affects 1 in 43 women (CRUK, 2013).

The majority of CRC and GC is sporadic, but approximately 5% of CRC is due to an inherited predisposition and up to 25% is familial. Recognising the level of risk within a family is vital for determining the correct level of screening required for those individuals.

Identifying those families in which genetics input could be helpful, whether for determining the appropriate screening, confirming the diagnoses in a family or carrying out some genetic testing, relies on a healthcare professional recognising certain 'clues' to a genetic predisposition. In this chapter a general overview of how to carry out a risk assessment for CRC, GC and related gynaecological cancers will be discussed. The learning objectives for Chapter 15 are:

- to be able to understand the relationship between increased risk and family history in relation to CRC, GC and related gynaecological cancers;
- to be able to understand what an average, moderate and high risk of CRC, GC and related cancers means;
- to be able to understand the subsequent risk management recommendations for people at each level of risk.

Obtaining a family history of CRC, GC and related gynaecological cancers

There are several factors which are suggestive of an inherited predisposition to CRC, GC and related gynaecological cancers and which need to be considered when assessing a family history. It is essential to obtain sufficient information to assess these factors and guidance on how to take a cancer family history can be found in Chapter 3.

In a CRC family history it is also important to look for gastric, endometrial, ovarian, urinary tract, pancreatic cancer, brain tumours and skin cancers.

Asking about relatives' screening can provide more information, and in a family with this clustering of cancers it is important to ask if people have developed bowel polyps. A history of colorectal polypectomies is also important, because these significantly lower the risk of CRC. Therefore, if someone regularly has polyps removed (which could have had cancerous potential had they been left) this may conceal a possible family history of CRC.

It is helpful to know whether female relatives have had a hysterectomy or oophorectomy, as this may mask an inherited syndrome by significantly reducing the risk of endometrial cancer (EC) or ovarian cancer (OC). There is also evidence that the use of oral contraceptives can lower the risk of these cancers (Maguire and Westhoff, 2011).

Several factors can increase the risk of CRC and GC, such as alcohol consumption and cigarette smoking (Trédaniel et al., 1997; Chan and Giovannucci, 2010). Some cancer treatments can also increase the risk of further primary cancers. For example, the use of tamoxifen following breast cancer increases the risk of EC (Bergman et al., 2000; Pukkala et al., 2002; Swerdlow and Jones, 2005) and this may alter the family risk assessment as EC can be linked genetically to CRC. In some families environmental factors may therefore cause cancers which are falsely suggestive of an inherited syndrome.

Specific questions relating to a family history of CRC, GC and related gynaecological cancers

◆ Have any relatives had a hysterectomy or oophorectomy?

◆ Has anyone had bowel screening, and if so have any polyps been found or removed?

Confirmation of a family history of CRC, GC and related gynaecological cancers

Colonoscopy reports for someone diagnosed with CRC are helpful to determine if the patient had multiple polyps or one primary tumour. This can alter the genetic testing recommended for the family.

The risk in a family with CRC, GC and related cancers can be significantly altered as the cancers are confirmed. For example, Miss S presented giving the family history illustrated in Table 15.1. This family history is high risk and meets the Amsterdam II criteria (Vasen et al., 1999), possibly indicating Lynch syndrome (LS) and necessitating tumour testing.

Table 15.1 Family history at initial presentation

Mother	Colorectal cancer	Age 45
Maternal aunt	Endometrial cancer	Age 35
Maternal grandfather	Colorectal cancer	In his 60s

Table 15.2 Revised family history following confirmation of the cancers

Mother	Colorectal cancer	Age 45	Confirmed
Maternal aunt	Cervical	Age 35	Confirmed
Maternal grandfather	Lung	Age 70	Confirmed

Miss S could potentially be at a 50% risk of LS, and therefore CRC, EC, OC and GC, requiring intensive screening (where available) and consideration of risk-reducing surgeries. However, upon confirming the cancers the family history changed (Table 15.2).

The revised family history means that Miss S can be reassured that the cervical and lung cancers are unlikely to have a genetic cause and are not involved in LS. This leaves one CRC in a first-degree relative under the age of 50. Tumour testing may still be indicated as this family meets the revised Bethesda criteria (Umar et al., 2004); however, the index of suspicion is significantly reduced. Miss S is at a low to moderate risk of CRC and a one-off colonoscopy at the age of 55 (Cairns et al., 2010) would be recommended. Screening based on the reported family history would have involved 2-yearly colonoscopies from 25 to 75 years of age, highlighting the importance of making a full assessment and confirming a reported family history, where possible, before implementing a screening plan.

Assessing a family history of CRC, GC and related gynaecological cancers

When assessing the risk of hereditary colorectal conditions, family histories may be suggestive of LS, a polyposis syndrome or both. Families at risk for LS may meet the Amsterdam or Bethesda criteria and these are generally used to recommend tumour testing (see Chapter 9).

Characteristics which are suggestive of LS include:

♦ affected relatives diagnosed with a LS-related cancer at a young age, i.e. CRC, GC, EC, OC, pancreatic cancer, sebaceous adenomas, urinary tract cancers or brain tumours;

♦ multiple relatives affected with LS-related cancers;

♦ multiple affected generations.

Some LS families will not have any cases of CRC. It is important to highlight those families with just gynaecological cancers or only GCs. Figure 15.1 shows an example of a family history that is suggestive of LS and has a high risk of CRC. The family meets the Amsterdam criteria showing three affected relatives in two generations with one relative diagnosed before the age of 50. Referral to genetics services is appropriate, with colonoscopy every 18–24 months (Cairns et al., 2010). Women also have a potentially increased risk of EC and OC.

Other families may be at high risk of CRC because of a possible polyposis syndrome. The risk of polyposis depends on the type and number of polyps found in an individual, the age at which polyps are found and the number of individuals affected. Most polyposis

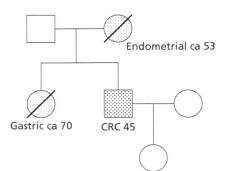

Figure 15.1 Example of a family history that meets the Amsterdam criteria (ca, cancer).

Endometrial ca 53

Gastric ca 70   CRC 45

syndromes are autosomal dominant and will cause multiple generations to be affected. However, *MUTYH*-associated polyposis (MAP) is recessive and therefore only one generation will be affected with polyps and/or early onset CRC. In general, individuals with ten or more polyps in their lifetime may benefit from a referral to genetics services (Jasperson, 2012).

Inherited GC

When assessing families for GC risk it is essential to obtain the histology of any GC or breast cancer in the family, as these are probably the most important clues. Lobular breast cancer and diffuse GC are suggestive of hereditary diffuse gastric cancer (HDGC), while other types do not suggest this condition. There will also usually be multiple affected generations. In addition, some GC may be caused by LS and these families will meet the characteristics of LS listed in Chapter 9.

Histology and tumour test results

Inherited cancer conditions can be associated with specific cancer characteristics which can be useful clues when used in conjunction with other information, such as age at diagnosis and number of affected relatives. When histology is suggestive of a particular syndrome it may be beneficial to consider a referral to genetics services. For example, it would be useful to refer a patient with mucinous signet ring CRC diagnosed at the age of 59 to genetics services for consideration of LS; however, if there were no mucin or signet ring features, a referral would not be helpful.

Table 15.3 summarises specific cancer histopathologies and their potential association with genetic syndromes. It is of course important to remember that this is just part of the overall picture, and regardless of histopathology a cancer may occur by chance or due to a different genetic mechanism.

The personal or family history of polyps is another important clue. In general less than 1% of polyps (Enders, 2012) will become cancerous, and they frequently occur by chance; however, different types of polyps can be associated with specific inherited conditions. Adenomas can be associated with LS, familial adenomatous polyposis and MAP,

Table 15.3 Histopathology and inherited CRC, GC and related gynaecological cancers

Origin of cancer	Histopathology	Syndrome to consider
Breast (Lynch et al., 2011)	Lobular	Hereditary diffuse gastric cancer
Gastric (stomach) (Lynch et al., 2011)	Diffuse (poorly cohesive clusters signet ring)	Hereditary diffuse gastric cancer
Gastric (Aarnio, 2012)	Intestinal	Lynch
Colorectal (Umar et al., 2004)	Mucinous/signet ring differentiation. Tumour-infiltrating lymphocytes. Crohn's-like lymphocytic reaction. Medullary growth pattern	Lynch
Endometrial (Broaddus et al., 2005)	Mixed endometrioid and non-endometrioid histology (Lynch). Lower uterine segment anatomical location (Lynch)	Lynch
Ovarian (Watson et al., 2001)	Surface epithelial including: serous, endometrioid, mucinous, clear cell, transitional cell	Lynch (*BRCA1/2*)

All surface epithelial ovarian cancers can be associated with Lynch syndrome. Non-epithelial cancers are unlikely to be related (e.g. germ cell tumours).

while hyperplastic polyps are very common in the general population, are usually small (<0.5 mm) and have a very low potential for malignancy (Aust and Baretton, 2010). It is well known that adenomas are precursors to carcinoma; however, it is now also understood that larger serrated polyps such as sessile serrated adenomas (SSAs) can have malignant potential. The number of polyps identified in an individual is also an important part of the risk assessment. As the number of polyps increases, the likelihood of an inherited syndrome also increases. Table 15.4 lists polyp pathology and associated inherited conditions.

Tumour testing can also alter an individual's cancer risk as it changes the likelihood that a family has LS. When microsatellite instability (MSI) and immunohistochemistry (IHC) for *MLH1*, *MSH2*, *MSH6* and *PMS2* are both normal it is very unlikely that the patient has LS. This is because the sensitivity of the two tests combined is high. IHC alone is 93% sensitive for all four genes (Hampel et al., 2005, 2008) while MSI alone has sensitivity in CRC of 89% (Lynch et al., 2011).

Familial risk

When LS is effectively ruled out or a family history is not suggestive of a known inherited condition there may still be a familial risk. This may be because there are other genes causing a moderately increased risk or because families share the same environmental factors. In general, a patient's risk of CRC increases with the number of affected relatives and earlier age at diagnosis. Guidelines published by Cairns et al. (2010) are used to categorise these families.

Table 15.4 Polyp pathology and associated inherited conditions[1]

Polyp type	Signs of concern	Potential syndrome
Hyperplastic	2+ >10 mm	Usually sporadic
	30+ polyps	Hyperplastic polyposis
Adenomas	>1 cm	Lynch syndrome
	>25% villous	Familial adenomatous polyposis
	High-grade dysplasia	*MUTYH*-associated polyposis
Sessile serrated adenoma	Multiple and large >1 cm	Hyperplastic polyposis or mixed polyposis
Mixed polyps		Hereditary mixed polyposis
Hamartomatous		Peutz–Jeghers syndrome
		PTEN
		Juvenile polyposis syndrome

[1] Source: data from Aust, D.E and Baretton, G.B., Serrated polyps of the colon and rectum (hyperplastic polyps, sessile serrated adenomas, traditional serrated adenomas, and mixed polyps) — proposal for diagnostic criteria, *Virchows Archv*, Volume 457, Issue 3, pp.291–297, Copyright © Springer-Verlag 2010.

Patients with a significantly elevated risk of CRC will usually have at least one affected first-degree relative, except in rare circumstances such as where the first-degree relative died at a young age. When both parents are affected these count as two affected first-degree relatives.

Families with three first-degree relatives diagnosed with CRC at any age (none before the age of 50) or two first-degree relatives diagnosed before the age of 60 are suggestive of a significant familial risk of CRC, and tumour testing should be used to evaluate the possibility of LS. Once LS has been excluded, these families are estimated to be at high moderate risk of CRC, which can be quantified as an estimated 10–17% or a 1 in 6 to 1 in 10 lifetime risk of death from CRC without screening. Individuals at high moderate risk should have a colonoscopy every 5 years from the ages of 50 to 75 (Cairns, 2010). Examples of high moderate-risk family histories are shown in Figs 15.2 and 15.3.

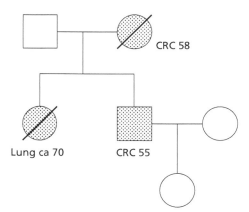

Figure 15.2 This family has two individuals diagnosed with colorectal cancer (CRC) before the age of 60. Therefore, this family has a high moderate risk of CRC (ca, cancer).

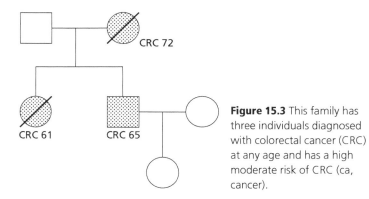

Figure 15.3 This family has three individuals diagnosed with colorectal cancer (CRC) at any age and has a high moderate risk of CRC (ca, cancer).

In families with two first-degree relatives diagnosed at the age of 60 or later or where one relative is diagnosed before the age of 50 (where LS has been excluded by tumour testing) the risk of death from CRC can be estimated to be 8% (1 in 12) (Cairns et al., 2010), and family members are therefore at low moderate risk. Examples of low moderate-risk family histories are shown in Figs 15.4 and 15.5.

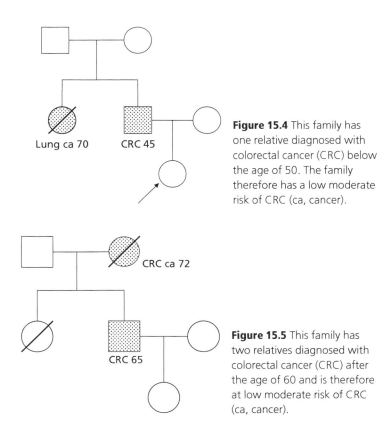

Figure 15.4 This family has one relative diagnosed with colorectal cancer (CRC) below the age of 50. The family therefore has a low moderate risk of CRC (ca, cancer).

Figure 15.5 This family has two relatives diagnosed with colorectal cancer (CRC) after the age of 60 and is therefore at low moderate risk of CRC (ca, cancer).

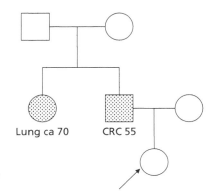

Figure 15.6 An example family with an average risk of colorectal cancer (CRC) (ca, cancer).

Lung ca 70   CRC 55

Table 15.5 Colorectal cancer (CRC) risk categorisation

Risk category	Lifetime risk of CRC death without surveillance	Odds ratio of CRC death without surveillance
Population risk	<8%	<1 in 12
Low moderate	8%	1 in 12
High moderate	10–17%	1 in 6 to 1 in 10
High	Varies dependent on syndrome <100%	<1

The risk for any patient who has only one relative diagnosed with colorectal cancer at the age 50 or later is not significantly elevated (it is less than 8% or 1 in 12) and no additional screening is required. All patients will be eligible for NHS bowel screening and should be informed about bowel awareness and be given general lifestyle and dietary advice. Figure 15.6 shows an example of an average-risk family history.

Table 15.5 summarises the categorisation of CRC family histories and the associated risk of death without surveillance.

When a patient with a family history of CRC, GC or related gynaecological cancer should be referred to genetics services and why

Cairns et al. (2010) suggested the following criteria to determine which family histories of gastrointestinal or gynaecological malignancies should be referred to a regional genetics centre for risk assessment:

1 A family history consistent with an autosomal dominant cancer syndrome (multiple affected generations).

2 Features of a polyposis syndrome in the individual or in a close relative (ten or more polyps or other characteristics of polyposis).

Table 15.6 CRC risk and family history[1]

CRC risk	Number of relatives affected	Age at diagnosis	Referral to genetics services
Population	▮ FDR with CRC	>50	No
Low moderate	▮▮ FDR with CRC	<50	Yes[2]
	▮▮ FDRs with CRC	>60	No
High moderate	▮▮ One FDR + one FDR/SDR with CRC/LSRC	<60	Yes[2]
		Any age	Yes[2]
	▮▮▮ FDR/SDR (at least one FDR) with CRC/LSRC		
High risk	▮▮▮ At least one FDR and one should be FDR of the other two, with CRC/LSRC	One <50	Yes[2]

FDR, first-degree relative; SDR, second-degree relative; CRC, colorectal cancer; LSRC, Lynch syndrome related cancer.

[1] Source: data from Cairns, S.R., et al, Guidelines for colorectal cancer screening and surveillance in moderate and high risk groups (update from 2002), *Gut*, Volume 59, Issue 5, pp. 666–689, Copyright © 2010.

[2] These families should be referred to genetics services for consideration of tumour testing. Where possible it is always preferable to refer the affected individual. Screening may be advised on the basis of present risk but the patient should be informed that it may alter as a result of testing.

3   A known mutation in a CRC susceptibility gene within the family.

4   Molecular (histological) features of a familial syndrome in a CRC in a first-degree relative (see Table 15.3 for more information).

Individuals who do not fulfil any of these four criteria should be excluded.

Table 15.6 summarises the categorisation of familial CRC risk (Cairns, 2010), giving a clearer idea of which family histories should be referred to genetics services. In addition, genetics services are always happy to receive queries regarding any patient should a healthcare professional have any concerns about a family history.

Summary

It is clear that family history is a very important tool in identifying those at increased risk of CRC, GC and associated cancers. It is therefore particularly important to ensure the accuracy of a family history. There are many clues indicating that a family history may be suggestive of an inherited risk, and both histology and tumour testing are particularly important when assessing such families. Once accurate risk assessments have been made these can be used to recommend appropriate screening, thereby lowering the risk of significant morbidity or mortality. Explaining these risk assessments and recommendations to both patients and professionals is an important part of the process.

References

Aarnio M 2012. Clinicopathological features and management of cancers in Lynch syndrome. *Pathol Res Int* **2012**: article ID 350309, doi: 10.1155/2012/350309.

Aust DE and Baretton GB 2010. Serrated polyps of the colon and rectum (hyperplastic polyps, sessile serrated adenomas, traditional serrated adenomas, and mixed polyps)—proposal for diagnostic criteria. *Virchows Arch.* **457**: 291–297.

Bergman L, Beelen ML, Gallee MP, et al. 2000. Risk and prognosis of endometrial cancer after tamoxifen for breast cancer. Comprehensive Cancer Centres' ALERT Group. assessment of liver and endometrial cancer risk following tamoxifen. *Lancet* **356**: 881–887.

Broaddus RR, Lynch HT, Chen LM, et al. 2006. Pathologic features of endometrial carcinoma associated with HNPCC: a comparison with sporadic endometrial carcinoma. *Cancer* **106**: 87–94.

Cairns SR, Scholefield JH, Steele RJ, et al. 2010. Guidelines for colorectal cancer screening and surveillance in moderate and high risk groups (update from 2002). *Gut* **59**: 666–689.

CRUK (Cancer Research UK) 2013. Cancer incidence statistics. Available at: <http://www.cancerresearchuk.org/cancer-info/cancerstats/incidence/> (last accessed 29 December 2013).

Chan AT and Giovannucci EL 2010. Primary prevention of colorectal cancer. *Gastroenterology* **138**: 2029–2043.

Citarda F, Tomaselli G, Capocaccia R, et al. 2001. Efficacy in standard clinical practice of colonoscopic polypectomy in reducing colorectal cancer incidence. *Gut.* **48**: 812–815.

Enders GH 2012. Colonic polyps. *Emedicine.* Available at: <http://emedicine.medscape.com/article/172674-overview> (last accessed 29 December 2013).

Hampel H, Frankel WL, Martin E, et al. 2005. Screening for the Lynch syndrome (hereditary nonpolyposis colorectal cancer). *N Engl J Med* **352**: 1851–1860.

Hampel H, Frankel WL, Martin E et al. 2008. Feasibility of screening for Lynch syndrome among patients with colorectal cancer. *J Clin Oncol* **26**: 5783–5788.

Jasperson K 2012. Genetic testing by cancer site. Colon (polyposis syndromes) *Cancer J* **18**: 328–333.

Lynch HT, Lynch JF, Shaw TG 2011. Hereditary gastrointestinal cancer syndromes. *Gastrointest Cancer Res* **4** (Suppl. 1): S9–S17.

Maguire K and Westhoff C 2011. The state of hormonal contraception today: established and emerging noncontraceptive health benefits. *Am J Obstet Gynecol* **205** (Suppl.): S4–S8.

Pukkala E, Kyyronen P, Sankila R, Holli K 2002. Tamoxifen and toremifene treatment of breast cancer and risk of subsequent endometrial cancer: a population-based case–control study. *Int J Cancer* **100**: 337–341.

Swerdlow AJ and Jones ME 2005. British Tamoxifen Second Cancer Study Group. Tamoxifen treatment for breast cancer and risk of endometrial cancer: a case–control study. *J Natl Cancer Inst* **97**: 375–384.

Trédaniel J, Boffetta P, Buiatti E, et al. 1997. Tobacco smoking and gastric cancer: review and meta-analysis. *Int J Cancer.* **72**: 565–573.

Umar A, Boland CR, Terdiman JP, et al. 2004. Revised Bethesda guidelines for hereditary nonpolyposis colorectal cancer (Lynch syndrome) and microsatellite instability. *J Natl Cancer Inst* **96**: 261–268.

Vasen HF, Watson P, Mecklin JP, Lynch HT 1999. New clinical criteria for hereditary nonpolyposis colorectal cancer (HNPCC, Lynch syndrome) proposed by the International Collaborative Group on HNPCC. *Gastroenterology* **116**: 1453–1456.

Watson P, Bützow R, Lynch HT, et al. (International Collaborative Group on HNPCC) 2001. The clinical features of ovarian cancer in hereditary nonpolyposis colorectal cancer. *Gynecol Oncol* **82**: 223–228.

Chapter 16

Cancer risk assessment and communicating risk. Summary

Lorraine Robinson and Patricia Webb

Introduction to section 4 summary

The chapters in Section 4 are concerned with balancing the fundamental tenets of the practice of risk assessment with the particular issues and principles of risk assessment for designated cancers.

Chapter 13. Cancer risk assessment and communicating risk. Introduction

The key concept of Chapter 13 centres on the notion of risk, which presents one of the main challenges to health professionals when talking with patients and their families. Each encounter needs to consider not only risk calculation but also the importance of communicating risk in a sensitive, honest and understandable way.

Guided activities for Chapter 13

- Identify your local genetics centre. In the UK a directory of regional genetics centres can be found at the website of the British Society for Genetic Medicine (BSGM) (<http://www.bsgm.org.uk/information-education/genetics-centres/>).

- In Europe, this information is more difficult to access but a good starting place is the website of the European Society of Human Genetics (ESHG) (<https://www.eshg.org/>).

- It is vital to ensure that you are using the most appropriate risk assessment tool available. Make contact with your genetics centre to identify and discuss the tools used for identifying risk. Take time to evaluate any local tools that are being used to ensure that they are fit for purpose, have been agreed with your genetics centre and have been updated to mirror current guidance.

- Go to the website of the National Genetics and Genomics Education Centre (<http://www.geneticseducation.nhs.uk>) where you will find resources to help you to identify, assess and communicate risk.

◆ Reflect on the current terminology you utilise in practice to communicate risk so that you are clear on the strategies used. Look at how your current practice fits with the multistep approach advocated by Julian-Reynier et al. (2003). Are there areas in which you and your colleagues need additional education and support with risk assessment and communication?

◆ From the articles by Hadley et al. (2008) and Hilgart et al. (2012), identify what has been shown to improve risk perception. How would you communicate risk to a patient in clear, succinct and understandable way? Work with a colleague to ensure that your explanation is accurate and comprehensible.

Chapters 14 and 15 Cancer risk assessments

Chapters 14 and 15 provide an overview of how to carry out a cancer risk assessment. Although the cancers discussed are common, there are unique characteristics that assist healthcare professionals in determining risk in families and individuals.

Guided activities for Chapters 14 and 15

◆ Familiarise yourself with the guidelines discussed in Chapters 14 and 15 and ensure you are clear about when a patient needs to be referred to genetics services, how to make a genetics referral and what information needs to be provided.

◆ Identify where you can access further training in the use of risk assessment tools. This may be through your genetics centre or the National Genetics and Genomics Education Centre (<http://www.geneticseducation.nhs.uk>). There may also be learning opportunities advertised on the website of the BSGM (<http://www.bsgm.org.uk>), the UK Cancer Genetics Group (<http://www.ukcgg.org>) and the ESHG (<https://www.eshg.org/>).

Guided practice for Chapters 14 and 15

The aim of this task is to develop confidence in communicating cancer risk and to practice this in a safe setting, helping you to navigate the National Institute for Health and Care Excellence (NICE) guidelines, use the Manchester scoring system and to become familiar with the best practice guidelines for colorectal cancer risk assessment.

We suggest that you undertake these tasks in triads with colleagues using the example family trees given in Fig 16.1 and 16.2. The task can be repeated using other examples from your own practice. Colleague 1 should act as the health professional, disclosing the risk assessment, but concentrating on practising listening skills and conveying information sensitively to the patient. Colleague 2 should act as a patient with a history of cancer, presenting the family history information. While acting as the patient, reflect on the emotions that may emerge and identify the importance of specific phrases and words that are helpful in understanding the information or make it difficult to understand. Colleague 3 should observe the interaction, identifying the key features of the session that could alter

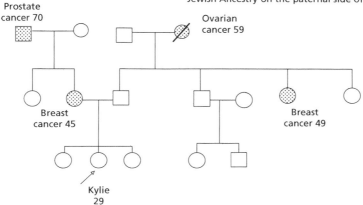

Figure 16.1 Breast/ovarian cancer family history exercise (the patient is Kylie).

Based on the maternal side of the family, Kylie is at near population risk of breast cancer, as although she has a first-degree relative diagnosed with breast cancer, this was diagnosed after the age of 40. The Manchester score is 7 (female breast cancer at age 40–49, score 6; prostate cancer over age 59, score 1).

On the paternal side of the family, the Manchester score is 19. The patient has two second-degree relatives, through a male, one with ovarian cancer (score 13) and the other with breast cancer under 50 (score 6). This patient could be referred to genetics based on the likelihood that the pattern of cancer could be due to a *BRCA* mutation. In addition, there is Jewish ancestry on this side of the family which increases the chances of specific mutations in the *BRCA* genes. However, it would therefore be sensible to suggest that her paternal aunt with breast cancer considers a genetics referral in the first instance.

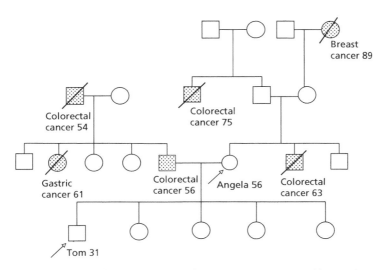

Figure 16.2 Colorectal cancer family history task (the patients are Tom and his mother Angela).

Angela is at near population risk of colorectal cancer, because although she has two relatives with colorectal cancer only one of them is a first-degree relative and he was diagnosed after the age of 50.

Tom is at high moderate risk of colorectal cancer because on his father's side he has one first-degree and two second-degree relatives with colorectal/Lynch syndrome related cancer. Genetics referral is indicated for Tom but ideally his father should be referred to genetics in the first instance.

the risk assessment. Practice giving feedback to Colleague 1, mirroring the approach that might be taken when talking to a patient. Focus on relaying the feedback sensitively and with empathy.

References

Hadley DW, Jenkins JF, Steinberg SM, et al. 2008. Perceptions of cancer risks and predictors of colon and endometrial cancer screening in women undergoing genetic testing for Lynch syndrome. *J Clin Oncol* **26**: 948–954.

Hilgart JS, Coles B, Iredale R 2012. Cancer genetic risk assessment for individuals at risk of familial breast cancer. *Cochrane Database Syst Rev* **2**: CD003721.

Julian-Reynier C, Welkenhuysen M, Hagoel L, et al. 2003. Risk communication strategies: state of the art and effectiveness in the context of cancer genetic services. *Eur J Hum Genet* **11**: 725–736.

Early detection of hereditary cancer

Chapter 17

Early detection of hereditary cancer. Introduction

Chris Jacobs

Introduction to early detection of hereditary cancer

People at risk of cancer due to their family history may have access to targeted cancer screening. The aim of screening is to identify disease at a pre-malignant or early stage, before symptoms are present, on the basis of evidence that detection of pre-invasive disease can prevent cancer or that treatment at an earlier stage can improve outcomes. Early detection of cancer is one of the primary reasons for undergoing risk assessment and genetic testing (Bleiker et al., 2013). Yet, in addition to the benefits, there are risks, limitations and challenges associated with screening that need to be considered by patients and health professionals.

The learning objectives for Chapter 17 are:

◆ to be able to discuss the aims and principles of screening for early detection or prevention of cancer;

◆ to be able to explain the key elements of an effective screening test;

◆ to be able to discuss the limitations and potential harms of screening;

◆ to consider the psychological impact of screening for individuals at high risk of cancer.

Aims of screening

Screening aims to prevent disease through early detection before symptoms arise. In order to be beneficial, screening must lead to treatment that is more effective than that which would have occurred once symptoms are manifest. Some types of screening (such as cervical smears to detect and treat dysplasia, and colonoscopy to detect and remove bowel polyps) involve detecting and removing precursors to cancer, while others (such as X-ray mammography for early detection of breast cancer) aim to detect cancer at an early stage.

Principles of screening for early detection of cancer

The fundamental principles of screening were established by Wilson and Junger (1968) for the World Health Organization. These principles (Box 17.1) continue to guide screening today, starting from the requirement that, overall, screening should do more good

Box 17.1 The World Health Organization principles of screening

1 Screening should be directed towards an important health problem.

2 There should be a simple, safe, precise and validated screening test.

3 Treatment started at an early stage should be of more benefit than treatment initiated later.

4 There should be evidence that the screening test is effective in reducing morbidity and mortality.

5 The benefit of screening should outweigh the physical and psychological harm caused by the test, diagnostic procedures and treatment.

6 The opportunity cost of the screening programme should be economically balanced in relation to expenditure on medical care as a whole.

7 There should be a plan for managing and monitoring the screening programme and an agreed set of quality assurance standards.

8 Potential screening participants should receive adequate information about benefits and disadvantages of participation.

than harm (Bretthauer and Kalager, 2013). Public demand for and confidence in screening is high, and enthusiasm for screening could potentially lead to unproven screening tests being adopted prematurely (Kemp and Potyk, 2005). This may be a particular problem within the private sector and in countries without a public health service. Understanding the principles of screening may be helpful when explaining to patients why population screening is not available for particular conditions and why enhanced screening is not available to everyone with a family history of cancer.

Ideally, before a screening programme is introduced, large randomised controlled trials will have been undertaken to assess the health and economic outcomes of screening for that particular disease. However, evaluating the incidence, mortality and long-term adverse effects of a screening test is challenging because of the long time period between the screening episode and the potential development of cancer as well as the relatively low incidence of even the most frequent cancers in the population. These studies therefore require a very large sample size and lengthy follow-up, making them extremely costly and challenging to conduct (Bretthauer and Kalager, 2013).

The performance of a screening test is assessed on its ability to separate diseased from healthy individuals and to identify those at higher risk compared with those at lower risk (Cuckle, 2004). The majority of people screened within a population screening programme will not develop the disease being screened for.

Screening may be targeted to individuals who are identified as being at increased risk of cancer due to family history or genetic susceptibility. For example, individuals at risk of colorectal cancer associated with Lynch syndrome will be screened within an individualised screening programme guided by best practice guidelines. Screening high-risk groups for some cancers may be justified when general population screening for the same cancer may be difficult to defend on grounds of cost or false-positive rates.

Key elements of a screening test

Before any screening modality is introduced, either within a large-scale screening programme or for more targeted high-risk screening, the validity, reliability, yield, acceptability, cost-effectiveness and availability of follow-up services need to be evaluated (Wilson and Junger, 1968).

A screening test needs to separate those with the condition from those without the condition and to detect a high proportion of those with the disease. The performance of a screening test is described using four indices: sensitivity, specificity, positive predictive value and negative predictive value:

- Sensitivity: this is the proportion of individuals who have the disease who are detected by the test (true positives). It is calculated as true positives divided by true positives + false negatives (individuals with the disease who have a negative test result) and is expressed as a percentage. An ideal test has 100% sensitivity.

- Specificity: this is the proportion of individuals who do not have the disease who are correctly classified as negative by the test (true negatives). It is calculated as true negatives divided by true negatives + false positives (individuals with no disease who have a positive test result) and is expressed as a percentage. An ideal test has 100% specificity. High specificity of a screening test is of vital importance, especially if a positive result triggers invasive diagnostic procedures (Brawley and Kramer, 2005).

- The positive predictive value (PPV) is the proportion of individuals with a positive test result who actually have cancer (true positives divided by true positives + false positives). An ideal test has 100% PPV.

- The negative predictive value (NPV) is the proportion of individuals with a negative test result who do not have cancer (true negatives divided by true negatives + false negatives). An ideal test has 100% NPV.

Limitations and potential harms of screening

It is important that individuals undergoing screening understand the risks and limitations associated with the test. As explained earlier, many, although not all, screening tests detect cancer early rather than prevent it from occurring. For individuals at increased risk this concept may be difficult to come to terms with, so much so that the option of prophylactic surgery may be preferable to screening. It is important that the risk of missing cancer through false-negative results and having unnecessary invasive procedures as a result of false-positive test results is made clear to patients prior to embarking on screening. Any risk associated with the screening test procedure itself also needs to be explained. Over-diagnosis of cancer or pre-invasive disease that would not have caused medical problems if left undetected can lead to significant harm through over-treatment. There has been much debate in recent years about the impact of over-diagnosis in population breast screening programmes (Duffy et al., 2005; Jorgensen, 2011).

The availability of high-risk screening in the UK

In the UK, following risk assessment women at moderate and high risk of breast cancer have access to X-ray mammography (XRM) via NHS breast units but outside of the NHS Breast Screening Programme. *BRCA1* and *BRCA2* mutation carriers and women at equivalent risk can access high-risk breast screening with XRM and magnetic resonance imaging (MRI) within the NHS higher-risk breast screening programme. Colorectal screening by colonoscopy is available within the NHS for moderate- and high-risk groups. High-risk ovarian screening is still under review, and there is currently no ovarian screening programme available within the NHS.

Psychological impact of screening on individuals at high risk of cancer

Screening of women at high risk of breast and ovarian cancer has been or is undergoing evaluation in large-scale studies. A systematic review of XRM in women at high risk of breast cancer concluded that women do not experience high levels of anxiety, although there may be a slight short-term increase in anxiety (Watson et al., 2005). A study in the United States assessing the clinical effectiveness of annual XRM in women under the age of 50 with a family history of breast cancer reported a decrease in worry about cancer and negative psychological consequences immediately after the screening result. Amongst women who were recalled, immediate psychological consequences were greater than in those not recalled, but after 6 months any cancer-specific distress had reduced (Tyndel et al., 2007). In a large UK study of breast screening for women with a *BRCA1* or *BRCA2* mutation (MARIBS), high levels of satisfaction and low levels of psychological morbidity were reported following MRI. However, intrusive MRI-related thoughts and distress were more likely to persist 6 weeks after the MRI. A significantly higher proportion of women reported that they intended to return for XRM than MRI (Hutton et al., 2011). A US study of screening high-risk women with MRI and XRM found that MRI did not have a detrimental psychological impact on *BRCA1/2* mutation carriers but a temporary increase in global anxiety was reported in women recalled for further imaging after a false-positive result (Spiegel et al., 2011).

A systematic review and meta-analysis of colorectal cancer screening found low levels of participation in colonoscopy screening (around 40%) in individuals at moderate risk of colorectal cancer (Ait Ouakrim et al., 2013) Amongst high-risk unaffected carriers who have undergone genetic testing, studies have reported a 53–100% uptake of colonoscopy screening (Bleiker et al., 2013). A review of the psychological factors affecting screening uptake concluded that recommendations from health professionals were a major consideration in screening decisions, with a relative's surgeon being the main source of information (Rees, 2008). Several studies found that awareness, knowledge and discussion of colorectal screening were positively associated with participation in screening (Rees, 2008).

A qualitative study of women's experiences of familial ovarian screening undertaken as part of the UK Familial Ovarian Cancer Screening Study (UKFOCSS), involving semi-structured interviews with 48 high-risk women, reported positive experiences in terms of peace of mind and the feeling that it was sensible to undergo screening, and negative experiences such as concern around the time of the test and dislike of the testing procedures (a transvaginal ultrasound scan and a blood test). Overall the positive experiences outweighed the negative (Lifford et al., 2013).

Therefore although some short-term anxiety is associated with breast, ovarian and colorectal screening in the high-risk population, there do not appear to be long-term psychological consequences.

Summary

Targeted screening for individuals with a cancer family history aims to prevent cancer or improve outcomes through detection of pre-invasive or early stage disease before symptoms become apparent. To ensure the principle that screening does more good than harm, the health and economic outcomes of a new screening test should be evaluated in large clinical trials. Studies of the psychological impact of screening in high-risk populations suggest that there are no long-term psychological consequences. It is important that the limitations as well as the benefits of targeted screening are discussed with patients before screening is commenced.

The chapters in this section describe the benefits and limitations of different methods of screening for breast cancer (Chapter 18), colorectal and gastric cancer (Chapter 19) and gynaecological cancers (Chapter 20) and evaluate the current position with regard to cancer screening in the UK and Europe.

References

Ait Ouakrim D, LockettT, Boussioutas, A, et al. 2013. Screening participation for people at increased risk of colorectal cancer due to family history: a systematic review and meta-analysis. *Fam Cancer* **12**: 459–472.

Bleiker EM, Esplen MJ, Meiser B, et al. 2013. 100 years Lynch syndrome: what have we learned about psychosocial issues? *Fam Cancer* **12**: 325–339.

Brawley OW and Kramer BS 2005. Cancer screening in theory and in practice. *J Clin Oncol* **23**: 293–300.

Bretthauer M and Kalager M 2013. Principles, effectiveness and caveats in screening for cancer. *Br J Surg* **100**: 55–65.

Cuckle H 2004. Principles of screening. *Obstet Gynaecol* **6**: 21–25.

Duffy SW, Agbaje O, Tabar L, et al. 2005. Overdiagnosis and overtreatment of breast cancer: estimates of overdiagnosis from two trials of mammographic screening for breast cancer. *Breast Cancer Res* **7**: 258–265.

Hutton J, Walker LG, Gilbert FJ, et al. 2011. Psychological impact and acceptability of magnetic resonance imaging and X-ray mammography: the MARIBS Study. *Br J Cancer* **104**: 578–586.

Jorgensen KJ, Keen JD, Gotzsche P 2011. Is mammography screening justifiable considering its substantial overdiagnosis rate and minor effect on mortality? *Radiology* **260**: 621–627.

Kemp C and Potyk D 2005. Cancer screening: principles and controversies. *Nurse Practitioner* **30**: 46–50.

Lifford KJ, Clements A, Fraser L, et al. 2013. A qualitative study of women's experiences of familial ovarian cancer screening. *Psycho-Oncology* **22**: 6576–6584.

Rees G 2008. Screening participation in individuals with a family history of colorectal cancer: a review. *Eur J Cancer Care (Engl)* **17**: 221–232.

Spiegel TN, Esplen MJ, Hill KA, et al. 2011. Psychological impact of recall on women with BRCA mutations undergoing MRI surveillance. *Breast* **20**: 424–430.

Tyndel S, Austoker J, Henderson BJ, et al. 2007. What is the psychological impact of mammographic screening on younger women with a family history of breast cancer? Findings from a prospective cohort study by the PIMMS Management Group. *J Clin Oncol* **25**: 3823–3830.

Watson EK, Henderson BJ, Brett J, et al. 2005. The psychological impact of mammographic screening on women with a family history of breast cancer—a systematic review. *Psycho-Oncology* **14**: 939–948.

Wilson JMG and Junger G 1968. *The principles and practice of screening for disease.* Geneva: World Health Organization.

Chapter 18

Early detection of hereditary breast cancer

Michael Michell

Introduction to early detection of hereditary breast cancer

The detection of small breast cancers by high-quality X-ray mammography in population screening programmes has been shown by large well-conducted prospective randomised trials to be effective in reducing deaths from breast cancer in the average-risk population. Breast screening programmes have been established in most European countries over the last 20 years. With increased awareness of genetics and risk factors for breast cancer amongst both the public and health professionals, there has been interest in the last 10 years in developing screening services for those with a significantly increased risk due to family history. X-ray mammography is used for screening younger women from the age of 40 years with a moderately increased risk of breast cancer. More recently, screening using magnetic resonance imaging (MRI) in young women with a high risk of breast cancer, combined with X-ray mammography from the age of 40 years, has been shown to be effective in the detection of small breast cancers. In this chapter, the breast screening services offered to women of both average and increased risk are described, together with the evidence base underpinning screening, the benefits and limitations of screening and the importance of robust quality assurance (QA).

The learning objectives for Chapter 18 are:

* to consider the benefits and limitations of current methods of screening for breast cancer;
* to be able to describe the current position with regard to breast screening in the UK and Europe.

Breast screening services

Normal-risk population

A national mammography screening programme was implemented in the UK following the publication in 1986 of the findings of an expert committee chaired by Sir Patrick Forrest (Forrest, 1986). The current UK policy for breast screening by mammography is:

1 Women aged 50–70 years are invited for screening once every 3 years. Women aged over 70 years may self-refer for screening. There is currently a trial taking place in the

UK to examine the effects of offering screening to women aged 47–50 and those aged 70–73 years (Moser et al., 2011).

2 The screening test is a lateral oblique and craniocaudal view mammogram of each breast.

The main stages of the screening process are invitation, basic screen, assessment and diagnosis, treatment:

1 Invitation: eligible women in the age range for screening are identified from the computerised records of women registered with general practitioners. Women are offered their first invitation for screening before the age of 53 and are sent further invitations every 3 years while they are within the age range for screening.

2 Basic screen: the basic screening mammogram is carried out in static units or mobile units, used in many rural areas. The screening images are read to identify any which show an abnormality suspicious for cancer. The images are read by specialist radiologists, appropriately trained clinicians or advanced practitioner radiographers and are double-read to improve accuracy.

3 Assessment and diagnosis: women whose basic screening mammogram shows an abnormality suspicious for cancer are recalled to a specialist, multidisciplinary clinic where facilities are available for triple assessment—clinical consultation and examination, standard and supplementary mammographic views, ultrasound and needle biopsy. In 90–95% women with breast cancer the diagnosis can be confirmed by needle biopsy and treatment is planned with appropriate support and counselling. Women who are found on further assessment to have normal breasts or benign change are reassured and discharged until their next routine screening examination.

Breast screening programmes using mammography have now been established in most European countries. Variations between the different national programmes such as the age range for invitation and the interval between screens have been recently reviewed by Giordano et al. (2012).

Screening for women with a family history of breast cancer

Services with varied protocols were developed in many parts of the UK up until 2007. The Cancer Reform Strategy (DoH, 2007) recommended that all women concerned about their risk of breast cancer should be offered the opportunity to have their risk formally assessed and to discuss management options in accordance with National Institute for Health and Care Excellence (NICE) guidelines for familial breast cancer (McIntosh et al., 2004). Updated NICE guidelines for familial breast cancer were published in 2013 (NICE, 2013). The NICE guidelines for screening women with a family history of breast cancer who have not had cancer themselves are shown in Table 18.1. The NICE guidelines for screening women with a personal and family history of breast cancer are shown in Table 18.2. The 2012 report *Improving outcomes: a strategy for cancer* (DoH, 2012) recommended that the NHS Breast Screening Programme (NHSBSP) should take on the management of surveillance

Table 18.1 Breast screening recommendations for women with a family history of breast cancer (BC) who have not had breast cancer (BC) themselves

Age (years)	Moderate risk	High risk				
	Untested women with 17– < 30% lifetime risk of BC	Untested women with ≥30% lifetime risk of BC and ≤30% chance of BRCA1/ BRCA2/ TP53 mutation	Untested women with >30% lifetime risk of BC and ≥30% chance of BRCA1/ BRCA2 mutation	Tested women with a known BRCA1/ BRCA2 mutation	Untested women with a >30% chance of TP53 mutation	Tested women with a known TP53 mutation
20–29	No screening	No screening	No screening	No screening	Annual MRI	Annual MRI
30–39	No screening	No MRI (consider annual XRM)	Annual MRI (consider annual XRM)	Annual MRI (consider annual XRM)	Annual MRI	Annual MRI
40–49	Annual XRM	Annual XRM	Annual MRI + XRM	Annual MRI + XRM	Annual MRI	Annual MRI
50–59	NHSBSP (consider annual XRM)	Annual XRM	Annual XRM (MRI only offered if breast density is high)	Annual XRM (MRI only offered if breast density is high)	NHSBSP (MRI only offered if breast density is high)	No XRM (consider annual MRI)
60–69	NHSBSP	NHSBSP	NHSBSP	Annual XRM	NHSBSP	No XRM (consider annual MRI)
70+	NHSBSP	NHSBSP	NHSBSP	NHSBSP	NHSBSP	No XRM

BC, breast cancer; MRI, magnetic resonance imaging; XRM, X-ray mammography; NHSBSP, NHS Breast Screening Programme.

National Institute for Health and Care Excellence (2013). Adapted with permission from CG164 *Familial breast cancer: Classification and care of people at risk of familial breast cancer and management of breast cancer and related risks in people with a family history of breast cancer.* London: NICE. Copyright © 2013, available from <http://guidance.nice.org.uk/CG164>. This information was accurate at time of press.

Table 18.2 Screening recommendations for women with a personal and family history of breast cancer (BC)

Age (years)	Women who remain at moderate risk of BC	Women who remain at high risk of BC	
		Known *BRCA1/BRCA2* mutation or >30% chance of *BRCA1/2* mutation	Known *TP53* mutation or >30% chance of *TP53* mutation
20–29	Follow-up screening for 5 years after diagnosis if appropriate as indicated by NICE (2009) guidelines	Follow-up screening for 5 years after diagnosis if appropriate as indicated by NICE (2009) guidelines	No XRM. Consider annual MRI
30–39	Follow-up screening for 5 years after diagnosis if appropriate then NHSBSP as indicated by NICE (2009) guidelines	Annual MRI	
40–49		Annual MRI + annual XRM	
50–59		Annual XRM (MRI only if breast density high)	
60–69		Annual XRM	
70 +		NHSBSP	No XRM

BC, breast cancer; MRI, magnetic resonance imaging; XRM, X-ray mammography; NHSBSP, NHS Breast Screening Programme.

National Institute for Health and Care Excellence (2013). Adapted with permission from CG164 *Familial breast cancer: Classification and care of people at risk of familial breast cancer and management of breast cancer and related risks in people with a family history of breast cancer*. London: NICE. Copyright © 2013, available from <http://guidance.nice.org.uk/CG164> and National Institute for Health and Care Excellence (2009). CG80 *Early and locally advanced breast cancer*. London: NICE. Copyright © 2009, available from <http://www.nice.org.uk/CG80>. This information was accurate at time of press.

of women at higher risk in order to provide a service with national standards and consistent high quality. The NHSBSP protocols for screening women at higher risk (including those who have not had breast cancer and those with a personal history of breast cancer) are shown in Table 18.3.

Screening for women at moderate risk

The recommended surveillance protocol for unaffected women at moderate risk of breast cancer is annual digital mammography from 40 to 49 years followed by 3-yearly mammography from 50 to 69 years (Table 18.1). Women with breast cancer who remain at moderate risk after breast cancer treatment are recommended to have 5 years of follow-up and then screening within the NHSBSP if appropriate (Table 18.2) (NICE, 2013).

There is no evidence from large-scale randomised controlled trials for the benefit of mammographic screening in this group equivalent to the evidence available for women aged 50 years and over. Evidence for the effect of screening in this group comes from observational studies (FH01 Management Committee, 2006 ; Duffy et al, 2013). Results from the FH01 study (FH01 Collaborative Teams, 2010) have shown that mammographically detected cancers in a group of moderate-risk women undergoing screening had significantly better prognostic features compared with a control group in the UK Age Trial and a cohort of Dutch women with a family history of breast cancer. It is estimated that the potential reduction in breast cancer mortality achieved by regular mammographic screening from 40 to 50 years for those with a relative risk of breast cancer of >3 is similar to the mortality reduction achieved in the normal-risk population aged over 50 years (NHS Cancer Screening Programmes, 2012a).

Screening for women at high risk

The current NICE guidelines (NICE, 2013) for screening women at high risk who have not had breast cancer are shown in Table 18.1. The guidelines (NICE 2013) also make recommendations for women with a personal history of breast cancer following treatment, which are shown in Table 18.2. The recommended screening depends on the likelihood that the woman carries a cancer-predisposing gene mutation.

Since the discovery of the *BRCA1*, *BRCA2* and the rarer *TP53* gene mutations in the 1990s and the recognition of a significant increased associated risk of breast cancer, much work has been carried out to identify a suitable and effective screening technique for young women at high risk, both carriers of a gene mutation and those who have not undergone genetic testing but have equivalent risk due to their family history. An effective screening technique needs to detect a large proportion of cancers either at a non-invasive stage or at an early stage of invasion when the cancer is small and the lymph nodes are clear. The significantly increased risk at a young age in this group requires a technique which is effective when a large proportion of the breast is composed of glandular tissue. Early studies of X-ray mammography alone in high-risk women in their 30s and 40s showed a low sensitivity and high interval cancer rates of 45–50% (Kerlikowske et al., 1996) (interval cancer is that which is diagnosed after a normal screening test and before a subsequent screen). A further factor which may influence the sensitivity of mammography in this group is the different mammographic appearance of cancers compared with that of sporadic cases diagnosed in the normal-risk population—many of the cancers found in the *BRCA1* group appear as well-defined masses (Hamilton et al., 2004).

Breast MRI has become established as an effective diagnostic technique for the further investigation and local staging of breast disease, used as an adjunct to standard X-ray mammography and ultrasound. The examination involves the patient lying in a prone position with special coils applied to the breasts. An intravenous injection of gadolinium, a low molecular mass contrast agent, is used to highlight lesions and their extent. The contrast agent leaks into the extracellular space in tissues with permeable vasculature, typical of the neo-angiogenesis found with malignant lesions. Thus, cancers are seen to enhance or light up on post-contrast scans and the pattern of enhancement can be measured in dynamic scan sequences providing further information about the nature of a lesion. Contrast-enhanced breast MRI has been shown to have a very high sensitivity for the demonstration of cancer, but has a lower specificity because many benign lesions show some enhancement. The assessment of lesions found on breast MRI involves the same multidisciplinary process as for standard screening. Many soft tissue lesions found on MRI will be visible on high-quality ultrasound and can be readily and accurately biopsied under ultrasound guidance. A few lesions detected by MRI will not be visible on standard mammographic and ultrasound imaging. In these cases, MRI-guided biopsy is necessary to obtain a diagnosis.

Prospective studies have been conducted in Europe and North America to evaluate the use of MRI in high-risk women and compare the accuracy of MRI with X-ray mammography (Lord et al., 2007; Warner et al., 2008; Leach, 2009; Lehman and Smith, 2009). The UK MARIBS study (Leach et al., 2005) was a large, multicentre study with 649 women aged 35–49 years with a strong family history of breast cancer or a high probability of *BRCA1*, *BRCA2* or *TP53* mutation. Thirty-five cancers were diagnosed and the sensitivity for MRI (77%; 95% confidence interval (CI) 60–90%) was significantly higher than for mammography alone (40%; 95% CI 24–58%). The highest sensitivity was for the two methods combined (94%; 95% CI 81–99%). In other published series comparing MRI with X-ray mammography, the sensitivity of MRI ranges from 71.1 to 94%, the sensitivity of X-ray mammography from 33 to 59%, and for the two methods combined the sensitivity is from 86.4 to 94%.

On the basis of the results of these studies, MRI is now offered to women at high risk who wish to undergo surveillance:

BRCA1/2 and equivalent risk

For carriers of *BRCA1* or *BRCA2* mutations and those at equivalent risk (including women who have a personal history of breast cancer), annual MRI is recommended from the age of 30 to 49 years. Annual X-ray mammography is recommended in addition from the age of 40 years (Table 18.3) (NHS Cancer Screening Programmes, 2013). Further surveillance is then decided on an individual basis according to the mammographic breast density—the sensitivity of mammography increases as the breast undergoes fatty involution with age.

This differs slightly from the NICE guidelines for familial breast cancer (NICE, 2013) where *BRCA1/2* carriers and untested women at greater than 30% probability of being a *BRCA1/2* carrier (with and without a personal history of breast cancer) are recommended to have annual MRI from ages 30 to 49 and annual mammograms from ages 40 to 69 followed by 3-yearly mammograms within the population screening programme (Tables 18.1 and 18.2).

TP53 and equivalent risk

For *TP53* carriers and those at equivalent risk (including women who have a personal history of breast cancer), annual MRI is offered from the age of 20 onwards (Table 18.3) (NHS Cancer Screening Programmes, 2013).

NICE guidelines for familial breast cancer recommend that *TP53* carriers with and without a personal history of breast cancer do not have mammograms at all. However, untested women with a greater than 30% chance of a *TP53* mutation are recommended to have annual MRI screening from ages 20 to 49 and then 3-yearly mammograms on the NHSBSP (NICE, 2013) (Table 18.1).

In other European countries it is recognised that special screening services, including the use of MRI, are effective in screening high-risk groups. These services are under

Table 18.3 NHS Breast Screening Programme protocols for the surveillance of women at higher risk of developing breast cancer

Group	Risk	Ages (years)	Surveillance protocol	Frequency	Notes
1	(a) *BRCA1* or (b) *BRCA2* carrier or (c) not tested, equivalent high risk	20–29	n/a	n/a	Review MRI annually on basis of background density
		30–39	MRI	Annual	
		40–49	MRI + mammography	Annual	
		50+	Mammography ± MRI	Annual	
2	*TP53* (Li–Fraumeni)	20+	MRI	Annual	No mammography
3a	A-T homozygotes	25+	MRI	Annual	No mammography
3b	A-T heterozygotes	40–49	Mammography	18-monthly	Routine screening from age 50
		50+	Mammography	Routine screening (3-yearly)	

MRI, magnetic resonance imaging; A-T, Ataxia telangiectasia.

Reproduced with permission from NHS Breast Screening Programme (NHSBSP) Publication No. 74, *Protocols for the surveillance of women at higher risk of developing breast cancer*, Version 4 © Crown Copyright 2013.

development and evaluation but there is no current Europe-wide agreed high-risk screening protocol (Perry et al., 2008).

Benefits, limitations and harmful effects of screening

Benefits

The principal benefit of screening for breast cancer is the prevention of deaths through the detection, diagnosis and treatment of breast cancers when they are small, when there is less chance of spread and when the outcome following treatment is better than for cancers diagnosed following symptoms. The effect of screening on breast cancer mortality has been measured in several large-scale prospective, randomised controlled trials carried out in Europe and North America (IARC, 2002; Tabar et al., 2003, 2011; Paci, 2012). The results of these trials have been analysed extensively, most recently by the Independent Breast Screening Review (The Independent UK Panel on Breast Cancer Screening, 2012). This review concluded from a meta-analysis of randomised trials with at least 13 years of follow-up data that the relative risk of death from breast cancer for women aged 50–69 years invited for screening is 0.80 (95% CI 0.73–0.89) compared with women not invited. Thus the relative risk reduction in breast cancer mortality in the groups invited for screening is estimated as 20% (95% CI 11–27%). The effect on women who attend for screening is likely to be greater than 20%. There have been significant improvements in the cancer detection rates in mammography screening programmes, mainly due to technical developments in mammography which have occurred since the trials were conducted—the effect of screening in current practice may well be higher than that observed in the trials.

Limitations and harmful effects

The limitations and harmful effects of screening are related to false-positive and false-negative results and over-diagnosis (Kopans et al., 2011; Raftery and Chorozoglou, 2011; Michell, 2012). False-positive results leading to recall for further assessment, and in some cases needle biopsy, and the inevitable associated anxiety occur because of the non-specific nature of some appearances found on both X-ray mammography and breast MRI scans. Specialist training and adequate experience of film readers are essential in order to mini-mise the number of such recalls while maintaining an adequate cancer detection rate. At the assessment clinic, specialist support is provided, led by the breast care nursing team. In most cases recalled to assessment, a definitive diagnosis of either cancer or benign change can be made through further imaging and very accurate image-guided needle biopsy tech-niques, using either ultrasound or X-ray stereotaxis. In modern practice with skilled mul-tidisciplinary teams using effective, accurate technology, it is very unusual for diagnostic surgical excision to be required to achieve a diagnosis.

Over-diagnosis

Over-diagnosis is defined as the detection by screening of breast cancer which would not otherwise have progressed to cause symptomatic disease within the natural lifespan of an individual woman. The variation in growth rate of breast cancers results in the detection of some very slowly progressive tumours for which the effect of mammography is to bring forward the time of diagnosis without any effect on the final outcome from the disease. The detection of such cases is inevitable in screening practice because the mammographic features of malignancy do not allow the screen film readers to reliably distinguish between low-grade indolent disease and high-grade aggressive disease. There has been extensive debate about the number of cases of over-diagnosis, and calculating the number is diffi-cult because of a paucity of data from trials. The Independent UK Panel on Breast Cancer Screening (2012) suggests over-diagnosis of about 11% as a proportion of breast cancer incidence during the screening period and for the remainder of the woman's lifetime, or about 19% as a proportion of cancers diagnosed during the screening period.

In September 2013 the NHSBSP published updated information for women to ensure that they are fully informed about both the benefits and harms of screening and are able to make an informed choice about whether to attend for screening (<http://www.cancer-screening.nhs.uk/breastscreen/publications/ia-02.html>).

QA in breast screening

A robust QA process is necessary for all breast cancer screening programmes in order to ensure that the benefits of screening are achieved within the target population and that the harmful effects of screening are minimised. National standards have been agreed for measuring performance at each stage of the screening process. Targets for participation and cancer detection rates are set at a level consistent with the reduction in breast cancer mortality achieved in randomised controlled trials of screening (NHS Cancer Screening

Table 18.4 Current (2013) national minimum standards for the NHS Breast Screening Programme

Objective	Criteria	Minimum standard	Achievable standard
1. To maximise the number of eligible women who attend for screening	The percentage of eligible women who attend for screening	≥70% of invited women to attend for screening	80%
2. To maximise the number of cancers detected	(a) The rate of invasive cancers detected in eligible women invited and screened	Prevalent screen ≥ 3.6 per 1000 Incident screen > 4.1 per 1000	Prevalent screen ≥ 5.1 per 1000
	(b) The rate of cancers detected that are *in situ* carcinoma[1]	Prevalent screen ≥0.5 per 1000 Incident screen > 0.6 per 1000	Incident screen >5.7 per 1000
	(c) Standardised detection ratio (SDR)	≥1.0	≥1.4
3. To maximise the number of small invasive cancers detected	The rate of invasive cancers less than 15 mm in diameter detected in eligible women invited and screened	Prevalent screen ≥ 2.0 per 1000 Incident screen ≥ 2.3 per 1000	Prevalent screen ≥ 2.8 per 1000 Incident screen ≥ 3.1 per 1000
4. To achieve optimum image quality	(a) High contrast spatial resolution	≥12 line pairs mm⁻1	
	(b) Minimal detectable contrast:		
	5–6 mm detail	≤1.2%	≤0.8%
	0.5 mm detail	≤5%	≤3%
	0.25 mm detail	≤8%	≤5%
	(c) Optical density		
5. To limit radiation dose	Mean glandular dose per exposure for a standard breast at clinical settings	≤2.5 mGy	
6. To minimise the number of women undergoing repeat examinations	The number of repeat examinations	≤3% of total examinations	≤2% of total examinations

Table 18.4 (continued) Current (2013) national minimum standards for the NHS Breast Screening Programme

Objective	Criteria	Minimum standard	Achievable standard
7. To minimise the number of women screened who are referred for further tests[2]	(a) The percentage of women who are referred for assessment	Prevalent screen < 10% Incident screen < 7%	Prevalent screen < 7% Incident screen < 5%
	(b) The percentage of women screened who are placed on short-term recall	<0.25%	<0.12%
8. To ensure that the majority of cancers, both palpable and impalpable, receive a non-operative tissue diagnosis of cancer	(a) The percentage of women who have a non-operative diagnosis of cancer by cytology or needle histology after a maximum of two visits	≥90%	≥95%
	(b) The percentage of women who have a non-operative diagnosis of DCIS by cytology or needle histology after a maximum of two attempts	≥85%	≥90%
9. To minimise the number of unnecessary operative procedures	The rate of benign biopsies	Prevalent screen < 1.5 per 1000 Incident screen < 1.0 per 1000	Prevalent screen < 1.0 per 1000 Incident screen < 0.75 per 1000
10. To minimise the number of cancers presenting between screening episodes in the women screened	The rate of cancers presenting in screened women:		
	(a) in the 2 years following a normal screening episode	Expected standard: 1.2 per 1000 women screened in the first 2 years	
	(b) in the third year following a normal screening episode	Expected standard: 1.4 per 1000 women screened in the third year	
11. To ensure that women are recalled for screening at appropriate intervals	The percentage of eligible women whose first offered appointment is within 36 months of their previous screen	≥90%	100%

Objective	Criteria	Minimum standard	Achievable standard
12. To minimise anxiety for women who are awaiting the results of screening	The percentage of women who are sent their result within 2 weeks	≥90%	100%
13. To minimise the interval from the screening mammogram to assessment	The percentage of women who attend an assessment centre within 3 weeks of attendance for the screening mammogram	≥90%	100%
14. To minimise diagnostic delay for women who are diagnosed non-operatively	Proportion of women for whom the time interval between non-operative biopsy and result is 1 week or less	≥90%	100%
15. To minimise the delay for women who require surgical assessment	Proportion of women for whom the time interval between the decision to refer to a surgeon and surgical assessment is 1 week or less	≥90%	100%
16. To minimise the delay between referral for investigation and first breast cancer treatment	The percentage of women who are admitted for treatment within 2 months of the date of referral[3]	≥90%	100%

[1] *In situ* carcinomas include ductal carcinoma *in situ* (DCIS), lobular carcinoma *in situ*, and microinvasive disease.

[2] Further tests include all second appointments, where procedures (including further views and/or clinical examination) beyond those normally undertaken at first appointment are carried out.

[3] Date of referral is the date of last read on the NBSS computer system

Reproduced with permission from the Department of Health, *Public health functions to be exercised by NHS England Service specification No. 24 Breast Screening Programme*, © Crown Copyright 2013, licensed under the Open Government Licence v2.0, available from <https://www.gov.uk/government/uploads/system/uploads/attachment_data/file/192975/24_Breast_Screening_Programme__service_specification_VARIATION__130,422_-NA.pdf>

Table 18.5 Screening results for 2010/2011 for women aged 45–74 years

Total number of women invited	2 862 370
Acceptance rate	73.4%
Total number of women screened	2 188 608
Total number recalled	90 141
% Women recalled for assessment	4.1
Number of cancers detected	17 258
Number of *in situ* cancers	3527
Number of invasive cancers < 15 mm diameter	7053

Adapted with permission from NHS Breast Screening Programme (NHSBSP), Annual Review 2012, Copyright © 2012 NSHBSP.

Programmes, 2010, 2011). Key performance targets and recent national screening results are shown in Tables 18.4 and 18.5.

More recently, QA guidelines for MRI screening have been published (NHS Cancer Screening Programmes, 2012b). The guidelines provide detailed technical standards to ensure that the MRI scans are of a consistent high quality. They also describe clinical standards to ensure that both the MRI scan reporting and the subsequent assessment of any abnormality detected is carried out by suitably trained and experienced radiologists to the required standard.

References

DoH (**Department of Health**) 2007. *Cancer reform strategy*. London: Department of Health.

DoH (**Department of Health**) 2012. *Improving outcomes: a strategy for cancer. Second annual report 2012*. London: Department of Health.

Duffy SW, Mackay J, Thomas S, et al. 2013. Evaluation of mammographic surveillance services in women aged 40–49 years with a moderate family history of breast cancer: a single arm cohort study. *Health Technol Assess* **17**(11). doi: 10.3310/HTA17110

FH01 Collaborative Teams 2010. Mammographic surveillance in women younger than 50 years who have a family history of breast cancer: tumour characteristics and projected effect on mortality in the prospective, single-arm, FH01 study. *Lancet Oncol* **11**: 1127–1134.

FH01 Management Committee 2006. The challenge of evaluating annual mammography screening for young women with a family history of breast cancer. *J Med Screen* **13**: 177–182.

Forrest P 1986. *Breast cancer screening. Report to the health ministers of England, Wales, Scotland & Northern Ireland*. London: Her Majesty's Stationery Office.

Giordano L, Von Karsa L, Tomatis M, et al. 2012. Mammographic screening programmes in Europe: organization, coverage and participation. *J Med Screen* **19** (Suppl. 1): 72–82.

Hamilton LJ, Evans AJ, Wilson AR, et al. 2004. Breast imaging findings in women with *BRCA1*- and *BRCA2*-associated breast carcinoma. *Clin Radiol* **59**: 895–902.

IARC 2002. *Breast cancer screening*. IARC Handbook of Cancer Prevention Volume 7. Lyon: IARC.

Kerlikowske K, Grady D, Barclay J, et al. 1996. Likelihood ratios for modern screening mammography. Risk of breast cancer based on age and mammographic interpretation. *J Am Med Assoc* **276**: 39–43.

Kopans DB, Smith RA, Duffy SW 2011. Mammographic screening and 'overdiagnosis'. *Radiology* **260**: 616–620.

Leach MO 2009. Breast cancer screening in women at high risk using MRI. *NMR Biomed* **22**: 17–27.

Leach MO, Boggis CR, Dixon AK, et al. 2005. Screening with magnetic resonance imaging and mammography of a UK population at high familial risk of breast cancer: a prospective multicentre cohort study (MARIBS). *Lancet* **365**: 1769–1778.

Lehman CD and Smith RA 2009. The role of MRI in breast cancer screening. *J Natl Compr Canc Netw* **7**: 1109–1115.

Lord SJ, Lei W, Craft P, et al. 2007. A systematic review of the effectiveness of magnetic resonance imaging

(MRI) as an addition to mammography and ultrasound in screening young women at high risk of breast cancer. *Eur J Cancer* **43**: 1905–1917.

McIntosh A, Shaw C, Evans G, et al. 2004. *Clinical guidelines and evidence review for the classification and care of women at risk of familial breast cancer* [updated 2006]. London: National Collaborating Centre for Primary Care/University of Sheffield.

Michell MJ 2012. Breast screening review—a radiologist's perspective. *Br J Radiol* **85**: 845–847.

Moser K, Sellars S, Wheaton M, et al. 2011. Extending the age range for breast screening in England: pilot study to assess the feasibility and acceptability of randomization. *J Med Screen* **18**: 96–102.

NHS Cancer Screening Programmes 2010. *Clinical guidelines for breast cancer screening assessment.* NHSBSP Publication no. 49, 3rd edn. Sheffield: NHS Cancer Screening Programmes.

NHS Cancer Screening Programmes 2011. *Quality assurance guidelines for breast cancer screening radiology.* NHSBSP Publication no. 59, 2nd edn. Sheffield: NHS Cancer Screening Programmes.

NHS Cancer Screening Programmes 2012a. *Report of the working party for higher-risk breast screening.* NHSBSP Occasional Report 12/04. Sheffield: NHS Cancer Screening Programmes.

NHS Cancer Screening Programmes 2012b. *Technical guidelines for magnetic resonance imaging for the surveillance of women at higher risk of developing breast cancer.* NHSBSP Publication no. 68. Sheffield: NHS Cancer Screening Programmes.

NHS Cancer Screening Programmes 2012c. *Screening for breast cancer in high risk women during pregnancy and lactation.* NHSBSP Occasional Report 12/02. Sheffield: NHS Cancer Screening Programmes.

NHS Cancer Screening Programmes 2012d. *NHS Breast Screening Programme annual review 2012.* Sheffield: NHS Cancer Screening Programmes.

NHS Cancer Screening Programmes 2013. *Protocols for the surveillance of women at higher risk of developing breast cancer.* NHSBSP Publication no. 74, version 4 June. Sheffield: NHS Cancer Screening Programmes.

NICE (National Institute for Health and Care Excellence) 2009. *Early and locally advanced breast cancer.* NICE Clinical Guideline 80. London: National Institute for Health and Care Excellence.

NICE (National Institute for Health and Care Excellence) 2013. *Familial breast cancer: classification and care of people at risk of familial breast cancer and management of breast cancer and related risks in people with a family history of breast cancer.* NICE Clinical Guideline 164. London: National Institute for Health and Care Excellence.

Paci E 2012. Summary of the evidence of breast cancer service screening outcomes in Europe and first estimate of the benefit and harm balance sheet. *J Med Screen* **19** (Suppl. 1): 5–13.

Perry N, Broeders M, De Wolf C, et al. 2008. European guidelines for quality assurance in breast cancer screening and diagnosis. Fourth edition—summary document. *Ann Oncol* **19**: 614–622.

Raftery J and Chorozoglou M 2011. Possible net harms of breast cancer screening: updated modelling of Forrest report. *Br Med J* **343**: d7627.

Tabar L, Yen MF, Vitak B, et al. 2003. Mammography service screening and mortality in breast cancer patients: 20-year follow-up before and after introduction of screening. *Lancet* **361**: 1405–1410.

Tabar L, Vitak B, Chen TH, et al. 2011. Swedish two-county trial: impact of mammographic screening on breast cancer mortality during 3 decades. *Radiology* **260**: 658–663.

The Independent UK Panel on Breast Cancer Screening 2012. *The benefits and harms of breast cancer screening: an independent review.* London: Cancer Research UK and Department of Health (England).

Warner E, Messersmith H, Causer P, et al. 2008. Systematic review: using magnetic resonance imaging to screen women at high risk for breast cancer. *Ann Intern Med* **148**: 671–679.

Chapter 19

Early detection of hereditary colorectal and gastric cancer

Abdulkani Yusuf and Kevin John Monahan

Introduction to early detection of hereditary colorectal and gastric cancer

Every year in the UK, colorectal cancer (CRC) is diagnosed in approximately 41 100 people and causes approximately 16 000 deaths. The occurrence of CRC is strongly related to age, with 93% of cases occurring in people over the age of 50. The overall lifetime risk of CRC in England and Wales is 1 in 18 for men and 1 in 20 for women (around 5%).

More than 90% of CRCs are adenocarcinomas arising from benign precursor adenomas. A small proportion may arise from other types of polyps including hyperplastic and serrated polyps. The National Polyp Study demonstrated that endoscopic removal of adenomas can prevent CRC occurring (Winawer et al., 1993). Endoscopic surveillance and polyp removal are vital tools in making CRC one of the most preventable of cancers. However, endoscopic procedures are associated with significant complications, and are only effective when performed in the 'right' high-risk populations and at the 'right' age. The identification of individuals who are at high risk due to genetic or environmental factors enables appropriate utilisation of endoscopic and other preventative measures. There is good evidence that endoscopic surveillance of patients with a high-risk genetic predisposition can prevent cancer (Jarvinen et al., 2000; Dove-Edwin et al., 2005, 2006).

People in the average-risk population (those with a lifetime risk of developing CRC of approximately 5%) are advised to enter the UK Bowel Cancer Screening Programme (BCSP) from the age of 60 to 75 years. The high-risk population will require further screening in addition to the BCSP. The British Society of Gastroenterology (BSG) and the Association of Coloproctology of Great Britain and Ireland (ACPGBI) developed guidelines in 2010 for the management of these conditions which include genetic predisposition, post-carcinoma patients and surveillance in inflammatory bowel disease (Cairns et al., 2010).

In this chapter we will discuss the role of different methods of screening for the prevention of CRC and gastric cancer (GC) in average-risk and high-risk populations. The learning objectives for Chapter 19 are:

◆ to consider the benefits and limitations of current methods of screening for CRC and GC;

◆ to be able to describe the current position with regard to CRC and GC screening in the UK.

Methods for CRC screening

Faecal occult blood testing (FOBT)

FOBT is based on the principle of detecting blood in the faeces that originated from CRC or large polyps. There are currently two main tests for detecting haemoglobin products in faeces: the guaiac-based test (gFOBT), which detects haem, and faecal immunochemical testing (FIT), which detects globin, a metabolite of haemoglobin (Young, 2004). FOBT is the initial screening test used in the UK BCSP, and six stool samples from three different bowel motions on three different occasions are required for this test. A positive FOBT is followed by invitation to a screening colonoscopy.

FOBT has been shown to reduce mortality from CRC in multiple prospective randomised studies from different countries, including the United States, the UK, Denmark and Sweden. These studies have suggested a reduction in mortality of 15–33% if the test is done annually or biennially and positive results are followed by colonoscopy (Kewenter et al., 1988; Mandel et al., 1993, 1999; Hardcastle et al., 1996; Kronborg et al., 1996).

Flexible sigmoidoscopy

Flexible sigmoidoscopy is an invasive procedure which allows direct endoscopic visualisation of rectum and the left side of the colon. The procedure does not require a full bowel preparation and can be performed without sedation. However, an enema is generally given shortly before the procedure for distal bowel cleansing. This procedure allows a biopsy to be taken and the resection of polyps. It is usually well tolerated and has a low complication rate.

There has recently been an increasing evidence that screening with flexible sigmoidoscopy reduces both the incidence of and mortality from CRC. The UK flexible sigmoidoscopy screening trial, which included 170 000 subjects with an 11-year follow-up, has shown that a single flexible sigmoidoscopy screening between the ages of 55 and 64 years reduced the incidence of CRC by 33% and mortality by 43% for those who attended for screening (Atkin et al., 2010).

A key limitation of flexible sigmoidoscopy is that the proximal colon is not examined and therefore proximal cancers and polyps can be missed, although the evidence that colonoscopy is effective for proximal bowel screening is unclear.

Colonoscopy

Colonoscopy is regarded as the gold standard procedure for detecting colonic abnormalities. It has a high sensitivity for detection of both adenomas and cancers (Table 19.1). The long-term results of the National Polyp Study (Zauber et al., 2012) confirm that removing pre-cancerous adenomas can not only reduce the risk of CRC but can also reduce the number of deaths from the disease by 53% after a mean follow-up period of 15.8 years. However, this study was not designed as a randomised controlled trial, and it recommended an intensive colonoscopic follow-up programme to screen the entire average-risk population, requiring massive resources.

Table 19.1 Sensitivity and specificity for different screening modalities

Screening test	Sensitivity for CRC (%)	Sensitivity for advanced adenomas (%)	Specificity for CRC (%)	Specificity for advanced adenomas (%)
FOBT				
gFOBT	11–64	11–41	91–98	n.a.
iFOBT	56–89	27–56	91–97	n.a.
Flexible sigmoidoscopy	60–70	50–81	60–70	50–80
Colonoscopy	95	95	95–99	90–95

FOBT, faecal occult blood testing; gFOBT, guaiac-based FOBT; iFOBT is the same as faecal immunochemical testing (FIT); n.a., not applicable.

Reproduced with permission from M. Bretthauer, Colorectal cancer screening, *Journal of Internal Medicine*, Volume 270, Issue 2, pp. 87–98, Copyright © 2011 The Association for the Publication of the Journal of Internal Medicine. Published by John Wiley & Sons, Ltd.

The perforation rate after polypectomy (polyp removal) is about 1:500. Post-polypectomy bleeding occurs in about a further 1:100. The rate of colonoscopy-related mortality has been reported as 0.83 per 10 000 procedures and 3.9 per 10 000 after polypectomy. The overall frequency of perforation, bleeding and death may be 0.3, 0.3 and 0.02%, respectively (Cairns et al., 2010). Therefore, there is an appreciable risk of complications from colonoscopy. For these reasons colonoscopy is performed as a primary test for high-risk groups only, with the average-risk population in the UK BCSP undergoing FOBT as an initial procedure (those with a positive FOBT may be regarded *per se* as a high-risk group).

Screening the average-risk population: the UK BCSP

The UK BCSP commenced in 2006. It comprises five programme hubs and approximately 90–100 local screening centres, each serving populations of 500 000 to 2 million people. Average asymptomatic risk groups are currently offered a 2-yearly FOBT followed by a colonoscopy where there are abnormal FOBT results.

There are separate bowel screening programmes in England, Wales, Scotland and Northern Ireland. In England and Wales, men and women aged between 60 and 74 years are offered a test every 2 years. In England people aged 75 and over can request to be tested. The National Bowel Screening Programme in Scotland screens men and women aged between 50 and 74 years. In Northern Ireland the screening programme is currently sending testing kits to people aged between 60 and 71.

In view of the results of the UK Flexible Sigmoidoscopy Trial, there are also plans to offer a once-only flexible sigmoidoscopy screening to people aged 55, and those over 55 will be able to request flexible sigmoidoscopy screening until they reach 60 years. Pilots began in 2013, and it is envisaged that full roll-out will be achieved in 2016.

Outcomes of the BCSP

By October 2008 almost 2.1 million people had been invited to participate in the UK BCSP, with tests being returned by 49.6% of men and 54.4% of women invited (Logan et al., 2012). The overall uptake in this first round of screening was only 40% in the London area but 55–60% outside London. Early Dukes stage cancer was found in 70% of those with cancer, thus increasing the likelihood of survival. Thus the BCSP is expected to achieve a 16% reduction in overall bowel cancer mortality.

Screening groups at increased risk for CRC

The UK BCSP targets an asymptomatic population of men and women aged 60–69. It is not designed to screen high-risk individuals with familial risk. These patients may be offered more rigorous screening such as colonoscopic surveillance from an early age.

Lynch syndrome

Lynch syndrome family members and gene carriers should have a colonoscopy every 18–24 months commencing from the age of 25. Surveillance should continue until the age of 75. If a mutation is found in a relative and the patient is not a carrier of the mutation, the patient should be given advice as per the general population (Cairns et al., 2010). Studies have shown that surveillance significantly reduces both CRC incidence and mortality (by 62% and 65–70%, respectively) (Jarvinen et al., 2000; de Jong et al., 2006). The use of chromoendoscopy with methylene blue/indigo carmine dye spray or narrow band imaging may enhance polyp detection in Lynch syndrome patients (East et al., 2007) (we favour the dye spray technique).

According to guidelines, members of Lynch families with two or more individuals with GC or mismatch repair gene carriers should have biennial gastroscopy commencing at the age of 50 years (Cairns et al., 2010). There is little evidence that GC screening or screening of other organs is effective in Lynch syndrome patients. Thus we recommend chemoprophyllaxis with aspirin to prevent extracolonic cancer in view of the results of the CAPP2 study (Burn et al., 2011).

Familial adenomatous polyposis (FAP)

Colorectal surveillance in FAP

Patients with typical FAP are advised to undergo prophylactic colectomy between the ages of 16 and 25 years. Annual flexible sigmoidoscopy and alternating colonoscopy may be offered to mutation carriers from diagnosis until their polyp load indicates a need for surgery. The cancer risk increases substantially after the age of 25, and so surgery should be undertaken before then unless polyps are sparse and there is no high-grade dysplasia. If colectomy and ileorectal anastomosis are performed, the rectum must be kept under review annually for life because the risk of cancer in the retained rectum is 12–29%. After restorative proctocolectomy the anorectal cuff should also be kept under annual review for life (Cairns et al., 2010).

Upper gastrointestinal surveillance in FAP

There is substantial risk of upper gastrointestinal (GI) tract malignancy in FAP. Although gastroduodenal polyposis is well recognised in FAP and surveillance is established practice in the overall management, there is limited evidence to estimate the potential benefit of surveillance. However, UK guidelines recommend 3-yearly upper GI endoscopy from the age of 30 years with the aim of detecting early curable cancers. Patients with large numbers of duodenal polyps should undergo annual surveillance (Cairns et al., 2010). The modified Spigelman classification may be used to determine when these patients should be referred for prophylactic pancreaticoduodenectomy (Spigelman et al., 1994).

MUTYH-associated polyposis (MAP)

Colonoscopy every 2–3 years is recommended from the age of 25 for bi-allelic *MUTYH* carriers. As a significant number of these patients also have adenomas in the upper GI tract, a 3–5-yearly gastroscopy is recommended (Cairns et al., 2010).

Peutz–Jeghers syndrome (PJS)

As PJS is rare, the evidence on effectiveness of surveillance is limited. The risk of CRC increases with age, being 39% at the age of 70. A 2-yearly colonoscopy as well as upper GI and small bowel surveillance is recommended from the age of 25 (Cairns et al., 2010). For upper GI and small bowel tumours surveillance, gastroscopy and intermittent small bowel MRI can be used.

Juvenile polyposis (JPS)

For at-risk individuals and mutation carriers, a 1–2-yearly colonoscopy from the ages of 15 to 18, and a gastroscopy from the age of 25, or earlier if the patient has presented with symptoms, is recommended. Screening intervals could be extended in at-risk individuals at the age of 35 (Cairns et al., 2010).

Screening for patients at moderately increased risk of CRC

Most referrals to secondary care consist of people with a family history of CRC without one of the high-risk genetic disorders discussed above. However, they often have an increased personal risk of the disease. Up to 9% of the population will have at least one first-degree relative (FDR; i.e. sibling, parent or child) and over 20% a second-degree relative (SDR; i.e. grandparent, uncle, aunt, grandchild) with CRC. For most of these there is no proven benefit for increased surveillance above that of the rest of the population (i.e. the BCSP). However a significant proportion may benefit from outpatient assessment for screening interventions and/or genetic testing.

The risk of CRC can be estimated empirically from the individual's current age, the age at onset of affected relatives and the family pedigree. The so-called moderate-risk group should be referred to secondary care for assessment, and would consist of individuals with two or more FDRs of any age, or one FDR diagnosed under the age of 50. The lifetime risk for these patients ranges from 1:6 to 1:12. Despite the increased risk of CRC in this group, any individual's absolute risk therefore remains small and the benefit of screening seems minimal below the age of 45 (Dove-Edwin et al., 2006).

We do not recommend additional screening above and beyond the BCSP to those who are not FDRs of an affected family member, as there is little evidence of benefit to these individuals (they have a risk of less than 1:12, i.e. about 8%, compared with the average population risk of 5%). The same principle exists for those with a single affected FDR diagnosed over the age of 50.

Gastric cancer

Screening for GC

Several screening methods, including barium meal, upper GI gastroscopy and serum pepsinogen, have been proposed for the detection of early asymptomatic GC. The latest report on GC from the UK National Screening Committee found that mass screening of the asymptomatic population is not recommended due to the low incidence of GC in the UK (Hillier and Fielder, 2009). However, other countries with a high incidence of GC, such as Japan, have adapted population-based screening programmes. In Japan, for example, population barium meal screening has been used since 1960. Although no randomised controlled trials have been reported, cohort and case–control studies generally show a decreased risk of mortality from GC in the screened subjects (Tsubono and Hisamichi, 2000).

The UK National Institute for Health and Care Excellence (NICE) guidelines (NICE, 2005; updated 2011) recommend referral for endoscopy or referral to upper GI cancer specialist for patients with dyspepsia associated with chronic GI blood loss, progressive dysphagia, progressive unintentional weight loss, persistent vomiting, iron deficiency anaemia, epigastric mass and abnormal barium swallow as well as patients aged 55 years or older with unexplained and persistent recent-onset dyspepsia.

Patients who meet the criteria for hereditary diffuse gastric cancer (HDGC) should be offered genetic counselling and testing for *CDH1* gene mutation, gastroscopy surveillance and prophylactic gastrectomy for those with confirmed *CDH1* mutation as the penetrance of the HDGC is high at 80% (Fitzgerald et al., 2010). There may be a role for gastroscopy surveillance in individuals who do not choose to undergo prophylactic gastrectomy.

Summary

CRC is a significant health problem but also a highly preventable disease. CRC develops slowly over many years through the adenoma–carcinoma sequence. There is therefore ample opportunity to prevent this through screening, which enables detection of early cancers and the removal of polyps that may develop into cancer.

The BCSP offers a biennial FOBT for the average-risk population, followed by colonoscopy if the FOBT is positive. Once-only flexible sigmoidoscopy will soon be offered to people at the age of 55 years in the UK and has been shown to significantly reduce both incidence and mortality from CRC. People with a higher risk are recommended to have an advanced screening protocol, usually performed with colonoscopy, which is the gold standard screening test for CRC.

People fulfilling the criteria for inherited cancer syndromes may need surveillance for CRC, upper GI cancers and other types of cancers, depending on the underlying genetic disorder. People with moderately elevated risk due to a family history without a high-risk genetic disorder can be referred to secondary care for assessment and screening.

GC is a major health concern internationally, but the incidence in the UK and other western countries is low. Mass screening of the population is not recommended in western countries. However, there are guidelines for surveillance for those with some inherited cancer syndromes.

References

Atkin WS, Edwards R, Kralj-Hans I, et al. 2010. Once-only flexible sigmoidoscopy screening in prevention of colorectal cancer: a multicentre randomised controlled trial. *Lancet* **375**: 1624–1633.

Bretthauer M 2011. Colorectal cancer screening. *J Intern Med* **270**: 87–98.

Burn J, Gerdes AM, Macrae F, et al. 2011. Long-term effect of aspirin on cancer risk in carriers of hereditary colorectal cancer: an analysis from the CAPP2 randomised controlled trial. *Lancet* **378**: 2081–2087.

Cairns SR, Scholefield JH, Steele RJ, et al. 2010. Guidelines for colorectal cancer screening and surveillance in moderate and high risk groups (update from 2002). *Gut* **59**: 666–690.

Dove-Edwin I, Sasieni P, Adams J, et al. 2005. Prevention of colorectal cancer by colonoscopic surveillance in individuals with a family history of colorectal cancer: 16 year, prospective, follow-up study. *Br Med J* **331**: 1047.

Dove-Edwin I, De Jong AE, Adams J, et al. 2006. Prospective results of surveillance colonoscopy in dominant familial colorectal cancer with and without Lynch syndrome. *Gastroenterology* **130**: 1995–2000.

East JE, Guenther T, Kennedy RH, et al. 2007. Narrow band imaging avoids potential chromoendoscopy risks. *Gut* **56**: 1168–1169.

Fitzgerald RC, Hardwick R, Huntsman D, et al. 2010. Hereditary diffuse gastric cancer: updated consensus guidelines for clinical management and directions for future research. *J Med Genet* **47**: 436–444.

Hardcastle JD, Chamberlain JO, Robinson MH, et al. 1996. Randomised controlled trial of faecal-occult-blood screening for colorectal cancer. *Lancet* **348**: 1472–1477.

Hillier SH and Fielder H 2009. *Screening for stomach cancer: a report for the National Screening Committee*. Screening Services, Public Health Wales.

Jarvinen HJ, Aarnio M, Mustonen H, et al. 2000. Controlled 15-year trial on screening for colorectal cancer in families with hereditary nonpolyposis colorectal cancer. *Gastroenterology* **118**: 829–834.

de Jong AE, Hendriks YM, Kleibeuker JH, et al. 2006. Decrease in mortality in Lynch syndrome families because of surveillance. *Gastroenterology* **130**: 665–671.

Kewenter J, Björk S, Haglind E, et al. 1988. Screening and rescreening for colorectal cancer. A controlled trial of fecal occult blood testing in 27,700 subjects. *Cancer* **62**: 645–651.

Kronborg O, Fenger C, Olsen J, et al. 1996. Randomised study of screening for colorectal cancer with faecal-occult-blood test. *Lancet* **348**: 1467–1471.

Logan RF, Patnick J, Nickerson C, et al. 2012. Outcomes of the Bowel Cancer Screening Programme (BCSP) in England after the first 1 million tests. *Gut* **61**: 1439–1446.

Mandel JS, Bond JH, Church TR, et al. 1993. Reducing mortality from colorectal cancer by screening for fecal occult blood. Minnesota Colon Cancer Control Study. *N Engl J Med* **328**: 1365–1371.

Mandel JS, Church TR, Ederer F, et al. 1999. Colorectal cancer mortality: effectiveness of biennial screening for fecal occult blood. *J Natl Cancer Inst* **91**: 434–437.

NICE (National Institute for Health and Care Excellence) 2005. *Referral for suspected cancer.* NICE Clinical Guideline 27 [modified April 2011]. London: National Institute for Health and Care Excellence.

Spigelman AD, Talbot IC, Penna C, et al. 1994. Evidence for adenoma-carcinoma sequence in the duodenum of patients with familial adenomatous polyposis. The Leeds Castle Polyposis Group (Upper Gastrointestinal Committee). *J Clin Pathol* **47**: 709–710.

Tsubono Y and Hisamichi S 2000. Screening for gastric cancer in Japan. *Gastric Cancer* **3**: 9–18.

Winawer SJ, AG MN, Ho ,et al. 1993. Prevention of colorectal cancer by colonoscopic polypectomy. The National Polyp Study Workgroup. *N Engl J Med* **329**: 1977–1981.

Young GP 2004. Fecal immunochemical tests (FIT) vs. office-based guaiac fecal occult blood test (FOBT). *Pract Gastroenterol* **XXVIII** (June): 46–56.

Zauber AG, Winawer SJ, O'Brien MJ, et al. 2012 Colonoscopic polypectomy and long-term prevention of colorectal-cancer deaths. *N Engl J Med* **366**: 687–696.

Chapter 20

Early detection of hereditary gynaecological cancers

Aleksandra Gentry-Maharaj and Usha Menon

Introduction to early detection of hereditary gynaecological cancer

Each year gynaecological cancers account for around 17% of new cancer cases in women and 14.6% of cancer deaths worldwide. In the UK, most deaths are from ovarian cancer (OC), with 7011 women diagnosed and 4295 deaths in 2010 (CRUK, 2010a). Although endometrial cancer (EC) is more common (8288 cases), it accounts for half the number of deaths (1937) compared with OC (CRUK, 2010b). Both cancers are more common in post-menopausal women in industrialised countries than in low to middle income countries.

A hereditary component has been described in about 5–10% of women with OC and about 5% with EC (Rosenthal and Jacobs, 2006). Women at increased risk are currently identified through their family history and fall largely into two groups, those with a family history of breast and/or OC or those with a family history of mainly colorectal cancer and EC (Lynch syndrome, LS). Women from hereditary breast and ovarian cancer (HBOC) families are usually defined as having a lifetime risk of OC of 10% or more, compared with 1–2% for the general population. However, risk is much higher in those with a mutation in the *BRCA1* or *BRCA2* genes, with the risk of developing OC by the age 75 being about 45% in *BRCA1* mutation carriers and 20% in *BRCA2* mutation carriers. A lower lifetime risk of OC has been described in those with mutations in the *RAD51C* gene (Coulet et al., 2013) and in women with LS (7–12%) who have mutations in mismatch repair genes (*MLH1*, *MSH2*, *MSH6*, *PMS1*, *PMS2*). However, the latter women have an increased lifetime risk of EC: 54% in *MLH1* mutation carriers, 21% in *MSH2*, 16% in *MSH6* (Bonadona et al., 2011) and 15% in *PMS2* mutation carriers (Senter et al., 2008). An increased risk of developing EC (from 1% at age 40 to 19% by age 60) is also reported in women with Cowden syndrome (CS) (incidence < 1/200 000) who have mutations in *PTEN*. Women with Peutz–Jeghers syndrome (PJS) (incidence < 1/25 000), where mutations are described in the *STK11* (*LKB1*) gene, have an increased risk of minimal deviation cervical adenocarcinoma ('adenoma malignum') and a predisposition to develop ovarian sex-cord stromal tumours.

The only proven management option to reduce the risk of gynaecological cancer is surgery to remove the ovaries, fallopian tubes (HBOC) and uterus (LS). However, a significant proportion of women opt not to undergo surgery because they have not completed their family, they have concerns regarding premature menopause despite evidence supporting the use of short-term hormone replacement therapy or they have fears about the surgery per se. Major efforts have therefore been made to explore the option of screening, which is the focus of this chapter. The learning objectives for Chapter 20 are:

+ to be able to consider the benefits and limitations of methods of screening for ovarian and endometrial cancer;

+ to be able to describe the current position with regard to ovarian and endometrial cancer screening in the UK and Europe.

The rationale for screening

OC has the worst survival rate of all gynaecological cancers: the 5-year survival rate declines sharply from 90% in early stage disease to 30–40% in advanced disease (Stage III/IV) (CRUK, 2010c). This has led to extensive efforts to detect the disease early through screening in the hope that it may impact on disease-specific mortality. Various screening strategies have been developed, the majority being based on serum cancer antigen 125 (CA125) and ultrasound. The survival benefit of screening was first reported in a randomised controlled trial (RCT) of 22 000 women (Jacobs et al., 1999). Since then, a number of trials of OC screening have been completed, with the Prostate Lung Colorectal Ovarian (PLCO) RCT showing no mortality benefit of OC screening. The results of the United Kingdom Collaborative Trial of Ovarian Cancer Screening (UKCTOCS), which is using an algorithm-based approach, should be available in 2014/2015 (Moyer, 2012). Similar low survival rates are seen in EC if it is detected at a late stage. However, overall 5-year survival is 77% as most women are diagnosed early (CRUK, 2010b). The incidence of EC has increased by 40% since the 1990s, further supporting the need for screening efforts (CRUK, 2010d).

Gynaecological cancer screening—the tests

Since it was first described in 1981 (Bast et al., 1981), serum CA125 has been the most studied marker. The widely adopted cut-off of 35 kU L^{-1} is based upon the distribution of CA125 values in healthy subjects (Bast et al., 1983). Varying cut-offs have been suggested for pre-menopausal women (50 kU L^{-1}), pre-menopausal women on oral contraceptives (40 kU L^{-1}) and post-menopausal women (35 kU L^{-1}). Eighty-five per cent of patients with epithelial OC have raised CA125 (>35 kU L^{-1}), with elevations in 50% of those with Stage I disease and >90% of those with Stage II–IV disease (Jacobs and Bast, 1989). CA125 is not expressed/produced by 20% of OCs (mainly mucinous and borderline tumours). CA125 levels are influenced by age and race and are increased in women with inflammatory disease, benign ovarian neoplasms or endometriosis and during menstruation and pregnancy. However, rising CA125 levels are seen mainly in OC and metastatic non-gynaecological malignancies such as breast, lung, endometrial and pancreatic cancer (Philpott et al., 2013).

Screening using CA125 with a cut-off of 30 kU L^{-1} in the general population has a low specificity (97%) and positive predictive value (PPV; 4.6%) compared with that required for screening (specificity 98.99%, PPV > 10%). Therefore, screening strategies have adopted pelvic ultrasound as a second-line test in women with raised CA125 levels; this improves PPV to 26.8% for detection of OC and fallopian tube (FT) cancer (Jacobs et al., 1993). The preferred approach is transvaginal ultrasound (TVS) as it gives a superior view of the pelvic organs and is also acceptable to post-menopausal women. Most OC screening trials define complex ovarian morphology as abnormal and use repeat scans (4–6 weeks) and clinical evaluation to manage abnormal findings (Menon et al., 2009). Ovarian cysts with solid areas or papillary projections are more likely to be associated with malignancy than those with increased septal thickness alone, unilocular ovarian cysts < 10 cm in diameter or inclusion cysts (Campbell, 2012). Lack of physiological change reduces false positives in post-menopausal women, but even in this population, small benign adnexal cysts or benign solid tumours up to 50 mm diameter are very common (Valentin et al., 2003).

Ovarian cancer screening in high-risk women

Over the past two decades a number of OC screening trials have been undertaken in women at high risk. Whether screening is of benefit in this group of women is yet to be determined. The initial strategy was annual screening using both serum CA125 and TVS as first-line tests. However, this was not effective in detecting early stage disease (Stirling et al., 2005). Results of annual screening from Phase I of the UK Familial Ovarian Cancer Screening Study (UKFOCSS) further confirm this. This study involved 3563 women who underwent annual screening with serum CA125 and TVS. Sensitivity for detection of incident OC/FT cancer within a year of the last screening was 81.3–87.5%, depending on whether occult cancers were classified as interval cancers or true positives. However, only 30.8% of screen-detected OC/FTCs were Stage I/II. There was preliminary evidence that advanced stage disease defined as ≥IIIC was more likely (85.7% versus 26.1%; $P = 0.009$) in those who had not been screened in the year before diagnosis compared with those who had (Rosenthal et al., 2013). As most cancers detected in this group of women are high-grade serous epithelial OCs which progress rapidly, a shorter screening interval is being investigated in UKFOCSS Phase II (Manchanda et al., 2009). Recent data suggest that high-risk women participating in frequent ovarian screening who are recalled for an abnormal result may experience transient cancer-specific distress but there is no significant effect on general anxiety/depression or overall reassurance.

UKFOCSS Phase II is using a sophisticated time-series algorithm to interpret serum CA125. An individual's age-specific incidence of OC and serial CA125 profile are used to estimate the 'risk of OC' (ROC) (Skates et al., 2003). Based on the ROC results, women are triaged into low, intermediate and elevated-risk. Those at intermediate risk have repeat CA125 test; those with elevated risk are referred for CA125 testing and TVS, and if either is positive, women are referred for clinical assessment by a gynaecological oncologist with a view to surgery (Menon et al., 2009). In the general population, for a target specificity of 98% for pre-clinical detection of OC, the ROC calculation achieved a sensitivity of 86%

(Skates et al., 2003). Four-monthly screening using ROC is being evaluated in UKFOCSS Phase II involving 5700 women. The ROC is also being evaluated prospectively in screening trials in women at high risk in the United States (Cancer Genetics Network, CGN, and Gynecologic Oncology Group, GOG). Addition of human epididymis protein 4 (HE4) to CA125 in screening may reduce false positives as its levels are lower in many of the benign conditions that elevate CA125, such as endometriosis.

In the UK there is currently no screening of high-risk women on the NHS. The recommendation for such women is referral for genetic counselling, OC symptom awareness National Institute for Health and Care Excellence (NICE) guidelines (NICE, 2011) and risk-reducing bilateral salpingo-oopherectomy in their early 40s on completion of their families. While surgery is the primary recommendation in the United States as well, screening using 6-monthly serum CA125 and TVS is still considered a reasonable approach for those who do not opt for risk-reducing salpingo-oophorectomy according to the guidelines of the National Comprehensive Cancer Network (NCCN, 2014).

Early detection using symptoms

Up to 90% of women experience symptoms (urinary symptoms in early stage disease; gastrointestinal symptoms, unusual fatigue, abdominal distension and weight change in advanced disease) prior to diagnosis (Bankhead et al., 2005). Symptom awareness is increasingly part of the counselling of high-risk women, with guidance on management of symptoms issued by the UK Department of Health (DoH, 2009). The 2011 NICE guidelines recommend sequential testing using serum CA125 followed by pelvic ultrasound in women with any of the following symptoms on a persistent or frequent basis: persistent abdominal distension/'bloating', feeling full and/or loss of appetite, pelvic/abdominal pain, increased urinary urgency and/or frequency, unexplained weight loss, fatigue or changes in bowel habit (NICE, 2011).

Future OC screening strategies

There is evidence that ovarian cancer is a heterogeneous disease and consists of Type I, slow-growing cancers with better prognosis (low-grade serous, endometrioid and transitional (Brenner) tumours, clear cell and mucinous carcinomas) and more aggressive Type II (high-grade serous, high-grade endometrioid, undifferentiated tumours and carcinosarcomas) (Kurman and Shih, 2010) with immediate implications for screening. It is likely that, for Type II cancers, early detection of low-volume disease rather than early stage disease is a more realistic target in screening. This is supported by modelling studies based on occult cancers in high-risk women, which suggest that the median diameter of a serous ovarian cancer when it progresses to Stage III/IV is about 3 cm (Brown and Palmer, 2009; Hori and Gambhir, 2011). Two further insights, that a proportion of high-grade serous OCs start as pre-malignant serous tubal intraepithelial cancerous lesions in the distal FT and spread to the ovary, especially in high-risk women (Crum et al., 2007), and that the origin of non-serous epithelial OC may lie elsewhere in the Mullerian epithelium

(Dubeau, 2008), are fuelling the search to discover cancer-specific tumour markers and high-resolution imaging modalities.

Screening for endometrial cancer

In the United States screening is currently recommended in women with LS or CS (Smith et al., 2012). Although the efficacy of such endometrial screening remains unproven, women are offered screening with annual TVS and endometrial biopsy with most guidelines recommending that screening starts at the age of 35 (Lindor et al., 2006). There is lack of consensus on the appropriate cut-off value for endometrial thickness in asymptomatic pre-menopausal women, and interval cancers are known to occur (Dove-Edwin et al., 2002; Rijcken et al., 2003). The superior performance of annual outpatient hysteroscopy and endometrial sampling over TVS was reported in a prospective observational cohort study of 41 women with LS (Manchanda et al., 2012) with four cases of endometrial cancer/atypical endometrial hyperplasia detected using this approach compared with two if TVS alone had been used. This confirms the guidance on the need for endometrial sampling in these women. This can be done either as a blind Pipelle endometrial biopsy (which has a 10% procedure failure rate) or using a hysteroscopy-directed approach (failure rate of 8–11%, but increasingly the gold standard). Screening for EC in the general population is not currently recommended in view of its good prognosis. Data from UKCTOCS indicated encouraging sensitivity of an endometrial thickness cut-off of 5 mm. However, the false positive rate was high (Jacobs et al., 2011). Although screening is currently recommended in the United States in women with LS (Smith et al., 2012), not all expert guidelines agree. The revised Mallorca guidelines state that 'given the lack of evidence of any benefit, gynaecological surveillance should preferably be performed as part of a clinical trial' (Vasen et al., 2013).

Summary

Currently there is no evidence that OC screening saves lives. Annual screening is not recommended in high-risk women. Shorter screening intervals of 3–6 months with interpretation of serum CA125 using time-series algorithms rather than cut-offs is being investigated in trials in the UK and United States that are likely to report in 2014. A definitive conclusion of whether screening has an impact on mortality will only be available following completion of the general population RCT, UKCTOCS, in 2015. Outpatient hysteroscopy seems to be the best approach to screening for women at risk of EC who have LS or CS. However, screening for endometrial cancer should preferably be performed as part of a clinical trial.

References

Bankhead CR, Kehoe ST, Austoker J 2005. Symptoms associated with diagnosis of ovarian cancer: a systematic review. *BJOG* **112**: 857–865.

Bast RC Jr, Feeney M, Lazarus H, et al. 1981. Reactivity of a monoclonal antibody with human ovarian carcinoma. *J Clin Invest* **68**: 1331–1337.

Bast RC Jr, Klug TL, St John E, et al. 1983. A radioimmunoassay using a monoclonal antibody to monitor the course of epithelial ovarian cancer. *New Engl J Med* **309**: 883–887.

Bonadona V, Bonaiti B, Olschwang S, et al. 2011. Cancer risks associated with germline mutations in MLH1, MSH2, and MSH6 genes in Lynch syndrome. *J Am Med Assoc* **305**: 2304–2310.

Brown PO and Palmer C 2009. The preclinical natural history of serous ovarian cancer: defining the target for early detection. *PLoS Med* **6**: e1000114.

Campbell S 2012. Ovarian cancer: role of ultrasound in preoperative diagnosis and population screening. *Ultrasound Obst Gynecol* **40**: 245–254.

Coulet F, Fajac A, Colas C, et al. 2013. Germline *RAD51C* mutations in ovarian cancer susceptibility. *Clin Genet* **83**: 332–336.

CRUK (Cancer Research UK) 2010a. *Ovarian cancer statistics* [online]. Available at: <http://www.cancerresearchuk.org/cancer-info/cancerstats/types/ovary/> (last accessed 23 April 2013).

CRUK (Cancer Research UK) 2010b. *Uterine cancer statistics* [online]. Available at: <http://www.cancerresearchuk.org/cancer-info/cancerstats/types/uterus/> (last accessed 23 April 2013).

CRUK (Cancer Research UK) 2010c. *Ovarian cancer survival statistics* [online]. Available at: <http://www.cancerresearchuk.org/cancer-info/cancerstats/types/ovary/survival/> (last accessed 23 April 2013).

CRUK (Cancer Research UK) 2010d. *Uterine (womb) cancer incidence statistics* [online]. Available at: <http://www.cancerresearchuk.org/cancer-info/cancerstats/types/uterus/incidence/> (last accessed 23 April 2013).

Crum CP, Drapkin R, Miron A, et al. 2007. The distal fallopian tube: a new model for pelvic serous carcinogenesis. *Curr Opin Obstet Gynecol* **19**: 3–9.

DoH (Department of Health) 2009. *Key messages for ovarian cancer for health professionals* [online]. Available at: <http://webarchive.nationalarchives.gov.uk/20130107105354/http://www.dh.gov.uk/en/Publicationsandstatistics/Publications/PublicationsPolicyAndGuidance/DH_110534> (last accessed 2 January 2014).

Dove-Edwin I, Boks D, Goff S, et al. 2002. The outcome of endometrial carcinoma surveillance by ultrasound scan in women at risk of hereditary nonpolyposis colorectal carcinoma and familial colorectal carcinoma. *Cancer* **94**: 1708–1712.

Dubeau L 2008. The cell of origin of ovarian epithelial tumours. *Lancet Oncol* **9**: 1191–1197.

Hori SS and Gambhir SS 2011. Mathematical model identifies blood biomarker-based early cancer detection strategies and limitations. *Sci Transl Med* **3**: 109ra116.

Jacobs I and Bast RC Jr 1989. The CA 125 tumour-associated antigen: a review of the literature. *Human Reprod* **4**: 1–12.

Jacobs I, Davies AP, Bridges J, et al. 1993. Prevalence screening for ovarian cancer in postmenopausal women by CA 125 measurement and ultrasonography. *Br Med J* **306**: 1030–1034.

Jacobs IJ, Skates SJ, Macdonald N, et al. 1999. Screening for ovarian cancer: a pilot randomised controlled trial. *Lancet* **353**: 1207–1210.

Jacobs I, Gentry-Maharaj A, Burnell M, et al. 2011. Sensitivity of transvaginal ultrasound screening for endometrial cancer in postmenopausal women: a case-control study within the UKCTOCS cohort. *Lancet Oncol* **12**: 38–48.

Kurman RJ and Shih IeM 2010. The origin and pathogenesis of epithelial ovarian cancer: a proposed unifying theory. *Am J Surg Pathol* **34**: 433–443.

Lindor NM, Petersen GM, Hadley DW, et al. 2006. Recommendations for the care of individuals with an inherited predisposition to Lynch syndrome: a systematic review. *J Am Med Assoc* **296**: 1507–1517.

Manchanda R, Rosenthal A, Burnell M, et al. 2009. Change in stage distribution observed with annual screening for ovarian cancer in BRCA carriers. *J Med Genet* **46**: 423–424.

Manchanda R, Saridogan E, Abdelraheim A, et al. 2012. Annual outpatient hysteroscopy and endometrial sampling (OHES) in HNPCC/Lynch syndrome (LS). *Arch Gynecol Obstet* **286**: 1555–1562.

Menon U, Gentry-Maharaj A, Hallett R, et al. 2009. Sensitivity and specificity of multimodal and ultrasound screening for ovarian cancer, and stage distribution of detected cancers: results of the prevalence screen of the UK Collaborative Trial of Ovarian Cancer Screening (UKCTOCS). *Lancet Oncol* **10**: 327–340.

Moyer VA 2012. Screening for ovarian cancer: U.S. Preventive Services Task Force reaffirmation recommendation statement. *Ann Intern Med* **157**: 900–904.

National Comprehensive Cancer Network 2014. *Guidelines for detection, prevention & risk reduction; Genetic/Familial High-Risk Assessment: Breast and Ovarian (version 01.2014).* Available at <http://www.nccn.org/professionals/physician_gls/f_guidelines.asp#detection> (last accessed 14 April 2014).

NICE (National Institute for Health and Care Excellence) 2011. *The recognition and initial management of ovarian cancer.* NICE Clinical Guideline 122. London: National Institute for Health and Care Excellence.

Philpott S, Rizzuto I, Fraser L, et al. 2013. Detection of non-ovarian cancers on Phase 2 of the UK Familial Ovarian Cancer Screening Study (UKFOCSS) [abstract]. *European Society of Gynaecological Oncology (ESGO) meeting, Liverpool.* Available at: <http://eacademy.esgo.org/esgo/2013/18th/37569/adam.n.rosenthal.detection.of.non-ovarian.cancers.on.phase.2.of.the.uk.html?history_id=478849> (last accessed 17 February 2014).

Rijcken FE, Mourits MJ, Kleibeuker JH, et al. 2003. Gynecologic screening in hereditary nonpolyposis colorectal cancer. *Gynecol Oncol* **91**: 74–80.

Rosenthal A and Jacobs I 2006. Familial ovarian cancer screening. *Best Pract Res. Clin Obst Gynaecol* **20**: 321–338.

Rosenthal AN, Fraser L, Manchanda R, et al. 2013. Results of annual screening in phase I of the United kingdom familial ovarian cancer screening study highlight the need for strict adherence to screening schedule. *J Clin Oncol* **31**: 49–57.

Senter L, Clendenning M, Sotamaa K, et al. 2008. The clinical phenotype of Lynch syndrome due to germ-line *PMS2* mutations. *Gastroenterology* **135**: 419–428.

Skates SJ, Menon U, Macdonald N, et al. 2003. Calculation of the risk of ovarian cancer from serial CA-125 values for preclinical detection in postmenopausal women. *J Clin Oncol* **21**: 206s–210s.

Smith RA, Cokkinides V, Brawley OW 2012. Cancer screening in the United States, 2012: a review of current American Cancer Society guidelines and current issues in cancer screening. *CA: Cancer J Clin* **62**: 129–142.

Stirling D, Evans DG, Pichert G, et al. 2005. Screening for familial ovarian cancer: failure of current protocols to detect ovarian cancer at an early stage according to the International Federation of Gynecology and Obstetrics system. *J Clin Oncol* **23**: 5588–5596.

Valentin L, Skoog L, Epstein E 2003. Frequency and type of adnexal lesions in autopsy material from postmenopausal women: ultrasound study with histological correlation. *Ultrasound Obst Gynecol* **22**: 284–289.

Vasen H, Blanco I, Aktan-Collan K, et al. 2013. Revised guidelines for the clinical management of Lynch syndrome (HNPCC): recommendations by a group of European experts. *Gut* **62**: 812–823.

Chapter 21

Early detection of hereditary cancer. Summary

Lorraine Robinson and Patricia Webb

Introduction to section 5 summary

Section 5 delivers a balanced account of the issues pertinent to the early detection of cancer for people in the general population and those at risk due to a family history. The scene was set in Chapter 17 with clear and concise definitions of the aims and standards associated with cancer screening for the early detection of cancer. Then Chapters 18–20 examined the particular issues associated with breast cancer, colorectal and gastric cancer, and ovarian and endometrial cancer.

Chapter 17. Early detection of hereditary cancer. Introduction

Chapter 17 introduces the pivotal concepts associated with effectiveness of screening, its limitations and the psychological issues therein. One of the important issues for practice is to develop a keen understanding of the relevant terminology.

Guided activities for Chapter 17

- Acquaint yourself with the WHO principles of screening that were established by Wilson and Junger (1968). How would you describe population screening to a colleague and/or patient. Why might you need to discuss this with a patient and their family?

- Identify the policy, processes and practice of your own organisation or local referral centre for cancer genetic screening for these specific cancers. Think about the effect and impact all of this has on individual patients and families and then ask to be an observer in a clinic to see it first hand. Of course the patient will need to give consent to your being present, so that may take some time to arrange. If not available for any reason, ask for some time from someone running a family history clinic and then learn the elements of family history-taking.

- Chapter 17 also provides an overview of the evidence about the psychological impact of screening. Read the relevant papers cited in the References to Chapter 17 then consider what the particular issues are (if any) for those at risk undergoing screening compared with the general population. Identify what support strategies are in place in your organisation for the support of patients undergoing screening.

Chapter 18. Early detection of hereditary breast cancer

Chapter 18 discusses the principles of breast cancer screening and the dilemmas and current debates surrounding over-diagnosis. The NHS Breast Screening Programme and the latest National Institute for Health and Care Excellence (NICE) guidance on familial breast cancer (NICE, 2013) underpin the chapter and its guidance.

Guided activities for Chapter 18

◆ Access the NHS Breast Screening programme website at <http://www.cancerscreening.nhs.uk/breastscreen/index.html>. Review the section 'Screening women at high risk', particularly the patient information. What questions might your patients raise about screening and how would you address these? Use the website resources as a source of information.

◆ Read *The benefits and harms of breast cancer screening: an independent review* (The Independent UK Panel on Breast Cancer Screening, 2012). Consider the main arguments for and against the NHS Breast Screening Programme; reflect on how you would discuss these with a woman at high risk who is unsure about the benefits of screening.

Further reading for Chapter 18

Lehman CD, Blume JD, Weatherall P, et al. 2005. Screening women at high risk for breast cancer with mammography and magnetic resonance imaging. *Cancer* 103: 1895–1905.

Chapter 19. Early detection of hereditary colorectal and gastric cancer

Chapter 19 provides an insightful overview of the UK Bowel Cancer Screening Programme. The approaches taken for individuals at high risk are explained and the decision-making issues for healthcare professionals are delineated. The contrast between the approaches for colorectal and gastric cancers is expounded.

Guided activities for Chapter 19

◆ Access the NHS Bowel Cancer Screening Programme website at <http://www.cancer-screening.nhs.uk/bowel/index.html>. Review the information resources available to patients about bowel screening. What additional information do you think a patient at high risk might need?

◆ Useful information about familial adenomatous polyposis and Lynch syndrome including issues of screening can be found at <http://www.macmillan.org.uk/Cancerinformation/Causesriskfactors/Genetics/Cancergenetics/Specificconditions/FAP.aspx> and <http://www.macmillan.org.uk/Cancerinformation/Causesriskfactors/Genetics/Cancergenetics/Specificconditions/lynchsyndrome.aspx>.

◆ Review the information provided to your patients; what else do you need to provide and/or review?

Chapter 20. Early detection of hereditary gynaecological cancers

Chapter 20 states that, at present, the only reliable approach to risk reduction for gynaeco-logical cancers is surgery. Against this backdrop, the efficacy of screening tests including CA125, pelvic and transvaginal ultrasound is explained with a detailed exploration of the research evidence and ongoing trials.

Guided activities for Chapter 20

◆ After having read Chapter 20 how would you explain to a patient at high risk why the use of CA125 as a screening test is not sufficient in isolation?

◆ Access and read the information on ovarian cancer screening on the Cancer Research UK website at <http://www.cancerresearchuk.org/cancer-help/type/ovarian-cancer/about/ovarian-cancer-screening>. This offers a good summary of the ovarian screen-ing situation for high-risk women and the UK Familial Ovarian Cancer Screening Study.

References

NICE (National Institute for Health and Care Excellence) 2013. *Familial breast cancer: classification and care of people at risk of familial breast cancer and management of breast cancer and related risks in people with a family history of breast cancer*. NICE Clinical Guideline 164. London: National Institute for Health and Care Excellence.

The Independent UK Panel on Breast Cancer Screening 2012. *The benefits and harms of breast cancer screening: an independent review*. London: Cancer Research UK and Department of Health (England).

Wilson JMG and Junger G 1968. *The principles and practice of screening for disease*. Geneva: World Health Organization.

Section 6

Reducing the risk of cancer

Chapter 22

Reducing the risk of cancer. Introduction

Chris Jacobs

Introduction to reducing the risk of cancer

For individuals at high risk of hereditary cancer there are a number of medical and surgical options available for reducing cancer risk as a result of advances in surgical techniques, knowledge about chemoprevention and growing evidence of survival benefit. However, significant psychological and physical morbidity is associated with both chemoprevention and surgery, and it is essential that the health benefits of risk-reducing measures outweigh the long-term costs to health and quality of life.

This chapter introduces the options for chemoprevention and risk-reducing surgery that are available for individuals at high risk of hereditary breast, ovarian, colorectal and gastric cancer and considers the importance of a multidisciplinary approach, including the input of cancer and genetics health professionals, in facilitating decision-making about risk-reducing options. The learning objectives for Chapter 22 are:

- to become aware of the chemoprevention and surgical measures available for reducing the risk of hereditary cancers;
- to consider the role of the multidisciplinary team in facilitating informed decision-making about risk-reducing options.

Chemoprevention

Cancer chemoprevention is 'the use of drugs or other agents to try to reduce the risk or delay the development or recurrence of cancer' (National Cancer Institute, 2013). In terms of hereditary cancer there have, until recently, been few options for chemoprevention. However, this area is moving forward and there is now some evidence of benefits of chemopreventive agents in reducing the cancer risk for breast, ovarian and colorectal cancer. Each of these chemopreventative agents will be discussed further in subsequent chapters in this section.

Tamoxifen has long been prescribed to women with oestrogen receptor (ER)-positive breast cancer to reduce the risk of contralateral disease. In England and Wales, recent guidelines from the National Institute for Health and Care Excellence (NICE, 2013) recommend that unaffected pre- and post-menopausal women at high risk of breast cancer are offered chemoprevention with the selective ER modulators (SERMs) tamoxifen or raloxifene for 5 years as a risk-reducing measure, provided this is not contraindicated and following discussion of the side effects and limitations of this treatment. The guidelines also recommend that health professionals consider tamoxifen or raloxifene for women at moderate risk of breast cancer.

Risk reduction associated with 5 years' use of tamoxifen is 38% and raloxifene is 23%, with risk benefit persisting for at least a further 5 years (Cuzick et al., 2013). NICE (2013) estimates a 25% uptake of chemoprevention. However, the side effects (including vasomotor symptoms, menstrual irregularity, increased risk of thromboembolic events and endometrial cancer) may make this option inappropriate or unacceptable to many women Patient information leaflets are available from the UK Cancer Genetics Group (see Chapter 26).

Aspirin has been shown to reduce the risk of colorectal cancer in both the general population and the high-risk population (Burn et al., 2011), although there are risks associated with the drug that need to be discussed prior to commencing treatment. As yet, the optimal dose for risk reduction is unknown but further research is under way to determine this (Burn et al., 2013).

The combined oral contraceptive pill has been shown to reduce the risk of ovarian cancer in *BRCA* mutation carriers as well as in the general population, providing a lifetime risk reduction of up to 50% (Narod et al., 1998). There is, however, an increased risk of breast cancer associated with use of the combined oral contraceptive pill. It is therefore not recommended that women at high risk of breast and ovarian cancer are prescribed the Pill for chemoprevention (NICE, 2013).

There are many issues to consider with regard to chemoprevention and full discussion of the risks, benefits and limitations with individuals who are considering this option and the provision of patient information leaflets, where available, is essential.

Risk-reducing surgery

Risk-reducing surgery aims to remove healthy tissue in an attempt to prevent the development of cancer. Advances in surgical techniques have reduced the morbidity associated with surgery. For example, the ability to perform laparoscopic risk-reducing bilateral salpingo-oophorectomy (BSO) usually eliminates the need for a laparotomy, shortens the in-patient stay and reduces post-operative discomfort and complications. Alongside this, there is growing evidence of cancer-specific and overall survival benefit associated with risk-reducing surgery for those at high risk of cancer.

Risk-reducing mastectomy with immediate reconstruction is available for women with a 30% or more lifetime risk of breast cancer following genetic assessment and family history verification, pre-operative counselling and under the management of the multidisciplinary team (NICE, 2013). A Cochrane review of risk-reducing mastectomy for the prevention of breast cancer (Lostumbo et al., 2010) concluded that, overall, while several studies indicate that risk-reducing mastectomy does effectively reduce the incidence and death from breast cancer (Hartmann, 1999; Meijers-Heijboer et al., 2001) there are various study biases and these findings should be interpreted with caution. The authors point out that it is essential that patients and clinicians understand the true risk for each individual when surgery is being considered.

The evidence of reduction of ovarian cancer risk (Rebbeck et al., 2002) and overall reduction in mortality (Domchek et al., 2010) afforded by prophylactic BSO, together with the lack of availability of evidence-based ovarian screening, means that surgery to remove the ovaries and fallopian tubes is offered to women with a *BRCA1* or *BRCA2* gene mutation from their late 30s or early 40s once they have completed their families. Add-back hormone replacement therapy is recommended in women with no personal history of breast cancer who undergo this surgery prior to the natural menopause in order to counterbalance the impact of surgical menopause on their quality of life and health (Finch and Narod, 2011).

For women with Lynch syndrome, the lack of availability of evidence-based endometrial and ovarian screening means that women at high risk may be offered a prophylactic hysterectomy (and BSO) from around the age of 40 once they have completed their families. This surgery has been shown to effectively reduce the cancer risks in women with Lynch syndrome (Schmeler et al., 2006), but recent consensus guidelines on the management of Lynch syndrome question whether the small gain in life expectancy associated with BSO outweighs the adverse effects in pre-menopausal women (Vasen et al., 2013).

Surveillance and risk-reducing surgery have greatly improved survival in familial adenomatous polyposis (FAP) (Vasen et al., 2008). The timing of risk-reducing surgery in FAP is guided by polyp numbers, size and dysplasia and informed decision-making (Cairns et al., 2010). Patients with a genetic predisposition to hereditary diffuse gastric cancer may also consider risk-reducing gastrectomy (Fitzgerald et al., 2010).

The importance of a multidisciplinary approach to facilitating informed decision-making about risk-reducing options

In order to make an informed decision about whether or not to opt for risk-reducing measures, individuals at high risk of cancer require up to date information, accurate risk assessment, assessment of their psychological and physical fitness for surgery and competing risks, and professional and family support. It is important that patients and health professionals are aware of: the individual's genetic risk; the level and pattern of risk of developing cancer without the risk-reducing treatment; the level of risk reduction afforded by the treatment; the side effects and potential complications of the risk-reducing treatment; the options available for reducing the risk, including the different surgical techniques that might be available elsewhere; the availability of screening for early detection and the risks and the limitations and benefits of these and the psychosocial morbidity associated with opting for or not opting for the risk-reducing measures. Access to current and accurate information and professional and peer support is essential for informed decision-making.

Facilitating decision-making about risk-reducing measures therefore requires input from the whole multidisciplinary team, including cancer, genetics and psychology health professionals. Families may inaccurately report that a gene mutation has been identified in a family member, either because of poor family communication or lack of understanding (Vos et al., 2011) and cases of fictitious cancer family histories have been reported (Evans et al., 1996). This highlights the importance of involvement of genetics health professionals before individuals embark on risk-reducing measures to investigate the family history, verify diagnoses, provide genetic counselling and undertake genetic testing where possible prior to undergoing risk-reducing measures. Consistency and communication between health professionals is extremely important as is establishing close links between genetics and cancer care through attendance at multidisciplinary meetings and joint clinics.

Summary

There are options for reducing the risk of cancer where the chance of developing cancer outweighs the risks associated with the risk management options. Involvement of health professionals in cancer care, psychology and genetics in discussions with patients who are considering these measures is vital. The issues surrounding risk reduction will be addressed in more detail for patients at risk of hereditary breast cancer in Chapter 24, hereditary colorectal and gastric cancer in Chapter 25 and hereditary gynaecological cancers in Chapter 26. The psychosocial issues involved in decisions about risk management are addressed in Chapter 34.

References

Burn J, Gerdes AM, Macrae F, et al. 2011. Long-term effect of aspirin on cancer risk in carriers of hereditary colorectal cancer: an analysis from the CAPP2 randomised controlled trial. *Lancet* **378**: 2081–2087.

Burn J, Mathers JC, Bishop DT 2013. Chemoprevention in Lynch syndrome. *Fam Cancer* **12**: 707–718.

Cairns, SR, Scholefield, JH, Steele, RJ, et al. 2010. Guidelines for colorectal cancer screening and surveillance in moderate and high risk groups (update from 2002). Gut **59**: 666–689.

Cuzick J, Sestak I, Bonanni B, et al. 2013. Selective oestrogen receptor modulators in prevention of breast cancer: an updated meta-analysis of individual participant data. *Lancet* **381**: 1827–1834.

Domchek SM, Friebel TM, Singer CF, et al. 2010. Association of risk-reducing surgery in BRCA1 or BRCA2 mutation carriers with cancer risk and mortality. *J Am Med Assoc* **304**: 967–975.

Evans DGR, Kerr B, Cade D, et al. 1996. Fictitious breast cancer family history. *Lancet* **348**: 1034.

Finch A and Narod SA 2011. Quality of life and health status after prophylactic salpingo-oophorectomy in women who carry a *BRCA* mutation: a review. *Maturitas* **70**: 261–265.

Fitzgerald RC, Hardwick R, Huntsman D, et al. 2010. Hereditary diffuse gastric cancer: updated consensus guidelines for clinical management and directions for future research. *J Med Genet* **47**: 436–444.

Hartmann LC 1999. Efficacy of bilateral prophylactic mastectomy in women with a family history of breast cancer. *New Engl J Med* **340**: 77–84.

Lostumbo L, Carbine NE, Wallace J 2010. Prophylactic mastectomy for the prevention of breast cancer. *Cochrane Database Syst Rev* Nov 10;(11): CD002748. doi: 10.1002/14651858.CD002748.pub3

Meijers-Heijboer H, Van Geel B, Van Putten WL, et al. 2001. Breast cancer after prophylactic bilateral mastectomy in women with a *BRCA 1* or *BRCA2* mutation. *N Engl J Med* **345**: 159–164.

Narod SA, Risch H, Moslehi R, et al. 1998. Oral contraceptives and the risk of hereditary ovarian cancer. Hereditary Ovarian Cancer Clinical Study Group. *N Engl J Med* **339**: 424–428.

National Cancer Institute 2013. *NCI dictionary of cancer terms.* Available at: <http://www.cancer.gov/dictionary?cdrid = 45487> (last accessed 31 July 2013).

NICE (National Institute for Health and Care Excellence) 2013. *Familial breast cancer: classification and care of people at risk of familial breast cancer and management of breast cancer and related risks in people with a family history of breast cancer.* NICE Clinical Guideline 164. London: National Institute for Health and Care Excellence.

Rebbeck TR, Lynch HT, Neuhausen SL, et al. 2002. Prophylactic oophorectomy in carriers of *BRCA1* or *BRCA2* mutations. *New Engl J Med* **346**: 1616–1622.

Schmeler KM, Lynch HT, Chen LM, et al. 2006. Prophylactic surgery to reduce the risk of gynecologic cancers in the Lynch syndrome. *N Engl J Med* **354**: 261–269.

Vasen HF, Möslein G, Alonso A, et al. 2008. Guidelines for the clinical management of familial adenomatous polyposis (FAP). *Gut* **57**: 704–713.

Vasen HF, Blanco I, Aktan-Collan K, et al. 2013. Revised guidelines for the clinical management of Lynch syndrome (HNPCC): recommendations by a group of European experts. *Gut* **62**: 812–823.

Vos J, Jansen AM, Menko F, et al. 2011. Family communication matters: the impact of telling relatives about unclassified variants and uninformative DNA-test results. *Genet Med* **13**: 333–341.

Chapter 23

Reducing the risk of breast cancer

Hisham Hamed and Jian Farhadi

Introduction to reducing the risk of breast cancer

Breast cancer is the most common cancer in women, with an annual incidence of more than 49 000 cases in the UK; exceeding the incidence of lung cancer in men and women combined (CRUK, 2011). It is second only to lung cancer as the major cause of cancer-related death in the world (CRUK, 2012). The direct cause(s) of the disease remains elusive. The discovery of the *BRCA1* and *BRCA2* mutations (Miki, 1994; Wooster, 1995) provided some understanding as to the pathogenesis of breast cancer, while posing more questions and presenting major challenges in the management of women who are carriers. It is estimated that 7% of breast cancer patients in the general population have an inherited basis for the disease (Claus, 1996).

The first part of this chapter will describe the principles of reducing the risk of breast cancer for women without a cancer diagnosis, the surgical risk-reducing measures available and the risks, benefits and limitations of these measures. The second part of the chapter will examine the options for breast reconstruction following risk-reducing mastectomy (RRM), highlighting the different techniques available and the issues surrounding these options.

The learning objectives for Chapter 23 are:

+ to be able to describe the available measures for reducing the risk of breast cancer;
+ to be able to discuss the risks, benefits and limitations of these measures.

Options for reducing the risk of breast cancer

Women at high risk of breast cancer due to a *BRCA1/2* gene mutation or based on verified family history have extremely difficult decisions to make, and therefore an understanding of the magnitude of risk is fundamental to informed decision-making. Health professionals have the responsibility and the challenge of conveying the relevant statistics in simple and clear language. Furthermore, women at high risk of breast cancer but with no previous history of the disease face complex decisions within limited choices in order to reduce their risk. There are few options available, and these have variable efficacy in reducing the risk of developing or dying from breast cancer: the options include risk reducing mastectomy (RRM), chemoprevention with agents such as tamoxifen, pre-menopausal bilateral oophorectomy and/or breast surveillance (see Chapter 18).

Chemoprevention

It has been observed that there is a modest decline in the incidence of breast cancer following early menopause and reduction in endogenous oestrogen. The risk of breast cancer is reduced by 50% in *BRCA1/2* mutation carriers following pre-menopausal bilateral oophorectomy (Rebbeck, 2002) and normal BRCA1 protein reduces epithelial proliferation in response to exposure to oestrogen. Several studies have shown a significant reduction in the risk of breast cancer in women with a family history or high risk of breast cancer following tamoxifen administration (King, 2001; Cuzick, 2002;). These particular studies showed a significant risk reduction in *BRCA2* carriers but not in those with a *BRCA1* mutation (although the total number of *BRCA1/2* carriers was small), suggesting that tamoxifen and other anti-oestrogen agents are only effective in reducing oestrogen receptor positive cancer. However, studies involving pre-menopausal bilateral oophorectomy showed significant reduction in the incidence of breast cancer in both *BRCA1* and *BRCA2* carriers. Furthermore, in a large study (Gronwald, 2006), the benefit of tamoxifen was seen equally in *BRCA1* and *BRCA2* carriers. The biological basis for the discrepancy between different studies is not yet clear. However, there is sufficient evidence to support the administration of tamoxifen for 5 years to reduce the risk of breast cancer in *BRCA1/2* carriers and in women at moderate and high risk following thorough discussion of the benefits, limitations and side effects (NICE, 2013).

Risk-reducing mastectomy

Surveillance relies on early detection, not prevention, of breast cancer, although it may reduce the risk of dying from the disease. However, it is estimated that as many as 25% of high-risk women who undergo regular surveillance will die of distant metastases despite a relatively early diagnosis (Klijn, 1997). Mastectomy has been established as the most effective means of reducing breast cancer risk. Several large studies have consistently shown that the reduction in breast cancer risk following bilateral mastectomy is as high as 90% (Hartmann, 2001; Meijers-Heijboer, 2001; Rebbeck, 2004). This risk reduction is shown to be even higher in women who have also undergone pre-menopausal oophorectomy (Rebbeck, 2002). Mastectomy may also be associated with a modest increase of number of life years gained (Schrag, 1997). As a result, an increasing number of carriers opt for bilateral RRM in preference to other measures. Mastectomy is considered to be mutilating surgery and it is not surprising that for some women it is not an option they can contemplate. Guidelines recommend that the option of RRM is discussed with women at high risk based on verified family history following genetic risk assessment (NICE, 2013). Women who choose not have RRM should not be solicited by health professionals to undergo surgery; two factors have been shown to contribute to poor outcome and recovery, namely inadequate and inferior-quality information and the clinician influencing the woman's decision (Josephson, 2000).

Women who embark on RRM have several important issues to address and should be given ample time to grasp, digest and reflect on the information and implications of the surgery and the opportunity to consult their surgeon as often as necessary. It is fundamental to the woman's welfare to have appropriate and adequate counselling in order to evaluate anxiety and stress levels and explore coping strategies. It is good practice for women to be referred to an onco-psychologist before undergoing surgery (Price, 2007), but at the very least all women considering RRM should be offered pre-operative counselling about the psychosocial and sexual consequences of surgery and have access to support groups or contact with other women who have undergone RRM (NICE, 2013).

RRM should be carried out by a specialist, skilled, accredited oncoplastic surgeon, and any woman considering this surgery should be referred for a genetic assessment prior to the surgery (NICE, 2013). It is important to convey to women contemplating this surgery that even a well-performed mastectomy does not eradicate all breast tissue, hence the term 'risk reducing' rather than prophylactic mastectomy. It is equally important to explain the potential post-operative complications and physical consequences, with particular reference to the risk of scarring and loss of sensation of the mastectomy flaps.

Surgical options for reducing breast cancer risk

Various mastectomy techniques are available, and all are oncologically safe and effective. However, there are some aesthetic aspects that must be taken in consideration and discussed with patients. Total mastectomy is associated with significant skin loss and therefore leads to inferior cosmetic results. This technique is rarely used now in risk-reducing surgery. The skin-sparing mastectomy (SSM) technique, which allows maximum preservation of breast skin, provides better cosmetic results than standard mastectomy. SSM is probably the most commonly used technique in RRM (Slavin, 1998). However, SSM does have the disadvantage of sacrificing the nipple. Nipple preservation (nipple-sparing or subcutaneous mastectomy, SCM) provides a superior aesthetic result to SSM with minimal compromise in risk reduction (Hartmann, 1999). Two studies (Hartmann, 1999; Rebbeck, 2004) found that all the post-mastectomy breast cancers that occurred in the study cohorts developed following SCM. Risk appears to be related to residual parenchymal tissue due to limited access rather than just due to preservation of the nipple areola complex. This observation highlights a very important issue; although mastectomy is carried out as a risk-reduction procedure and in the absence of breast cancer, it should not be compromised in exchange for aesthetics. Adequate access and careful dissection are fundamental oncological principles. This potential drawback of SCM should be clearly shared with women embarking on mastectomy with nipple preservation, together with the fact that preserved nipples are functionless and devoid of sensation.

One study found invasive breast cancer in 0.1–7.7% of the breasts removed for risk reduction (Heemskerk-Gerritsen, 2007). It is good practice therefore to carry out a thorough physical examination and breast imaging with bilateral mammography and magnetic resonance imaging to identify asymptomatic or occult breast cancer prior to surgery. Post-operative histological examination of the breast tissue should be carried out according to agreed protocols and by specialist pathologists, and the possibility of breast cancer being diagnosed histologically following surgery should be discussed with women pre-operatively (McIntosh et al., 2004).

The risks, benefits and limitations of surgical risk reduction

The decision to undergo mastectomy with all the evidence of successful risk reduction is far from straightforward. *BRCA1/2* mutation carriers of any age live every day with the fear of being told that they have breast cancer and young women under the age of 30 are no exception. Predictive genetic testing is offered to women as young as 18 years of age. Young women sometimes request mastectomy, despite understanding that their risk levels do not rise significantly until their late 20s. There are no guidelines to ascertain the acceptable minimum age for RRM. For young women there are compounding factors such as career, marriage, starting a family and breast-feeding. These issues add significant weight to the complexity of the decision-making, coupled with persistent anxiety.

Several studies have reported adverse effects of RRM on body image and sexual relationships (Mulvihill, 1982; Frost, 2000). In a small study, 13/15 (87%) women reported that the cosmetic results were better than expected, but 8/15 (53%) reported that they felt the reconstruction was not part of their bodies (Josephson, 2000). In another study, 7/45 (16%) women required psychiatric help following RRM (Hopwood, 2000). Frost (2000) reported high levels of satisfaction in women who did not have reconstruction. However, despite the fact that mastectomy is irreversible, studies have overwhelmingly found that women who have undergone RRM report satisfaction with the decision, having no regrets and lower levels of anxiety and fear about developing breast cancer (Stefanek, 1995; Borgen, 1998; Hatcher, 2001).

Breast reconstruction

The aim of breast reconstruction is the maintenance of quality of life following mastectomy. There have been a number of advances in breast reconstruction over the past few years, leading to safer and more reliable surgery. With an increase in the available options, the advantages and disadvantages of each technique can be combined with individual patient characteristics to achieve the best results (Table 23.1). In patients undergoing RRM, reconstruction is always performed at the same time.

In broad terms, current options can be divided into use of prosthetic material or autologous (patient derived) tissue. Prosthetic options include single-stage implant reconstruction or a staged tissue expander followed by implant reconstruction. Autologous reconstructions involve harvesting tissue from one area of the body and transferring it to the mastectomy site. The flap of tissue may retain its original blood supply (pedicled flap) or be joined to a new blood supply at the recipient site (free flap) requiring microvascular anastomoses. Pedicled flaps include the latissimus dorsi (LD) and transverse rectus abdominis myocutaneous (TRAM) flaps. Free flaps include the deep inferior epigastric perforator (DIEP), superior gluteal artery perforator (SGAP), transverse myocutaneous gracilis (TMG) and its modification the profunda artery perforator (PAP) flap (Fig. 23.1).

Table 23.1 Advantages and disadvantages of different breast reconstruction techniques

Procedure	Advantage	Disadvantage	Comment
Two stage with expander/implant	Quick, simple, no donor site	Two operations, symmetry	High rate of capsular contracture
One stage with ADM	Quick, simple, no donor site	High rate of seroma and infection	Lower rate of capsular contracture
Latissimus dorsi flap	No microsurgery	Shoulder dysfunction, need for implant	Scar, seroma
Pedicled TRAM	No microsurgery	Abdominal hernia	
DIEP flap	Good tissue match, no implant	Microsurgical expertise needed	Failure rate of 2%
SGAP flap	For slim patient	Complex flap raising	Indentation of buttock
TMG/PAP flap	Easy flap harvest	Pain, seroma	Good for very slim patients with small breasts

ADM, acellular dermal matrix; TRAM, transverse rectus abdominis myocutaneous; DIEP, deep inferior epigastric perforator; SGAP, superior gluteal artery perforator; TMG, transverse myocutaneous gracilis; PAP, profunda artery perforator.

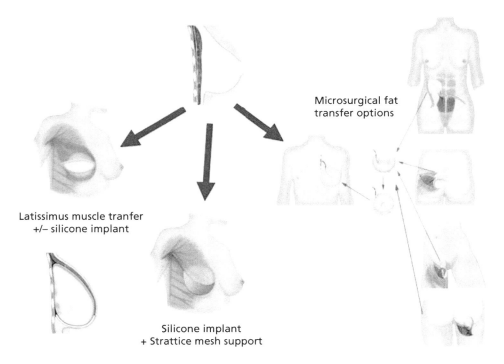

Microsurgical fat transfer options

Latissimus muscle tranfer +/− silicone implant

Silicone implant + Strattice mesh support

Figure 23.1 Breast reconstruction options. This figure shows all the different options for immediate breast reconstruction that are currently available (2014).

Image courtesy of Jian Fahardi

Prosthetic reconstruction

Implants

The advent of silicone breast implants in the late 1960s allowed the option of post-mastectomy implant-based reconstruction. The implant is inserted under the pectoralis major muscle as a single-stage operation. Implant reconstruction is a simple, short operation with no flap-associated morbidity.

Tissue expander/implant reconstruction

In a SSM the initial tissue expander is placed under the chest muscle to gain full coverage of the implant later. The expander can be subsequently inflated within an out-patient clinic setting to the desired volume. A second-stage operation is then performed to exchange the expander for a matched implant. An advantage of the expander technique is the ability to adjust the final volume. This technique involves two operations with the associated complications for implant placement. A major disadvantage to any implant-based reconstruction technique is the increased risk of fibrosis. Fibrosis and contracture around the implant compromise the aesthetic outcome of the reconstruction and may necessitate further revision surgery.

Acellular dermal matrix

Most recently, acellular dermal matrix (ADM) has been used as an adjuvant product in prosthetic reconstructions. ADM is a sterile, acellular surgical mesh. It consists of dermis (human, porcine or foetal bovine) which is stripped from its cellular components to make it biochemically inert. ADM acts in a number of ways to enhance implant reconstruction. It acts as a scaffold for the ingrowth of cells needed to regenerate and heal the surgical wound locally and can provide additional soft tissue cover for prosthetic devices. The additional tissue cover is hypothesised to reduce implant-related complications such as rippling and contour deformity, but one of the main advantages is the possibility of a one-stage breast reconstruction with an implant without the introduction of an expander. Furthermore, the use of ADM has reduced capsular contracture rates to 2–3% in non-irradiated breast reconstruction (Spear, 2012).

Autologous reconstruction

Autologous reconstructions are based on the concept that a patient's own tissue is most likely to mimic breast tissue lost during mastectomy. Abdominal tissue is most commonly utilised, as the texture and consistency of the subcutaneous tissue matches well to breast tissue, but tissue may be harvested from other sites. In addition, the harvested skin will age with the patient and create natural ptosis and a good aesthetic outcome.

Free flaps can have post-operative vascular complications if the donor or recipient vessels are compromised.

Latissimus dorsi (LD) flap

The flap is raised from the large muscle of the back and is tunnelled through the axilla to the pectoral region. The flap remains attached to its vascular pedicle, the thoracodorsal pedicle, which is robust and therefore guarantees low flap necrosis and failure rates. LD flaps can also be used to cover implants if more breast volume is desired.

Deep inferior epigastric perforator (DIEP) flap

The DIEP flap has gained increasing popularity amongst plastic surgeons as the abdominal perforator flap of choice for immediate breast reconstructions. It is a modification of the free TRAM flap. The TRAM flap can be either harvested as a pedicled flap using the superior epigastric vessels or a free abdominal flap using inferior epigastric vessels (Hartampf, 1982). The flap is based on the rectus abdominis muscle and its overlying skin and subcutaneous tissue. Harvesting the flap results in an iatrogenic weakness in the abdominal wall which is repaired using a synthetic mesh. Despite mesh repair, patients are at risk of developing abdominal wall herniation at this site (Serletti, 2006). Since the introduction of the DIEP flap, the TRAM flap is less often used.

The DIEP flap is based upon the perforating vessels of the abdominal tissue and therefore avoids the need to dissect fascia and muscle (Granzow et al., 2006), thus reducing the risk of abdominal wall herniation and bulging. Raising the DIEP flap involves careful microdissection of the perforating branches to provide a suitable pedicle for anastomosis in the chest. In light of this, operating times for a bilateral reconstruction are often in excess of 8 hours and heavily rely on the skill of the surgeon. The flap requires a sufficient amount of abdominal tissue and is therefore not suitable for those patients with a low body mass index (BMI). Similarly, patients with very high BMI, diabetes or those who are heavy smokers are known to have increased post-operative complications (Seidenstuecker et al., 2011). The abdominal flap harvest is similar to an abdominoplasty procedure and offers patients the simultaneous advantage of a tummy tuck, which remains an attractive option for post-menopausal women.

Transverse myocutaneous gracilis (TMG) flap and profunda perforator artery (PAP) flap

The TMG flap is derived from the inner thigh, and as such is a useful option for reconstruction in thinner, small to moderately breasted patients. As a free flap it relies on the proximal pedicle of the gracilis muscle and consists of the whole muscle and an elliptical transverse cutaneous paddle. The flap is relatively quick to raise due to the fairly constant anatomy. Thigh lift is an addition benefit from the procedure. The PAP flap is a further development of the TMG flap in which an adipocutaneous free flap is based on a perforator from the adductor magnus (Allen, 2012).

Superior gluteal artery perforator (SGAP) flap

This flap is based on the superior gluteal artery perforating vessels which supply the overlying subcutaneous tissue and skin in the gluteal region. Perforators are identified and dissected through the gluteus muscle, and as such, a limited pedicle length can be achieved. Dissection is often time-consuming and challenging. The gluteal muscle is preserved and therefore donor site morbidity is low with minimal post-operative pain. The nature of the donor tissue is firm and hence it provides good texture and projection to reconstructed breasts (Werdin et al., 2010).

Nipple reconstruction

A range of surgical techniques are available for nipple reconstruction. All aim to use a small section of skin to re-create a nipple using a single pedicled local flap. The results are variable with little evidence to recommend one technique over another (Farhadi et al., 2006).

Summary

BRCA1/2 mutation carriers who know they have a very high risk of breast cancer are faced with difficult and complex decisions. There are various risk-reduction options, ranging from surveillance and chemoprevention to mastectomy. The latter is the most difficult choice of all but it confers maximum risk reduction. The complexity of the decision requires multidisciplinary team management and the full support of all involved. Mastectomy has been shown to significantly reduce anxiety, but there are other complex psychological issues associated with altered body image. There are a variety of modalities available for breast reconstruction, making it possible to offer implant-based as well as autologous options. It is important to offer every woman a comprehensive consultation in which all options are discussed. The greater availability and choice of mastectomy technique and advances in reconstructive surgery have assisted with minimising post-surgical psychological morbidity and restoring normality to the lives of these women.

References

Allen RJ, Haddock NT, Ahn CY, Sadeghi A 2012. Breast reconstruction with the profunda artery perforator flap. *Plast Reconstr Surg* **129**: 16e–23e.

Borgen PI, Hill AD, Tran KN, et al. 1998. Patients regrets after bilateral prophylactic mastectomy. *Ann Surg Oncol* **5**: 603–606.

Claus EB, Shildkraut JM, Thompson WD, et al. 1996. The genetic attributable risk of breast and ovarian cancer. *Cancer* **77**: 2318–2324.

CRUK (Cancer Research UK) 2011. Available at: <http://www.cancerresearchuk.org/cancerinfo/cancerstats/incidence/commoncancers/#Ten3> (last accessed 13 April 2014).

CRUK (Cancer Research UK) 2012. Available at: <http://www.cancerresearchuk.org/cancer-info/cancerstats/world/incidence/> (last accessed 13 April 2014).

Cuzick J, Forbes J, Baum M, et al. 2002. First result from the International Breast Cancer Interventional Study (IBIS-I): a randomized prevention trial. *Lancet* **360**: 817–824.

Farhadi J, Maksvytyte GK, Schaefer DJ, et al. 2006. Reconstruction of the nipple-areola complex: an update. *J Plast Reconstr Aesthet Surg* **59**: 40–53.

Frost MH, Schaid DJ, Slezak JM, et al. 2000. Long term satisfaction and psychological and social functions following bilateral prophylactic mastectomy. *J Am Med Assoc* **284**: 319–324.

Granzow JW, Levine JL, Chiu ES, Allen RJ 2006. Breast reconstruction with the deep inferior epigastric perforator flap: history and an update on current technique. *J Plast Reconstr Aesthet Surg* **59**: 571–579.

Gronwald J, Tung N, Foulkes WD, et al. 2006. Tamoxifen and contralateral breast cancer in *BRCA1* and *BRCA2* carriers: an update. *Int J Cancer* **118**: 2281–2284.

Hartmann LC, Schaud DJ, Woods JE, et al. 1999. Efficacy of bilateral prophylactic mastectomy in women with a family history of breast cancer. *N Engl J Med* **340**: 77–84.

Hartmann LC, Sellers TA, Schaid DJ, et al. 2001. Efficacy of bilateral prophylactic mastectomy in *BRCA1* and *BRCA2* gene mutation carriers. *J Natl Cancer Inst* **93**: 1633–1642.

Hartrampf CR, Scheflan M, Black PW 1982. Breast reconstruction with a transverse abdominal island flap. *Plast Reconstr Surg* **69**: 216–225.

Hatcher M, Fallowfield L, A'hern R 2001. The psychological impact of bilateral prophylactic mastectomy. prospective study using questionnaire and semistructured interviews. *Br Med J* **13**: 76–79.

Heemskerk-Gerritsen BAM, Brekelmans CTM, Menke-Pluymers MBE, et al. 2007. Prophylactic mastectomy in *BRCA1/2* mutation carriers and women at risk of hereditary breast cancer: long term experience at the Rotterdam family cancer clinic. *Ann Surg Oncol* **12**: 3335–3344.

Hopwood P, Lee A, Shemon A, et al. 2000. Clinical follow up after bilateral risk reducing (prophylactic) mastectomy: mental health and body image outcomes. *Psycho-Oncology* **9**: 462–472.

Josephson U, Wickman M, Sandelin K 2000. Initial experience of women from hereditary breast cancer families after bilateral prophylactic mastectomy: a retrospective study. *Eur J Cancer* **26**: 351–356.

King MC, Wienand S, Hale K, et al. 2001. Tamoxifen and breast cancer incidence among women with inherited mutations in *BRCA1* and *BRCA2*. (NSABP-P1) Breast Cancer Prevention Trial. *J Am Med Assoc* **286**: 2251–2256.

Klijn JGM, Janin N, Cortes-Funes H, et al. 1997. Should prophylactic surgery be used in women at high risk of breast cancer? *Eur J Cancer* **33**: 2149–2159.

McIntosh A, Shaw C, Evans G, et al. 2004 [updated 2006]. *Clinical guidelines and evidence review for the classification and care of women at risk of familial breast cancer.* NICE Clinical Guideline 014. London: National Collaborating Centre for Primary Care/University of Sheffield. Available at: <http://www.nice.org.uk/nicemedia/live/10993/30233/30233.pdf>.

Meijers-Heijboer H, Van Geel B, Van Putten WJL, et al. 2001. Breast cancer after prophylactic bilateral mastectomy in women with a *BRCA1* or *BRCA2* mutation. *N Engl J Med* **345**: 159–164.

Miki Y, Swansen J, Shattuck-Eidens D, et al. 1994. A strong candidate for breast and ovarian cancer susceptibility gene *BRCA1*. *Science* **266**: 66–71.

Mulvihill JJ, Safyer AW, Bening JK 1982. Prevention in familial breast cancer: counseling and prophylactic mastectomy. *Prevent Med* **11**: 500–511.

NICE (National Institute for Health and Care Excellence) 2013. *Familial breast cancer: classification and care of people at risk of familial breast cancer and management of breast cancer and related risks in people with a family history of breast cancer.* NICE Clinical Guideline 164. London: National Institute for Health and Care Excellence.

Price AM, Butow PN, Lo SK, et al. 2007. Predictor of cancer worry in unaffected women from high risk breast cancer families: risk perception is not the primary issue. *J Genet Counsel* **16**: 635–644.

Rebbeck TR, Lynch HT, Neuhaussen SL, et al. 2002. Prophylactic oophorectomy in carriers of *BRCA1* or *BRCA2* mutations. *N Engl J Med* **346**: 1616–1622.

Rebbeck TR, Friebel T, Lynch H, et al. 2004. Bilateral prophylactic mastectomy reduces breast cancer risk in *BRCA1* and *BRCA2* mutation carriers. The PROSE Study. *J Clin Oncol* **22**: 1055–1062.

Schrag D, Kuntz KM, Garber JE, et al. 1997. Decision analysis—effects of prophylactic mastectomy and oophorectomy on life expectancy among women with *BRCA1* and *BRCA2* mutations. *N Engl J Med* **336**: 1465–1471.

Seidenstuecker K, Munder B, Mahajan AL, et al. 2011. Morbidity of microsurgical breast reconstruction in patients with comorbid conditions. *Plast Reconstr Surg* **127**: 1086–1092.

Serletti JM 2006. Breast reconstruction with the TRAM flap. Pedicled and free. *J Surg Oncol* **94**: 532–537.

Slavin SA, Schnitt SJ, Duda RB, et al. 1998. Skin-sparing mastectomy and immediate reconstruction: oncologic risk and aesthetic results in patients with early stage of breast cancer. *Plast Reconstr Surg* **102**: 49–62.

Spear SL, Sher SR, Al-Attar A. 2012. Focus on technique: supporting the soft-tissue envelope in breast reconstruction. *Plast Reconstr Surg* **130**(Suppl 2): 89S–94S.

Stefanek RK 1995. Bilateral prophylactic mastectomy: issues and concerns. *J Natl Cancer Inst Monogr* **17**: 37–42.

Werdin F, Peek A, Martin NC, Baumeister S 2010. Superior gluteal artery perforator flap in bilateral breast reconstruction. *Ann Plast Surg* **64**: 17–21.

Wooster R, Bingell G, Lancaster J, et al. 1995. Identification of breast cancer susceptibility gene *BRCA2*. *Nature* **378**: 789–792.

Chapter 24

Reducing the risk of colorectal and gastric cancer

Eric Alexandre Chung and Mark George

Introduction to reducing the risk of colorectal and gastric cancer

In the UK the lifetime risk rate for colorectal cancer (CRC) is about 5% and for gastric cancer (GC) 1.5%. These risks arise from an interaction between environment, lifestyle and inherited factors, ranging from no inherited predisposition to cancer to inherited conditions that will almost certainly lead to the development of cancer. The aim of this chapter is to review environmental and lifestyle risk factors that are associated with CRC and GC, and to focus on measures that can be taken to reduce the risk of these cancers. The learning objectives for Chapter 24 are:

- to be able to describe the measures available for reducing the risk of CRC and GC;
- to be able to discuss the risks, benefits and limitations of these measures.

Environmental and lifestyle risk factors for CRC and GC

Since Sir Percivall Pott's observation in 1775 of an association between scrotal cancer in chimney sweeps and exposure to soot, it has been known that environmental and lifestyle factors can affect cancer rates. There is increasing appreciation that although there may be uncontrollable factors associated with the development of cancers, lifestyle modifications can reduce the risk of developing CRC and GC. Understanding these risk factors can lead to strategies for reducing the overall risk.

Obesity

Throughout the developed world there has been a huge increase in rates of obesity since the 1980s. There is increasing epidemiological evidence that obesity is associated with a greater risk of colonic adenomas and cancers. Studies show an increased prevalence of adenomas in subjects who are abdominally obese. A prospective study of 46 000 male health professionals in the United States revealed an association of bowel cancer with short- and long-term weight gain (Thygesen et al., 2008). Individuals with a high body mass index (BMI) and large waist and hip sizes have increased rates of CRC (Harriss et al., 2009). Obesity results in measurable metabolic alterations, such as hyperinsulinaemia, hyperleptinaemia and increased visceral adiposity. Hyperinsulinaemia promotes cellular proliferation and inhibits cellular apoptosis in colonic cancer cell lines. This may be mediated by the insulin growth factor (IGF) system, and high amounts of IGF-1 itself have been implicated in increased levels of CRC (Giovannucci, 2001). Leptin and adiponectin are adipose-derived hormones that play a role in regulating appetite and metabolism. Obesity is associated with raised levels of leptin and reduced levels of adiponectin. Altered levels of these hormones effect angiogenesis, tumourigenesis and cell proliferation and may contribute to the development of cancer (Tilg and Moschen, 2006). Raised visceral fat activates nuclear transcription factors which can lead to transcription of tumourigenesis-promoting genes (Donohoe et al., 2010). There is little information on the effects of obesity reduction on CRC.

There are few data on the effect of obesity on GC, though meta-analysis has indicated that obesity is associated with an increased risk of GC, and this increases with increasing BMI (Yang et al., 2009).

Diet

The typical western diet includes high levels of red and processed meat. There is an association between consumption of red meat and CRC (Oba et al., 2006). The mechanism behind this association may be the formation of mutagenic compounds, namely heterocyclic amines and polycyclic aromatic hydrocarbons. These form as haem molecules change when meat is cooked at a high temperature; together with nitrates found in processed meats these are converted to carcinogenic N-nitroso compounds which affect the colon. There appears to be no increased risk associated with poultry and fish intake; in fact, fish consumption is associated with a decreased risk of CRC (Wu et al., 2012).

Caffeine and high-fat dairy foods are associated with reduced levels of CRC. The benefit of dairy products could be related to their high levels of calcium and vitamin D (Sun et al., 2011). Another characteristic of western diets is a low level of dietary fibre. Fibre, antioxidants, folate, flavones and other micronutrients may have a protective effect against colorectal cancer (Lin, 2009). Diets low in sources of these compounds, such as fruits and vegetables, are associated with an increased risk of CRC (Terry et al., 2001). The evidence for the benefit of fibre alone is mixed.

High cholesterol intake is associated with a large increased relative risk of CRC and the use of statins has been shown to have an effect on lowering CRC rates (Bardou et al., 2010).

A copious literature exists on the role of diet in the pathogenesis of GC. Diets high in starch and low in protein increase the risk of GCs, possibly from damage to gastric mucosa through acid-catalysed nitrosation in the stomach. Such diets tend to have a low fruit and vegetable content. A negative correlation exists between use of a refrigerator, fruit consumption and GC mortality and there is a positive correlation with sodium intake (Park et al., 2011). High dietary levels of salted fish, soy sauce, pickles and cured meat enhance rates of infection with *Helicobacter pylori* and increase the risk of GC via mucosal injury (Wang et al., 2009). Nitrates are found naturally in foods, coming from fertilisers, being added in processing and in cured or flame-cooked meats. Nitrate consumption, with subsequent conversion of nitrates to *N*-nitroso compounds by gastric acid, increases the risk of GC (Liu and Russell, 2008). High consumption of smoked foods containing polycyclic aromatic hydrocarbons has also been associated with increased risk of GC.

Smoking

Smoking has been shown to have an association with CRC, and meta-analyses have shown an increased absolute risk of CRC (Botteri et al., 2008). Smokers develop symptoms of CRC earlier in life than non-smokers and also have a higher rate of polyp recurrence than non-smokers. There is an association with tumour subtypes, with studies showing high expression of mutations in oncogenes such as *p53* and *KRAS* in tumours from smokers (Diergaarde et al., 2003).

Smoking has a dose-dependent effect on the risk of developing GC, and combined with alcohol there is a synergistic effect increasing that risk. Smokers who have had surgery with curative intent for GC have an increased risk of recurrence and death compared with non-smokers (Smyth et al., 2012).

Alcohol

There is disagreement regarding the level of alcohol consumption that is associated with CRC risk, with some studies suggesting the risk is raised with three drinks a day (Mizoue et al., 2008) and others showing CRC risk increases with higher levels of alcohol intake (Cho et al., 2004). An explanation for this might be the reduced folate levels in heavy drinkers (Gellad and Provenzale, 2010). Cessation of drinking reduces this risk in a time-dependent manner (Liang et al., 2009).

Heavy alcohol intake, particularly of strong beverages, increases the risk of developing GC. The process behind this is thought to be due to the irritant effects of ethanol on the stomach and its conversion to acetaldehyde, which is carcinogenic. Individuals with mutations in alcohol and acetaldehyde dehydrogenase genes are prone to developing upper gastrointestinal (GI) tract cancers (Mikko, 2012).

Exercise

Low levels of physical activity are common in developed societies and the WHO world health report of 2002 identified this as a risk to healthy life (WHO, 2002). Studies have shown that any amount of regular exercise can reduce the level of CRC by up to 60% compared with inactive individuals (Coyle, 2009). Exercise has been associated with a reduction in adenomatous polyps (Rosenberg et al., 2006). It has been postulated that the protective effect of exercise is related to a faster colonic transit time with reduced exposure to carcinogens, altered immune function, altered gut hormones and increased prostaglandin levels (Quadrilatero and Hoffman-Goetz, 2003). Raised levels of insulin and IGF are associated with CRC, and there is a rise in these factors in people who are physically inactive.

There is limited evidence that physical inactivity has any association with the development of GC.

Inflammation and infection

Patients with inflammatory bowel disease (IBD) have an increased risk of CRC. With ulcerative colitis (UC) this risk increases with time: the incidence of cancer is less than 1% within 10 years of disease onset but rises to 10–15% in the second decade and to over 20% after 20 years. After 10 years of symptoms, the risk of cancer increases by approximately 1% per year, similar to the risks with Crohn's colitis. Colonic surveillance for flat dysplasia or dysplasia-associated lesions or masses (DALM) is done to reduce the risk of CRC in IBD. Screening using dye spraying and/or random biopsies to look for areas of dysplasia/DALMs, with subsequent colonoscopy if required, is recommended 10 years following diagnosis (Mowat et al., 2011). No evidence exists that particular colonic infections or a specific spectrum of colonic bacterial colonisation is associated with the development of CRC (Wogan et al., 2012)

Over 80% of GCs have been attributed to *Helicobacter pylori* infection. *Helicobacter pylori* infection is a Gram-negative microaerophilic bacterium found in the gastric mucosa of patients with gastritis. One Japanese study demonstrated its presence in all patients with peptic ulceration who went on to develop GCs, whereas those who were not infected did not develop GC (Uemura et al., 2001). The number of data implicating *H. pylori* as a cause of GC has resulted in it being classified as a carcinogen. Approximately 50% of the world's population is infected, with high levels of infection being found in developing Asian countries (Fock and Ang, 2010). For *H. pylori* to cause cancer, the host must provide the right environment and be genetically susceptible. The gastric epithelium progresses through atrophic gastritis, intestinal metaplasia and dysplasia to carcinoma, and *H. pylori* secretes products that damage the gastric mucosa, including urease, proteases, phospholipase, ammonia and acetaldehyde (Kim et al., 2011). This culminates in oxidative stress with the production of reactive oxygen and nitrogen species and oxidative DNA damage. Other cited mechanisms for damage include the formation of mutagenic compounds through inflammatory mediators and disruption of mismatch repair pathways (Nagini, 2012). Reducing the risk of developing GC involves eradicating *H. pylori* in all patients with atrophy and/or intestinal metaplasia and in first-degree relatives of GC patients, together with endoscopic and histological surveillance. Eradication therapy has been shown to reduce the risk of GC and can be used as part of a screening treatment.

Preventative measures

Studies have shown that some compounds reduce risk by acting as chemopreventative agents.

Aspirin and non-steroidal anti-inflammatory drugs (NSAIDs)

There is increasing evidence for the use of aspirin and NSAIDs to reduce rates of CRC and GC in the general population. Aspirin has been shown to reduce the incidence of CRC with increased benefit associated with duration of treatment (Das et al., 2007), but as yet no clearly established strategy has been developed for its use. A daily dose of 75 mg appears to be sufficient for risk reduction in the general population (Rothwell et al., 2011). The protective effect is thought to be mediated by restoring anti-tumour activity by the permanent inactivation of platelet cyclooxgenase (COX) 1. The use of aspirin has also been shown to reduce the risk of developing CRC in patients with known Lynch syndrome (LS). The mechanism behind this has been hypothesised to be a reduction in the effect of mutations in mismatch repair genes. Studies of medical treatments are incomplete and risk reduction with medical therapy has yet to become mainstream in treating LS. Celecoxib use has been shown to reduce the risk of recurrence of adenoma (Cooper et al., 2010).

Antioxidants, trans-resveratrol and calcium

Studies suggest that antioxidants could act as chemopreventative agents to reduce the risk of CRC. Vitamins A, C and E, selenium, zinc and folate have been shown to reduce CRC in epidemiological studies and pre-clinical models (Bonelli et al., 2013), and low serum vitamin D levels are associated with adenoma formation (Yin et al., 2011). Trans-resveratrol is a natural phytoalexin found in grapes, red wine, berries and nuts. It provides anti-cancer health benefits by inhibiting cell proliferation and inducing apoptosis *in vitro* and reducing pre-neoplastic lesions and the incidence of tumours in trials (Juan et al., 2012). Diets high in dairy products are protective for CRC and there is some evidence that calcium supplements maybe protective (Vargas and Thompson, 2012).

Risk-reducing surgery

Colectomy

Prophylactic colectomy should be discussed with carriers of LS mutations who have had a tumour resection, given the high risk of their developing further cancers (Vasen et al., 2013). A decision about whether to opt for regular surveillance or surgery needs discussion on an individual basis. Surgical options are subtotal colectomy and ileo-rectal anastomosis or stoma, or proctocolectomy with restorative ileo-anal pouch formation. The risk of developing rectal cancer after a subtotal colectomy is quoted as 12% at 12 years and therefore annual endoscopic surveillance should be performed when the rectum is not removed.

With a diagnosis of familial adenomatous polyposis (FAP), prophylactic surgery is offered prior to the development of cancer. Indications for immediate surgery are the presence of a high polyp burden, large polyps or symptoms. Often there is an elective delay to surgery, as teenagers wish to finish schooling first. No strict guidelines exist about the age at which surgery should be performed, and the decision is made on an individual basis. The operations offered are similar to those for LS. Surgery leaving the rectum intact will require ongoing surveillance, as will any procedure where a cuff of rectal mucosa is left, such as when stapled anastomoses are performed. Mucosectomy with a hand-sewn anastomosis avoids this problem but can result in poorer function. Follow-up is required in all patients. In those with ileo-rectal anastomoses or ileo-anal pouch formation annual digital rectal examinations and flexible sigmoidoscopy should be performed.

Polypectomy

Polypectomy should be carried out every 2 years in individuals affected with juvenile polyposis syndrome or attenuated FAP. Colectomy is indicated if the polyps are too large or numerous to be managed in this way (Latchford et al., 2012a).

FAP is associated with the development of polyps in the upper GI tract, and half of those affected go on to develop gastric polyps. These have a low potential for malignancy. Duodenal polyps are more common, with 10% being severe and half of those eventually becoming malignant (Groves et al., 2002). Endoscopic surveillance starts from the age of 20, with repetition depending upon the severity of the polyps. There are high recurrence rates after polypectomy (polyp removal) and the procedure is associated with high perforation rates. Argon-beam therapy is safer. Surgical treatment is reserved for severe disease due to the high morbidity associated with pancreatico-duodenectomy.

Gastrectomy in hereditary diffuse gastric cancer (HDGC)

This rare condition is caused by a germline mutation in the *CDH1* gene. Individuals with mutations in this gene are at high risk of developing HDGC and account for about 1% of all cases and 50% of familial cases. In family members where a *CDH1* mutation has been identified there are no unified recommendations for surveillance. Six-monthly endoscopy should be performed by experienced endoscopists using dye spray and random biopsies to identify early cancers (Fitzgerald and Caldas, 2004).

Prophylactic gastrectomy is controversial given the high mortality and morbidity associated (Shaw et al., 2005). No conclusive studies have yet been done to ascertain the benefits of gastrectomy versus surveillance. However, there is greater than 80% penetrance in carriers of mutations and gastrectomy should be strongly considered in carriers of *CDH1* mutations. It is recommended that gastrectomy be undertaken in these cases when the individual is over the age of 20 (Fitzgerald et al., 2010). The recommended operation is a total gastrectomy with Roux-en-Y reconstruction. Pouch reconstruction is offered in some centres. Morbidity following gastrectomy is high, and support needs to be in place for patients following surgery.

Summary

A wide range of environmental and lifestyle factors are associated with the incidence of CRC and GC. Taking action on the factors that are known to increase the risk, for example obesity, should lead to a reduction in incidence. Further work needs to be done to clarify the factors that affect risk and for this information to be used to educate and guide the public into adopting changes in their diet, exercise regimes and lifestyle in order to reduce the incidence of these cancers. Awareness, treatment and management of those diseases that carry an associated cancer risk by doctors and other healthcare professionals is essential for reducing the incidence of CRC and GC in patients.

References

Bardou M, Barkun A, Martel M 2010. Effect of statin therapy on colorectal cancer. *Gut* **59**: 1572–1585.

Bonelli L, Puntoni M, Gatteschi B, et al. 2013. Antioxidant supplement and long-term reduction of recurrent adenomas of the large bowel. A double-blind randomized trial. *J Gastroenterol* **48**: 698–705.

Botteri E, Iodice S, Bagnardi V, et al. 2008. Smoking and colorectal cancer: a meta-analysis. *J Am Med Assoc* **300**: 2765–2778.

Cho E, Smith-Warner SA, Ritz J, et al. 2004. Alcohol intake and colorectal cancer: a pooled analysis of 8 cohort studies. *Ann Intern Med* **140**: 603–613.

Cooper K, Squires H, Carroll C, et al. 2010. Chemoprevention of colorectal cancer: systematic review and economic evaluation. *Health Technol Assess* **14**: 1–206.

Coyle YM 2009. Lifestyle, genes, and cancer. *Methods Mol Biol* **472**: 25–56.

Das D, Arber N, Jankowski JA 2007. Chemoprevention of colorectal cancer. *Digestion* **76**: 51–67.

Diergaarde B, Vrieling A, Van Kraats AA, et al. 2003. Cigarette smoking and genetic alterations in sporadic colon carcinomas. *Carcinogenesis* **24**: 565–571.

Donohoe CL, Pidgeon GP, Lysaght J, Reynolds JV 2010. Obesity and gastrointestinal cancer. *Br J Surg* **97**: 628–642.

Fitzgerald RC and Caldas C 2004. Clinical implications of E-cadherin associated hereditary diffuse gastric cancer. *Gut* **53**: 775–778.

Fitzgerald RC, Hardwick R, Huntsman D, et al. 2010. Hereditary diffuse gastric cancer: updated consensus guidelines for clinical management and directions for future research. *J Med Genet* **47**: 436–444.

Fock KM and Ang TL 2010. Epidemiology of Helicobacter pylori infection and gastric cancer in Asia. *J Gastroenterol Hepatol* **25**: 479–486.

Gellad ZF and Provenzale D 2010. Colorectal cancer: national and international perspective on the burden of disease and public health impact. *Gastroenterology* **138**: 2177–2190.

Giovannucci E 2001. Insulin, insulin-like growth factors and colon cancer: a review of the evidence. *J Nutr* **131**: 3109S–3120S.

Groves CJ, Saunders BP, Spigelman AD, Phillips RK 2002. Duodenal cancer in patients with familial adenomatous polyposis (FAP): results of a 10 year prospective study. *Gut* **50**: 636–641.

Harriss DJ, Atkinson G, George K, et al. 2009. Lifestyle factors and colorectal cancer risk (1): systematic review and meta-analysis of associations with body mass index. *Colorectal Dis* **11**: 547–563.

Juan ME, Alfaras I, Planas JM 2012. Colorectal cancer chemoprevention by trans-resveratrol. *Pharmacol Res* **65**: 584–591.

Kim SS, Ruiz VE, Carroll JD, Moss SF 2011. *Helicobacter pylori* in the pathogenesis of gastric cancer and gastric lymphoma. *Cancer Lett* **305**: 228–238.

Latchford AR, Neale K, Phillips RK, Clark SK 2012. Juvenile polyposis syndrome: a study of genotype, phenotype, and long-term outcome. *Dis Colon Rectum* **55**: 1038–1043.

Liang PS, Chen TY, Giovannucci E 2009. Cigarette smoking and colorectal cancer incidence and mortality: systematic review and meta-analysis. *Int J Cancer* **124**: 2406–2415.

Lin OS 2009. Acquired risk factors for colorectal cancer. *Methods Mol Biol* **472**: 361–372.

Liu C and Russell RM 2008. Nutrition and gastric cancer risk: an update. *Nutr Rev* **66**: 237–249.

Mikko S 2012. Interactions of alcohol and tobacco in gastrointestinal cancer. *J Gastroenterol Hepatol* **27** (Suppl. 2): 135–139.

Mizoue T, Inoue M, Wakai K, et al. 2008. Alcohol drinking and colorectal cancer in Japanese: a pooled analysis of results from five cohort studies. *Am J Epidemiol* **167**: 1397–1406.

Mowat C, Cole A, Windsor A, et al. 2011. Guidelines for the management of inflammatory bowel disease in adults. *Gut* **60**: 571–607.

Nagini S 2012. Carcinoma of the stomach: a review of epidemiology, pathogenesis, molecular genetics and chemoprevention. *World J Gastrointest Oncol* **4**: 156–169.

Oba S, Shimizu N, Nagata C et al. 2006. The relationship between the consumption of meat, fat, and coffee and the risk of colon cancer: a prospective study in Japan. *Cancer Lett* **244**: 260–267.

Park B, Shin A, Park SK, et al. 2011. Ecological study for refrigerator use, salt, vegetable, and fruit intakes, and gastric cancer. *Cancer Causes Control* **22**: 1497–1502.

Quadrilatero J and Hoffman-Goetz L 2003. Physical activity and colon cancer. A systematic review of potential mechanisms. *J Sports Med Phys Fitness* **43**: 121–138.

Rosenberg L, Boggs D, Wise LA, et al. 2006. A follow-up study of physical activity and incidence of colorectal polyps in African-American women. *Cancer Epidemiol Biomarkers Prev* **15**: 1438–1442.

Rothwell PM, Fowkes FG, Belch JF, et al. 2011. Effect of daily aspirin on long-term risk of death due to cancer: analysis of individual patient data from randomised trials. *Lancet* **377**: 31–41.

Shaw D, Blair V, Framp A, et al. 2005. Chromoendoscopic surveillance in hereditary diffuse gastric cancer: an alternative to prophylactic gastrectomy? *Gut* **54**: 461–468.

Smyth EC, Capanu M, Janjigian YY, et al. 2012. Tobacco use is associated with increased recurrence and death from gastric cancer. *Ann Surg Oncol* **19**: 2088–2094.

Sun Z, Wang PP, Roebothan B, et al. 2011. Calcium and vitamin D and risk of colorectal cancer: results from a large population-based case-control study in Newfoundland and Labrador and Ontario. *Can J Public Health* **102**: 382–389.

Terry P, Giovannucci E, Michels KB, et al. 2001. Fruit, vegetables, dietary fiber, and risk of colorectal cancer. *J Natl Cancer Inst* **93**: 525–533.

Thygesen LC, Gronbaek M, Johansen C, et al. 2008. Prospective weight change and colon cancer risk in male US health professionals. *Int J Cancer* **123**: 1160–1165.

Tilg H and Moschen AR 2006. Adipocytokines: mediators linking adipose tissue, inflammation and immunity. *Nat Rev Immunol* **6**: 772–783.

Uemura N, Okamoto S, Yamamoto S, et al. 2001. *Helicobacter pylori* infection and the development of gastric cancer. *N Engl J Med* **345**: 784–789.

Vargas AJ and Thompson PA 2012. Diet and nutrient factors in colorectal cancer risk. *Nutr Clin Pract* **27**: 613–623.

Vasen HF, Blanco I, Aktan-Collan K, et al. 2013. Revised guidelines for the clinical management of Lynch syndrome (HNPCC): recommendations by a group of European experts. *Gut* **62**: 812–823.

Wang XQ, Terry PD, Yan H 2009. Review of salt consumption and stomach cancer risk: epidemiological and biological evidence. *World J Gastroenterol* **15**: 2204–2213.

Wogan GN, Dedon PC, Tannenbaum SR, Fox JG 2012. Infection, inflammation and colon carcinogenesis. *Oncotarget* **3**: 737–738.

World Health Organization 2002. *The world health report 2002: reducing risks, promoting healthy life.* Geneva: World Health Organization.

Wu S, Feng B, Li K, et al. 2012. Fish consumption and colorectal cancer risk in humans: a systematic review and meta-analysis. *Am J Med* **125**: 551–559 e5.

Yang P, Zhou Y, Chen B, et al. 2009. Overweight, obesity and gastric cancer risk: results from a meta-analysis of cohort studies. *Eur J Cancer* **45**: 2867–2873.

Yin L, Grandi N, Raum E, et al. 2011. Meta-analysis: serum vitamin D and colorectal adenoma risk. *Prev Med* **53**: 10–16.

Chapter 25

Reducing the risk of gynaecological cancers

Adam Rosenthal

Introduction to reducing the risk of gynaecological cancer

This chapter focuses on risk-reduction strategies for preventing ovarian cancer (OC), fallopian tube cancer (FTC) and endometrial cancer (EC) in at-risk women. These strategies are principally surgical, but other risk-modifying options are also discussed. The learning objectives for Chapter 25 are:

- to be able to describe the measures available for reducing the risk of OC, FTC and EC;
- to be able to discuss the risks, benefits and limitations of these measures.

Principles of risk-reducing gynaecological surgery

Risk-reducing gynaecological surgery is surgery to prevent gynaecological cancers in at-risk women. The term 'risk-reducing' is preferred to 'prophylactic' as the former correctly implies that not all cancers are preventable; for example, risk-reducing salpingo-oophorectomy (RRSO) for women at increased risk of *BRCA1*- and *BRCA2*-associated FTC and OC cannot prevent subsequent primary peritoneal cancer (PPC). In addition, RRSO can reduce (but not eliminate) the risk of subsequent breast cancer when performed before the age of natural menopause (Domchek et al., 2010).

It is crucial for healthcare professionals and women considering risk-reducing surgery to understand that it is being suggested to prevent future ill-health rather than to treat an established problem. Because penetrance is incomplete, cancer may never develop even if surgery is not performed. However, as there are no tests which can predict whether a particular woman will develop cancer or not, it is safer to assume that she could develop cancer. Therefore, she should manage her risk as she sees fit in the light of the actual and potential consequences of surgery. In particular, she needs to balance the risks of rare but serious complications against the risks of not undergoing surgery. Fortunately, the majority of such women are young and fit. If they are confirmed as being at high cancer risk, then their risk of harm from surgery will be far less than if they do not undergo surgery.

In order for healthcare professionals to advise a high-risk woman, and for her to make an informed choice, it is vital that risk assessment is as accurate as possible. This is discussed in detail in Chapters 13–16.

Two types of risk-reducing surgery are offered for gynaecological cancers:

1 RRSO for women at risk of OC and FTC

2 risk-reducing total hysterectomy and bilateral salpingo-oophorectomy (RR-THBSO) for women at risk of EC and OC.

It should be emphasised that in those with *BRCA1/2* mutations it is thought that the majority of gynaecological cancers are high-grade serous cancers which originate at the distal end of the fallopian tube (Dubeau, 2008) rather than in the ovaries. These women have an increased risk not only of OC but also of FTC and PPC. This has important implications for the type of surgery performed and the way in which the removed organs are analysed.

In addition, because the consequences of risk-reducing surgery, particularly when performed pre-menopausally, are potentially serious, women should be encouraged to undergo genetic assessment to clarify their risk prior to surgery. This can avoid unnecessary surgery in women whose risk is not sufficiently high.

Occult cancers detected as a result of risk-reducing surgery

Women undergoing risk-reducing surgery must be aware of the small possibility of finding an occult (asymptomatic) cancer. This can be minimised by obtaining a transvaginal ultrasound and cancer antigen 125 (CA125) blood test prior to RRSO, and in addition an endometrial biopsy prior to RR-THBSO. However, even normal results cannot completely exclude occult OC, FTC, peritoneal or other cancer (e.g. metastatic breast cancer). For this reason, a woman should be counselled that if an occult cancer is found it may be necessary for her to undergo further surgery to stage and treat the cancer. The risk of finding an occult cancer depends on genetic status and age; older post-menopausal *BRCA1* mutation carriers have a higher risk than younger pre-menopausal women of unknown mutation status (Manchanda et al., 2011).

The SEE-FIM (sectioning and extensively examining the fimbrial end) histopathology protocol (Crum et al., 2007) for analysis of the removed tubes and ovaries is recommended to avoid missing an occult cancer. This protocol involves more extensive sampling of the at-risk tissue than standard histopathological analysis. In addition, a finding of the precancerous lesion 'tubal intra-epithelial carcinoma' (TIC) in a woman of unknown mutation status makes it feasible to offer gene testing for which she might otherwise be ineligible. TIC is less likely to be missed if the SEE-FIM protocol is used.

Primary peritoneal cancer

Women undergoing RRSO must be warned about the possibility of developing PPC. There are two reasons for this:

1 symptoms suggestive of PPC (persistent bloating, pelvic or lower abdominal pain, feeling full quickly after eating) should not be ignored and warrant urgent referral to a gynaecologist;

2 women who are not aware of this and who develop PPC may be concerned that their RRSO was inadequate.

Timing of surgery

Whilst risk-reducing surgery should be offered to high-risk women, the decision about when surgery should be performed is complex, because surgery inevitably results in infertility and premature menopause when performed before the age of the natural menopause. However, delaying surgery until after the natural menopause risks development of OC/FTC/EC and is not recommended. The risk of developing pre-menopausal OC is as high as 27% in *BRCA1* mutation carriers and 4% in those with *BRCA2* mutations (Rosenthal et al., 2013). In addition, whilst RRSO reduces the risk of subsequent breast cancer in *BRCA1/2* carriers who undergo surgery in their early 40s, delaying RRSO until after the natural menopause confers no such benefit (Eisen et al., 2005; Domchek et al., 2010).

Clearly, surgery is not appropriate until after a woman has completed her family. Women may consult a gynaecologist for advice when they are young and/or prior to child-bearing. They should be informed that delaying child-bearing beyond the age of 35 increases the risk of subfertility, foetal chromosomal abnormalities and pregnancy-related problems. In addition, in *BRCA1* mutation carriers delaying RRSO to facilitate childbearing in the late 30s is associated with a real risk of developing OC/FTC. Because the age of onset of OC/FTC in *BRCA2* carriers is later, and the penetrance lower than in *BRCA1* carriers, surgery can usually be delayed until after the age of 40, providing ample time for the majority of women to complete their families. If a woman comes from a family without a proven mutation but her risk has been assessed as equivalent to that of a *BRCA1/2* carrier, then it is safest to assume they are a *BRCA1* rather than *BRCA2* carrier, as this will prompt earlier surgery and prevent early onset cancers in this particularly high-risk group. Women with Lynch syndrome (LS) can usually delay RR-THBSO until after the age of 40, again because of the usual age of onset of gynaecological cancers in LS and the relatively low OC penetrance compared with *BRCA1* carriers.

When making decisions around timing of surgery, knowing the absolute risk of developing a cancer in any given year can be helpful. The figures from Antoniou et al. (2003) (Table 25.1) are particularly helpful as they report the absolute risk a woman of a specific age has of developing OC in the next year if she delays RRSO. Depending on the woman's age and mutation, these risks are usually low enough to reassure most women that they have a very small risk of developing cancer before they have completed their families.

A key issue affecting the timing of a woman's surgery is her willingness to take hormone replacement therapy (HRT). Women undergoing pre-menopausal RRSO are likely to suffer considerable physical and/or psychological symptoms as a result of abrupt surgical menopause. Symptoms may include the following: vasomotor symptoms (hot flushes, night sweats), mood and sleep disturbance, loss of libido, reduced vaginal lubrication, musculoskeletal pain, dry skin, headaches, urinary tract infections and palpitations. HRT is not only the treatment most likely to successfully alleviate these symptoms, but it is also likely to reduce the detrimental effects of premature menopause on bone strength and cardiovascular health. Nevertheless, women undergoing RRSO must be aware that even if they are fully compliant with HRT there is no guarantee that all symptoms will be alleviated.

Table 25.1 Annual percentage incidence of ovarian cancer (OC) in mutation carriers according to age

Age (years)	*BRCA1* carrier OC risk (%)	*BRCA2* carrier OC risk (%)
20–24	0.001	0.001
25–29	0.002	0.002
30–34	0.18	0.004
35–39	0.28	0.01
40–44	0.87	0.08
45–49	1.49	0.14
50–54	0.96	0.60
55–59	1.19	0.75

Adapted from *The American Journal of Human Genetics*, Volume 72, Issue 5, Antoniou et al., Average risks of breast and ovarian cancer associated with BRCA1 or BRCA2 mutations detected in case series unselected for family history: a combined analysis of 22 studies, pp. 1117–1130, Copyright © 2003 The American Society of Human Genetics, with permission from Elsevier.

In addition, whilst there is now evidence that RRSO results in reduced all-cause mortality in *BRCA1* (Domchek et al., 2010; Finch et al., 2014) and *BRCA2* (Finch et al., 2014) mutation carriers, median and mean follow-up was only 4.3 and 5.6 years in these studies, respectively. It therefore remains possible that all-cause mortality might increase when this population is followed up for longer, if it suffers increased risks of osteoporosis or ischaemic heart disease.

The benefits of RRSO for subsequent risk of breast cancer are now well established, but only occur in women undergoing RRSO under the age of 50 (Eisen et al., 2005; Domchek et al., 2010). The younger the age at which a woman has surgery, the greater the reduction in risk of breast cancer, but this must be balanced against the potential risks of osteoporosis and heart disease associated with RRSO when younger. Clearly, if a woman has undergone or is planning to undergo risk-reducing mastectomy, then the benefit of RRSO on subsequent risk of breast cancer is not likely to influence the age at which she undergoes RRSO. Taking HRT until the age of natural menopause does not appear to reduce the benefit of RRSO on subsequent breast cancer risk (Rebbeck et al., 2005), and it is important that women are aware of this as they should not be dissuaded from taking HRT until the age of natural menopause.

Hormonal considerations

All women without a prior history of breast cancer need to take HRT until the age of natural menopause (around 51 years) if they undergo pre-menopausal RRSO as recommended by the National Institute for Health and Care Excellence (NICE) guidelines (NICE, 2013). HRT reduces menopausal symptoms and helps reduce the risk of osteoporosis and heart disease that results from premature menopause (Shuster et al., 2010).

No two women will respond in the same way to RRSO, nor can they be expected to respond in the same way to HRT. There are a multitude of HRT preparations, and in addition to the type of hormone provided, doses and routes of administration of HRT can alter efficacy. Consequently, women who express dissatisfaction with a particular type of

HRT should be encouraged to try different doses or preparations before stopping it. It is worth noting that the levonorgestrel intrauterine system (IUS) can be inserted at the time of RRSO and results in lower systemic absorption than other forms of progestogenic HRT. Therefore use of the IUS combined with oestrogen-only HRT has theoretical advantages in terms of side effects and subsequent risk of breast cancer.

Women should be aware that there are a variety of non-hormonal treatments for menopausal symptoms and bone and cardiovascular protection, but most of these are not as effective as HRT. Therefore, given the safety of HRT when used until natural menopausal age, women should be encouraged to persevere with it in preference to other potentially less effective treatments. These can be used if HRT fails to alleviate specific symptoms or if there is evidence of worsening cardiovascular or bone health despite the use of HRT.

Although there is an absence of evidence of harm in giving HRT to *BRCA* carriers with previous breast cancer, current guidelines (Finch et al., 2012) suggest that even those with triple-negative tumours should not take HRT following RRSO. However, if quality of life from menopausal symptoms which have not responded to non-hormonal treatments is intolerable, then the use of low-dose HRT should be discussed with the woman's oncologist on an individual patient basis.

Surgical considerations

When undertaking surgery, the benefits of the procedure must clearly outweigh the risks. This is particularly important with risk-reducing surgery, which is being done to prevent future ill-health rather than to treat disease. Consequently any complication may result in reduced quality of life, with no counterbalancing benefit to current health.

In order to guide decision-making, it is helpful to answer three questions:

1 Is the woman's cancer risk high enough to justify surgery?

2 Are there patient-specific factors (e.g. serious comorbidities/previous major abdominal surgery) which increase the risk of the procedure?

3 Having taken questions 1 and 2 into account, is the woman statistically more likely to come to harm if she undergoes surgery than if she does not?

Question 1 is usually best answered by the clinical genetics team. They have the knowledge, experience and infrastructure to clarify risk. It is particularly important to have confirmation of risk status when contemplating surgery on a woman whose mutation status is unknown. Surgeons should keep up to date with the area of clinical genetics relevant to their practice and should contact the genetics team if their risk assessments differ, for example when new information on the woman's family history has come to light since the team last assessed her risk.

Patient-specific factors

Laparoscopic bilateral salpingo-oophorectomy in a young, fit, thin patient with no prior abdominal surgery can usually be achieved successfully with minimal risk of complications, and with current 'enhanced-recovery' programmes is frequently a day-case procedure. However, not all patients conform to this surgical ideal and there are a number of patient-specific factors, which can increase the risks of surgery, occasionally to a point where surgery should not be offered even to a woman with a mutation. These factors can be grouped under two headings:

1 Significant comorbidities limiting the patient's ability to withstand general anaesthesia and surgery (e.g. chronic obstructive pulmonary disease, angina). In such cases, assessment by an anaesthetist is necessary before taking any decision to go ahead with surgery.

2 Factors which make surgery technically challenging (e.g. obesity or known adhesions). Women anticipated to pose such challenges are best operated on by experienced laparoscopic surgeons.

Irrespective of patient factors, all women undergoing risk-reducing surgery via a planned laparoscopic approach must be consented for possible laparotomy, both immediate (in the event of technical difficulties or intra-operative complications) or delayed (in the event of a late-presenting complication).

Type of surgical intervention

As with all surgery, the least invasive procedure possible to achieve the desired aim (exclusion of occult malignancy and prevention of future malignancy) should be performed. Consequently, RRSO is all that is required for women at risk of OC/FTC only. In this situation, hysterectomy should only be performed for concurrent treatment of benign gynaecological pathology which cannot be managed by non-surgical or less invasive surgical treatments. Examples of this would include women with large symptomatic fibroids or severe pelvic endometriosis, where previous conservative measures have failed. Hysterectomy is associated with a greater risk of complications (e.g. ureteric injury) compared with RRSO alone, and should only be performed when there is an additional valid indication. This author does not consider avoidance of progestogens in women requiring HRT nor prevention of subsequent uterine cancers in women taking tamoxifen to be valid indications. This is because the absolute risks of taking combined rather than oestrogen-only HRT (Beral et al., 2003), or developing a tamoxifen-related cancer (Davies et al., 2013) are not sufficiently high to justify a major surgical procedure.

The only clinical genetic indication for hysterectomy is a proven germline mutation in a mismatch repair gene associated with LS, or in the absence of gene testing, a family history suggestive of LS where the proband is a first-degree relative of an affected individual or where there is evidence of paternal transmission via the proband's father despite the proband not having an affected first-degree relative. RR-THBSO in LS should be considered as a sole procedure, or at the time of any colorectal cancer surgery. Recent data on EC penetrance in Cowden syndrome (Riegert-Johnson et al., 2010) suggest that hysterectomy may be justifiable for this rare syndrome.

Hysterectomy should wherever possible be performed laparoscopically (total laparoscopic or laparoscopic-assisted vaginal hysterectomy) as this facilitates the obtaining of peritoneal washings and complete removal of tubes and ovaries, which can be difficult to

---

Box 25.1 Recommended points of information when consenting for risk-reducing gynaecological surgery

Premenopausal women only

- Surgery results in infertility and premature menopause
- HRT is advised until age of natural menopause unless there is a personal history of breast cancer

All women

- General surgical risks (anaesthetic risks, bleeding, blood transfusion, infection, organ injury, thrombo-embolic disease)
- Possibility of conversion to open surgery or re-operation in the event of complications
- Risk of subsequent peritoneal cancer and other cancers which surgery cannot prevent
- Risk of finding occult cancer and/or the need for a second staging operation

---

achieve via the vaginal route. Peritoneal washings at the time of surgery are mandatory, as they can affect the staging of any occult FTC/OC, and could indicate the presence of occult PPC (Manchanda et al., 2012a).

Box 25.1 summarises points to raise and discuss with women prior to consenting for risk-reducing surgery.

Screening for familial gynaecological cancers

This is discussed in Chapter 20. Screening cannot currently be recommended as a safe alternative to RRSO nor RR-THBSO in *BRCA* mutation carriers (Rosenthal et al., 2013) and LS (Manchanda et al., 2012b), respectively.

Lifestyle modifications

Many modifiable epidemiological risk factors for OC have been described in the general population. In terms of reproductive history, increasing parity, breast-feeding, use of the combined oral contraceptive pill (COCP) and tubal ligation (sterilisation) are all known to protect against OC. This would appear to hold true in *BRCA1* mutation carriers but is less clear in *BRCA2* carriers (McLaughlin et al., 2007; Antoniou et al., 2009). Clearly, decisions to have children or undergo sterilisation are complex, and neither measure should be advocated purely as a means of reducing the risk of OC. However, it can be encouraging for women to know that they may have reduced their OC risk if they have had children or used the Pill. High-risk women considering tubal ligation should be aware of two issues. Firstly, adhesions following sterilisation could occasionally render subsequent RRSO more challenging, thus increasing the risk of complications. Secondly, if she is unwilling to undergo removal of her ovaries, consideration should be given to sterilisation via salpingectomy rather than tubal ligation alone. Although this slightly increases the procedural time and risks compared with tubal ligation, it should give greater protection against the development of cancer in *BRCA1/2* carriers (Dubeau, 2008).

Despite early data to the contrary, infertility treatments do not appear to pose a significantly increased risk of OC, particularly if they succeed (Jensen et al., 2009). Given the association between *BRCA1* and subfertility (Oktay et al., 2010), this information may be reassuring for women contemplating assisted conception.

The issue of the COCP is complex, as this has been associated with an increased risk of breast cancer in the general population (Collaborative Group on Hormonal Factors in Breast Cancer, 1996). Risk is thought to depend on current or recent COCP use and disappears 10 years after stopping it. This risk needs to be balanced against the following:

1 The COCP remains one of the most reliable and convenient forms of contraception.

2 *BRCA1/2* carriers already have a very high lifetime risk of breast cancer and will usually undergo surveillance if they do not undergo risk-reducing mastectomy.

3 Recent data (Iodice et al., 2010) on COCP formulations since 1975 have not demonstrated an increased risk of breast cancer in *BRCA1/2* carriers.

4 In the general population, the COCP offers significant reduction in the risk of OC (and also EC) (Beral et al., 2007), which usually carries a worse prognosis than breast cancer, especially if the woman undergoes breast cancer screening. There are also data from the *BRCA* population, suggesting a reduced risk of OC with COCP use (McLaughlin et al., 2007; Antoniou et al., 2009).

Given these points, rather than specifically advocating the COCP to reduce the risk of OC, it would seem reasonable to explain the advantages and disadvantages of the Pill to women at increased risk of OC and/or breast cancer and let them decide if they want to use it for contraception.

Other modifiable OC risk factors include lack of physical activity, obesity (also a risk factor for EC), smoking and asbestos exposure. Clearly, avoidance of these factors offers many other benefits, and maintaining a healthy weight and avoiding smoking should be encouraged in all women irrespective of their risk of OC. Data on the use of perineal talc as a risk factor for OC are conflicting. It is at worst only a minor risk factor and is easily avoided.

Use of aspirin (Burn et al., 2011) or the levonorgestrel IUS (Wan and Holland, 2011) may reduce the risk of EC in women with LS, but more evidence of efficacy is required.

It is important to note that modifying the above risk factors and protective factors cannot be guaranteed to negate the very high risk of OC and/or EC due to predisposing germline mutations. Consequently, high-risk women must understand that lifestyle modifications cannot be considered a safe alternative to RRSO.

Summary

Risk-reducing surgery is the only proven method of preventing OC, FTC and EC. It can reduce the risk of breast cancer if performed pre-menopausally and has been shown to reduce all-cause mortality in *BRCA1* and *BRCA2* carriers, but needs to be timed appropriately for a woman's risk level and taking into account her fertility wishes and willingness to take HRT. In addition to the risks of surgery, women need to be aware of the small possibility of an occult cancer being found and the small residual risk of PPC. Wherever possible, surgery should be via the laparoscopic route and performed in centres with access to expert histopathological analysis. Hysterectomy is not necessary unless LS is the proven or likely diagnosis or the woman has other gynaecological problems justifying the procedure. Screening cannot currently be recommended as a safe alternative to risk-reducing surgery. The COCP reduces the risk of OC and EC but increases risk of breast cancer in current/recent users. Women should be informed of these facts before they decide whether they wish to use this highly effective form of contraception. Similarly, breast-feeding may reduce the risk of OC and should be encouraged for its other benefits to mother and child. Aspirin or the levonorgestrel IUS may reduce the risk of EC, but more evidence of efficacy is required. There is evidence of a small detrimental effect of obesity and smoking on the risk of OC, and avoidance of these risk factors is beneficial for numerous additional reasons.

References

Antoniou A, Pharoah PD, Narod S, et al. 2003. Average risks of breast and ovarian cancer associated with *BRCA1* or *BRCA2* mutations detected in case series unselected for family history: a combined analysis of 22 studies. *Am J Hum Genet.* **72**: 1117–1130.

Antoniou AC, Rookus M, Andrieu N, et al. 2009. Reproductive and hormonal factors, and ovarian cancer risk for *BRCA1* and *BRCA2* mutation carriers: results from the International BRCA1/2 Carrier Cohort Study. *Cancer Epidemiol Biomarkers Prev* **18**: 601–610.

Beral V and the Million Women Study Collaborators 2003. Breast cancer and hormone-replacement therapy in the Million Women Study. *Lancet* **362**: 419–427.

Beral V and the Million Women Study Collaborators 2007. Ovarian cancer and hormone replacement therapy in the Million Women Study. *Lancet* **369**: 1703–1710.

Collaborative Group on Hormonal Factors in Breast Cancer 1996. Breast cancer and hormonal contraceptives: collaborative reanalysis of individual data on 53 297 women with breast cancer and 100 239 women without breast cancer from 54 epidemiological studies. *Lancet* **347**: 1713–1727.

Burn J, Gerdes AM, Macrae F, et al. 2011. Long-term effect of aspirin on cancer risk in carriers of hereditary colorectal cancer: an analysis from the CAPP2 randomised controlled trial. *Lancet* **378**: 2081–2087.

Crum CP, Drapkin R, Miron A, et al. 2007. The distal fallopian tube: a new model for pelvic serous carcinogenesis. *Curr Opin Obstet Gynecol* **19**: 3–9.

Davies C, Pan H, Godwin J, et al. 2013. Long-term effects of continuing adjuvant tamoxifen to 10 years versus stopping at 5 years after diagnosis of oestrogen receptor-positive breast cancer: ATLAS, a randomised trial. *Lancet* **381**: 805–816.

Domchek SM, Friebel TM, Singer CF, et al. 2010. Association of risk-reducing surgery in *BRCA1* or *BRCA2* mutation carriers with cancer risk and mortality. *J Am Med Assoc* **304**: 967–975.

Dubeau L 2008. The cell of origin of ovarian epithelial tumours. *Lancet Oncol* **9**: 1191–1197.

Eisen A, Lubinski J, Klijn J, et al. 2005. Breast cancer risk following bilateral oophorectomy in *BRCA1* and *BRCA2* mutation carriers: an international case-control study. *J Clin Oncol* **23**: 7491–7496.

Finch A, Evans DG, Narod SA 2012. *BRCA* carriers, prophylactic salpingo-oophorectomy and menopause: clinical management considerations and recommendations. *Women's Health* **8**: 543–555.

Finch AP, Lubinski J, Møller P, et al. 2014. Impact of oophorectomy on cancer incidence and mortality in women with a *BRCA1* or *BRCA2* mutation. *J Clin Oncol.*

Iodice S, Barile M, Rotmensz N, et al. 2010. Oral contraceptive use and breast or ovarian cancer risk in *BRCA1/2* carriers: a meta-analysis. *Eur J Cancer* **46**: 2275–2284.

Jensen A, Sharif H, Frederiksen K, et al. 2009. Use of fertility drugs and risk of ovarian cancer: Danish Population Based Cohort Study. *Br Med J* **338**: b249.

McLaughlin JR, Risch HA, Lubinski J, et al. 2007. Reproductive risk factors for ovarian cancer in carriers of *BRCA1* or *BRCA2* mutations: a case–control study. *Lancet Oncol* **8**: 26–34.

Manchanda R, Abdelraheim A, Johnson M, et al. 2011. Outcome of risk-reducing salpingo-oophorectomy in *BRCA* carriers and women of unknown mutation status 2011. *BJOG* **118**: 814–824.

Manchanda R, Drapkin R, Jacobs I, et al. 2012a. The role of peritoneal cytology at risk-reducing salpingo-oophorectomy (RRSO) in women at increased risk of familial ovarian/tubal cancer. *Gynecol Oncol* **124**: 185–191.

Manchanda R, Saridogan E, Abdelraheim A, et al. 2012b. Annual outpatient hysteroscopy and endometrial sampling (OHES) in HNPCC/Lynch syndrome (LS). *Arch Gynecol Obstet* **286**: 1555–1562.

NICE (National Institute for Health and Care Excellence) 2013. *Familial breast cancer: classification and care of people at risk of familial breast cancer and management of breast cancer and related risks in people with a family history of breast cancer.* NICE Clinical Guideline 164. London: National Institute for Health and Care Excellence.

Oktay K, Kim JY, Barad D, et al. 2010. Association of *BRCA1* mutations with occult primary ovarian insufficiency: a possible explanation for the link between infertility and breast/ovarian cancer risks. *J Clin Oncol* **28**: 240–244.

Rebbeck TR, Friebel T, Wagner T, et al. 2005. Effect of short-term hormone replacement therapy on breast cancer risk reduction after bilateral prophylactic oophorectomy in *BRCA1* and *BRCA2* mutation carriers: the PROSE Study Group. *J Clin Oncol* **23**: 7804–7810.

Riegert-Johnson DL, Gleeson FC, Roberts M, et al. 2010. Cancer and Lhermitte–Duclos disease are common in Cowden syndrome patients. *Hered Cancer Clin Pract.* **8**(1): 6.

Rosenthal AN, Fraser L, Manchanda R, et al. 2013. Results of annual screening in the UK Familial Ovarian Cancer Screening Study (UK FOCSS Phase 1) highlight need for strict adherence to screening schedule. *J Clin Oncol* **31**: 49–57.

Shuster LT, Rhodes DJ, Gostout BS, et al. 2010. Premature menopause or early menopause: long-term health consequences. *Maturitas* **65**: 161–166.

Wan YL and Holland C. 2011. The efficacy of levonorgestrel intrauterine systems for endometrial protection: a systematic review. *Climacteric* **14**: 622–632.

Chapter 26

Reducing the risk of cancer. Summary

Lorraine Robinson and Patricia Webb

Introduction to section 6 summary

Section 6 addresses the principles of risk reduction for breast cancer, colorectal and gastric cancers and gynaecological cancers. Chemoprevention and surgery are the main approaches discussed and the involvement of the multidisciplinary team (MDT) in decision-making and patient support is emphasised.

Chapter 22. Reducing the risk of cancer. Introduction

Guided activities for Chapter 22

- Consider the importance of the MDT in facilitating decisions about risk-reducing measures. Summarise the key issues that need to be attended to by the MDT. Arrange to observe a MDT meeting at which risk-reducing strategies for your patient group are discussed. Reflect with a colleague on your observations and how the involvement of the MDT enhanced the patient experience.

- Media watch: documentaries, news stories and blogs regularly report the stories of people undergoing risk-reducing surgery (mainly risk-reducing mastectomy). Take some time to review this material; what impact do you think this might have on an individual thinking about risk-reducing surgery? What do you feel is the impact of celebrity stories and stories of everyday people—are they the same? What responsibility do you believe you have as a healthcare professional in your encounters with the media?

Chapter 23. Reducing the risk of breast cancer

The significant lifetime risk conferred by being a *BRCA1/2* mutation carrier is described alongside the efficacy of breast cancer risk-reduction strategies. The evidence is appraised, and, while the negative impact of mastectomy is analysed, the positive effect of such surgery is examined in an objective account of the significant issues.

Guided activities for Chapter 23

- First read Chapters 22 and 23, then scan cancer information websites for the most up to date information and research.

- The Macmillan website (<http://www.macmillan.org.uk>) presents a blog on double mastectomy as a preventative measure for breast cancer for women carrying *BRCA1* and *BRCA2* gene mutations. Also look also at the information provided on ovarian and prostate cancer.

- Breakthrough Breast Cancer (<http://www.breakthrough.org.uk>) provides an online video on how women should check their breasts, which is also available as an Android or iPhone app. For those without the technology, there is also a leaflet with identical information.

- Check the information provided for individual tests/examinations used regularly to detect breast cancer in your own centre or your nearest referral centre and determine whether or not it is user-friendly and easy to understand as well as being attractive to look at. Look particularly at information on biopsy procedure, mammography and ultrasound and manual examination of the breasts.

- Check the risk-reduction options and consider how you would tailor information about these to individuals in your care. Look carefully at the recent National Institute for Health and Care Excellence (NICE) guidelines for breast cancer (NICE, 2013), including the evidence upon which these are based.

- Access the patient information leaflets referred to in Chapter 22 regarding chemoprevention for women at moderate and high risk of breast cancer (<http://www.ukcgg. org/news-events/news/breast-cancer-chemoprevention-leaflets>). Consider how you might discuss this option with a patient with a family history of breast cancer.

Chapter 24. Reducing the risk of colorectal and gastric cancer

The environmental and lifestyle issues that contribute to the development of colorectal and gastric cancer are outlined. It is essential that healthcare professionals promote these issues as they have a pivotal role in reducing cancer risk, not only for the general population but also for those who are at high risk.

Guided activities for Chapter 24

- What lifestyle advice would you consider giving your patients who are at risk of colorectal cancer? See <http://www.bowelcanceruk.org.uk/> and <http://www.macmillan.org.uk/ Cancerinformation/Causesriskfactors/Healthandlifestyle.aspx> for further information.
- How would you explain the rationale for risk-reducing surgery to a patient with FAP?

Chapter 25. Reducing the risk of gynaecological cancers

The complexity of decisions surrounding risk-reducing surgery for women at high risk of gynaecological cancers is discussed. Lifestyle changes may be important in reducing risk but it is stressed that surgery is the only sure cancer preventative measure.

Guided activities for Chapter 25

◆ How would you advise a 30-year-old nulliparous *BRCA2* mutation carrier about how she could manage her risk of developing ovarian cancer? Think about lifestyle and environmental issues; see <http://www.macmillan.org.uk/Cancerinformation/Causesriskfactors/Genetics/Cancergenetics/Specificconditions/Ovariancancer.aspx> for helpful information.

◆ Read the NHS and Breakthrough Breast Cancer patient-focused document for women undergoing risk-reducing breast and gynaecological surgery (<http://www.nhs.uk/ipgmedia/national/Breakthrough%20Breast%20Cancer/Assets/Riskreducingsurgery-aguideforwomenathighriskofdevelopingbreastcancerBBC6pages.pdf>).

◆ Access and review the document 'Hereditary ovarian cancer' produced by Ovarian Cancer Action (<http://www.ovarian.org.uk/media/24365/2011_hereditary_leaflet.pdf>). How is risk reduction explained? What questions might be raised by your patient group?

Further reading for Chapter 25

Finch A, Beiner M, Lubinski J, et al. 2006. Salpingo-oophorectomy and the risk of ovarian, fallopian tube and peritoneal cancers in women with *BRCA1* or *BRCA2* mutation. *J Am Med Assoc* 296: 185–192.

Rebbeck TR, Kauff ND, Domchek SM 2009. Meta-analysis of risk reduction estimates associated with risk reducing salpingo-oophorectomy in *BRCA1* and *BRCA2* mutation carriers. *J Natl Cancer Inst* 101: 80–87.

Reference

NICE (**National Institute for Health and Care Excellence**) 2013. *Familial breast cancer: classification and care of people at risk of familial breast cancer and management of breast cancer and related risks in people with a family history of breast cancer*. NICE Clinical Guideline 164. London: National Institute for Health and Care Excellence.

Section 7

Managing hereditary cancer

Chapter 27

Managing hereditary cancer. Introduction

Chris Jacobs

Introduction to managing hereditary cancer

Until recently, individuals with cancer have tended to be referred for genetic counselling and testing once their cancer treatment has been completed, often at the instigation of another family member. For some individuals with cancer, confirmation of a cancer-predisposing gene mutation can be helpful in explaining the cause of the disease. For others, a diagnosis of hereditary cancer can rekindle feelings about the cancer diagnosis as well as raising concerns about future risks for themselves and their relatives.

Advances in genetic testing techniques and developments in cancer treatment have enabled genetic testing to be offered close to diagnosis in order to inform cancer management, raising additional issues for patients and their families and also for health professionals in cancer care and genetics. This chapter focuses on the practical, clinical and psychosocial impacts of genetic testing close to cancer diagnosis. The learning objectives for Chapter 27 are:

- to become aware of the impact of a cancer-predisposing gene mutation on cancer management;
- to consider the psychosocial implications of genetic testing close to cancer diagnosis;
- to be able to discuss the challenges of genetic testing close to diagnosis.

The impact of a cancer-predisposing gene mutation on cancer management

The targeting of cancer treatment is increasingly important in the stratified management of patients with breast, ovarian and colorectal and related cancers. Identifying a cancer-predisposing gene mutation also raises awareness of the risk of future cancers and risk management issues and enables accurate risk assessment and targeted risk management for relatives.

The National Institute for Health and Care Excellence (NICE) guidelines for familial breast cancer recommend that women with breast cancer who are eligible for genetics referral are offered a choice of accessing genetic testing during or after initial cancer management (NICE, 2013) although genetic testing at diagnosis is not recommended outside of a clinical trial.

There are some management implications of identifying a mutation close to diagnosis for patients with cancer which are discussed further in Chapters 28–30. For example, identification of a *BRCA1/2* mutation in a woman with breast cancer can alter surgical decision-making. Some women opt for a double mastectomy in order to reduce the future possibility of developing contralateral breast cancer. The presence of a *BRCA1/2* mutation may also increase a woman's eligibility for clinical trials. In women with ovarian cancer, genetic testing may be offered to target chemotherapy and identify eligibility for clinical trials (Trainer et al., 2010). For those with colorectal and related cancers, tumour testing for microsatellite instability (MSI) and immunohistochemistry (IHC) staining may be undertaken at diagnosis in order to target genetic testing, but as yet there is insufficient evidence for the use of MSI in guiding chemotherapy (Iacopetta and Watanabe, 2006). At present, confirmation of a cancer-predisposing gene mutation mainly has implications for future cancer risks for the patient and their relatives and eligibility for clinical trials. There are arguments for offering genetic testing at diagnosis where testing will alter cancer management or where the risk of recurrence and poor prognosis may prevent some families from accessing genetic testing after treatment is completed, for example to women with ovarian cancer (Daniels et al., 2009). As understanding of the aetiology of hereditary cancers increases, identification of a cancer-predisposing gene close to diagnosis or during treatment is likely to become more important in targeting cancer treatment to the individual's biological profile.

The psychosocial impact of genetic testing close to cancer diagnosis

Studies investigating the psychological impact of genetic testing on patients with cancer have mainly focused on women with breast cancer tested after some time after completing their cancer treatment (see Chapter 33). Some studies have investigated motivation for and acceptability of testing close to breast cancer diagnosis. An exploratory study using focus groups to understand whether women would want information about genetic testing close to breast cancer diagnosis and the views of the health professionals treating them, reported that offering genetic testing at the same time as a woman was coping with the emotional overload of a new cancer diagnosis and making decisions about treatment would be too stressful. However, some members of both groups thought that offering genetic testing around the time of breast cancer diagnosis would be important if the results could alter treatment decisions (Ardern-Jones et al., 2005). Similarly, in-depth interviews with women newly diagnosed with ovarian cancer found that they considered the concept of genetic testing at diagnosis acceptable if the primary motivation for testing was to increase their treatment options (Meiser et al., 2012). These studies suggest that testing close to diagnosis would be acceptable if there is a benefit to treatment.

Several qualitative studies have explored the psychosocial impact of testing close to diagnosis but at the time of these studies genetic testing took 6 months or more to complete. A qualitative study of nine women with newly diagnosed breast cancer interviewed following their genetic counselling appointment found that the women were satisfied with the timing of the appointment. However, those who had already completed surgery for their breast cancer lacked understanding of the purpose and implications of the genetic counselling or genetic testing and felt that the genetics information was of little use in the context of their own diagnosis (Vadaparampil et al., 2008). In a Dutch study, women found to carry a *BRCA1/2* gene mutation who were tested less than a year from their breast cancer diagnosis reported a lower level of well-being than those who had a longer time between diagnosis and testing (van Roosmalen et al., 2004). Schlick-Bakker et al. (2008) assessed psychological distress amongst breast cancer patients approached for genetic counselling about *BRCA1/2* at the start of adjuvant radiotherapy during the first year after diagnosis. The study concluded that patients who were actively approached did not show more long-term distress than patients who were not eligible for genetic counselling.

The psychosocial and behavioural impacts of genetic testing close to cancer diagnosis, however, have not yet been thoroughly investigated. A US study found that 48% of newly diagnosed breast cancer patients who received a positive *BRCA1/2* test result opted for bilateral mastectomy as their definitive breast cancer treatment, as did 24% of those who received uninformative test results and 4% of those who declined genetic testing altogether (Schwartz et al., 2004). A qualitative study of the attitudes, experiences and information needs of 26 women with breast cancer towards genetic testing at diagnosis (Wevers et al., 2011) found that it was highly acceptable (Meiser et al., 2011). In a pilot study of 26 women with breast cancer undergoing genetic testing close to diagnosis, 10 had a *BRCA1/2* mutation. Six of those with a *BRCA1/2* mutation had immediate bilateral mastectomy compared with three of the women in whom no *BRCA1/2* mutation was identified. Of the 26 women who underwent testing at diagnosis, five reported frequent worries about cancer recurrence but none reported that anxiety interfered with daily functioning (Wevers et al., 2012). Multicentre randomised clinical trials are under way to investigate the behavioural and psychosocial effects of rapid genetic testing in newly diagnosed breast cancer patients (Watts et al., 2012; Wevers et al., 2012).

There is less research into the psychosocial impact of testing close to diagnosis for other cancers. A systematic review of studies into the psychological impact of genetic testing in patients with colorectal cancer (CRC) found no studies evaluating testing in newly diagnosed individuals (Landsbergen et al., 2009b). A cross-sectional study of psychological distress in 81 patients treated for CRC just after MSI testing in the Netherlands between 2007 and 2009 found less psychological distress in patients undergoing testing within a year of diagnosis than in those tested at a later stage (Landsbergen et al., 2011). A qualitative study by the same authors found that CRC patients considered that the positive aspects of genetic testing close to diagnosis outweighed the negative ones (Landsbergen et al., 2009a). The authors concluded that in general genetic testing during CRC treatment may not be harmful. Further research in this area is required.

Practical challenges for health professionals in cancer care and genetics in managing genetic testing of newly diagnosed cancer patients

As targeted treatments and rapid genetic testing become more widely available, genetic testing close to diagnosis will increasingly become a part of routine cancer care. This will raise many challenges for both cancer and genetics health professionals, such as the education of cancer health professionals, communication and collaboration between cancer and genetics services, communication of genetic information in the cancer care setting, management of testing and decision-making within the time frames for surgery, interpretation of genetic test results. New models for genetic counselling, robust and streamlined pathways between cancer care and genetics services, excellent communication and a collaborative and multidisciplinary approach to the management of carriers will be required.

Summary

Identifying a cancer-predisposing mutation currently mainly impacts on future cancer risks and risks for relatives; however, there can be an impact on the management of a current cancer. Demand for genetic testing close to diagnosis is likely to increase as new genes are identified and targeted treatments become available. Genetic testing of cancer patients does not appear to cause long-term distress. However, testing close to diagnosis is relatively new and the psychological impact of this has not yet been fully investigated. Further research in this area is under way. Genetic testing for hereditary cancer close to diagnosis raises challenges for health professionals in cancer care and genetics as well as for patients. Close collaboration, multidisciplinary working and robust pathways between genetics and cancer care will need to be developed.

Chapters 28–30 discuss the management of hereditary breast, colorectal and gynaecological cancers.

References

Ardern-Jones A, Kenen R, Eeles R 2005. Too much, too soon? Patients and health professionals' views concerning the impact of genetic testing at the time of breast cancer diagnosis in women under the age of 40. *Eur J Cancer Care* **14**: 272–281.

Daniels MS, Urbauer DL, Stanley JL, et al. 2009. Timing of *BRCA1/BRCA2* genetic testing in women with ovarian cancer. *Genet Med* **11**: 624–628.

Iacopetta B and Watanabe T 2006. Predictive value of microsatellite instability for benefit from adjuvant fluorouracil chemotherapy in colorectal cancer. *Gut* **55**: 1671–1672.

Landsbergen KM, Prins JB, Brunner HG, Hoogerbrugge N 2009a. Genetic testing offered directly after the diagnosis of colorectal cancer: a pilot study on the reactions of patients. *Genetic Counsel* **20**: 317–325.

Landsbergen KM, Prins JB, Brunner HG, et al. 2009b. Genetic testing for Lynch syndrome in the first year of colorectal cancer: a review of the psychological impact. *Fam Cancer* **8**: 325–337.

Landsbergen KM, Prins JB, Brunner HG, Hoogerbrugge N 2011. Shortened time interval between colorectal cancer diagnosis and risk testing for hereditary colorectal cancer is not related to higher psychological distress. *Fam Cancer* **10**: 51–57.

Meiser B, Gleeson M, Kasparian N, et al. 2012. There is no decision to make: experiences and attitudes toward treatment-focused genetic testing among women diagnosed with ovarian cancer. *Gynecol Oncol* **124**: 153–157.

Meiser B, Mitchell G, Zilliacus E, et al. 2011. Rapid genetic testing for breast cancer risk. *Fam Cancer* **10**: S81.

NICE (National Institute for Health and Care Excellence) 2013. *Familial breast cancer: classification and care of people at risk of familial breast cancer and management of breast cancer and related risks in people with a family history of breast cancer.* NICE Clinical Guideline 164. London: National Institute for Health and Care Excellence.

van Roosmalen MS, Stalmeier PFM, Verhoef LCG, et al. 2004. Impact of *BRCA1/2* testing and disclosure of a positive test result on women affected and unaffected with breast or ovarian cancer. *Am J Med Genetics A* **124A**: 346–355.

Schlich-Bakker KJ, Ausems MG, Schipper M, et al. 2008. *BRCA1/2* mutation testing in breast cancer patients: a prospective study of the long-term psychological impact of approach during adjuvant radiotherapy. *Breast Cancer Res Treat* **109**: 507–514.

Schwartz MD, Lerman C, Brogan B, et al. 2004. Impact of *BRCA1/BRCA2* counseling and testing on newly diagnosed breast cancer patients. *J Clin Oncol* **22**: 1823–1829.

Trainer AH, Meiser B, Watts K, et al. 2010. Moving toward personalized medicine: treatment-focused genetic testing of women newly diagnosed with ovarian cancer. *Int J Gynecol Cancer* **20**: 704–716.

Vadaparampil ST, Quinn GP, Brzosowicz J, Miree CA 2008. Experiences of genetic counseling for *BRCA1/2* among recently diagnosed breast cancer patients: a qualitative inquiry. *J Psychosoc Oncol* **26**: 33–52.

Watts KJ, Meiser B, Mitchell G, et al. 2012. How should we discuss genetic testing with women newly diagnosed with breast cancer? Design and implementation of a randomized controlled trial of two models of delivering education about treatment-focused genetic testing to younger women newly diagnosed with breast cancer. *BMC Cancer* **12**: 320.

Wevers MR, Ausems MG, Verhoef S, et al. 2011. Behavioral and psychosocial effects of rapid genetic counseling and testing in newly diagnosed breast cancer patients: design of a multicenter randomized clinical trial. *BMC Cancer* **11**: 6.

Wevers MR, Hahn DEE, Verhoef S, et al. 2012. Breast cancer genetic counseling after diagnosis but before treatment: a pilot study on treatment consequences and psychological impact. *Patient Educ Counsel* **89**: 89–95.

Chapter 28

Managing hereditary breast cancer

Jennifer Glendenning, Ashutosh Kothari,
Amanda Shewbridge and Andrew Tutt

Introduction to managing hereditary breast cancer

Following a diagnosis of primary breast cancer, accurate and timely identification of an underlying genetic mutation may have a significant impact on an individual's therapeutic pathway. Currently, confirmed carrier status primarily affects decisions related to choice of the type and extent of surgery. However, when genetic predisposition is first suspected at presentation, primary cytotoxic sequencing provides additional time for confirmatory testing and processing the large amount of information offered to carriers in relation to potential future cancer risks and oncoplastic surgical options. Although standard systemic therapy recommendations in the adjuvant/neoadjuvant setting are not currently influenced by carrier status, the prognostic information afforded by the magnitude of the pathological response to therapy, particularly in those with triple-negative histology, may help in the assessment of competing risks regarding both new primaries and metastatic relapse which can affect the timing of risk-reducing surgery in subsequently confirmed carriers. In addition confirmed carrier status may make the patient eligible for novel targeted agents, particularly in the research context or at metastatic relapse.

The learning objectives for Chapter 28 are:

- to be able to understand the factors suggesting that an individual may exceed the 10% risk threshold and qualify for genetic testing even in the absence of significant family history;

- to be able to describe the strategies for sequencing therapy that may permit genetic testing without incurring significant treatment delay or compromising options for future surgical reconstruction;

- to be able to recognise the additional psychological burden incurred by individuals who have potential or confirmed carrier status and know about the support strategies that may be of benefit as women consider both therapeutic and risk-reducing interventions.

Accommodating genetic testing in the early breast cancer timeframe

Early recognition of individuals with clinical features suggesting an underlying genetic predisposition and the provision of formal risk assessment and confirmatory testing without incurring detrimental therapeutic delay are key challenges for the multidiscipli-nary team. The combination of detailed family history, age, cancer phenotype and ancestry are well-established indicators of risk and help in selecting a high-risk population that may benefit from testing for a *BRCA* mutation. In women with both hormone- and HER2 receptor-negative invasive breast cancer or medullary cancer aged under 40–50 years at diagnosis, the overall frequency of *BRCA1* mutations is high, and this strong phenotypic association permits recognition of individuals with triple-negative breast cancer (TNBC) who exceed the 10% risk threshold criterion even in the absence of other familial risk fac-tors (Gonzalez-Angulo et al., 2011; Robertson et al., 2012; NICE, 2013). The current US National Comprehensive Cancer Network hereditary breast and ovarian cancer guide-lines continue to recommend referral for genetics review of all women aged under 60 with TNBC, with recent data from a prospective population based study lending support to this age cut-off (National Comprehensive Cancer Network, 2013; Sharma et al., 2013). A family or personal history of multiple primary tumours, particularly sarcoma, breast, brain or adrenocortical carcinoma, raises suspicion of germline *TP53* mutation (Gonzalez et al., 2009).

Diagnosis of breast cancer is itself stressful, and early referral for genetic testing has the potential to add greatly to this (Meiser et al., 2008; Zilliacus et al., 2012). Factors such as cancer-related distress, fear of recurrence, body image and anxiety are the primary drivers behind patients' decisions following a breast cancer diagnosis (Spittler et al., 2012) and coordinated care between disciplines is essential in reducing anxiety for patients. Follow-ing a positive result, patients potentially face an additional decision burden that extends beyond management of the index breast to include risk-reducing surgery on the contralat-eral breast. In addition, since many women may not have completed their family at the time of diagnosis, there may be the additional strain of discussing a fertility preservation strategy before chemotherapy. Depending on individual circumstances, each of these fac-ets needs to be considered at a very early stage in the treatment pathway. Primary surgery is usually the preferred option when individuals wish to preserve their fertility. Although in some centres results from rapid genetic testing are possible within weeks, affected in-dividuals may benefit from additional time to comprehend the magnitude of the infor-mation provided before they feel in a position to finalise decisions regarding therapeutic options. Where it is known from the outset that adjuvant chemotherapy will be required, in the absence of suspected germline *TP53* mutation, neoadjuvant sequencing may 'buy time' for testing without compromising patient outcome or delaying the first definitive treatment. The optimal timing for referral to a specialist genetics clinic following breast cancer diagnosis remains unclear and should therefore be guided by the individual needs of each patient (NICE, 2013).

Management of the index breast

In early breast cancer, the surgical strategy favours breast conservation and adjuvant ra-diotherapy in preference to mastectomy where possible. Radiotherapy is contraindicated in the context of germline *TP53* mutation due to the risk of radiation-induced second malignancy, and in these patients mastectomy is generally considered to be the recommended surgical approach (Heymann et al., 2010). In *BRCA* mutation carriers presenting with conservable disease, adjuvant radiotherapy following breast conservation appears safe with no reported increase in either acute or late toxicity (Pierce et al., 2000, 2006; Shanley et al., 2006) nor added contralateral risk attributable to radiation scatter (Pierce et al., 2010). *BRCA* mutation carriers who elect for conservation and radiotherapy in preference to mastectomy may be reassured that differences in either systemic recurrence or overall survival have not been reported. However, the data suggest that carriers treated with breast-conserving surgery (BCS) and radiotherapy may be at increased risk of local recurrence as the first failure compared to those who underwent mastectomy (cumulative estimated risk 23.5% versus 5.5% at 15 years, $P < 0.001$) (Pierce et al., 2010). Although this excess risk may be mitigated in part by chemotherapy (local recurrence 11.9% after BCS and chemotherapy), factors including the timeframe to second presentation, location outside the index quadrant and histological differences from the initial primary suggest that this potentially represents second primary disease for which prior adjuvant radiotherapy has had no risk-reducing impact.

   Based on these data, patients who have had initial BCS may consider subsequent mastectomy with a view to minimising their risk of future ipsilateral disease. Patients with breast cancer opting for autologous deep inferior epigastric artery perforator (DIEP) micro-vascular reconstruction may consider having contralateral risk-reducing mastectomy (RRM) surgery at the same time, as this reconstructive option can only ever be used once. The intention to give radiotherapy may affect the mastectomy and reconstructive options best suited to an individual. Following implant reconstruction, the risk of post-radiotherapy capsular contracture may be as high as 40%, but radiotherapy may also affect the texture and volume of autologous reconstructions and increase the risk of fat necrosis (Kronowitz and Robb, 2009). In situations where second ipsilateral primary risk reduction is deemed important from the outset, mastectomy may be preferred over BCS as the first surgical procedure, and in the absence of initial locally advanced disease (T stage ≥ 3 or significant nodal disease) obviates the need for adjuvant radiotherapy and the potential for adverse impact on the cosmetic appearance of the reconstruction. The recently updated National Institute for Health Care and Excellence (NICE) guidance (NICE, 2013) recommends that all women considering a RRM should have the opportunity to discuss their options for breast reconstruction (immediate and delayed) with a member of a surgical team who has the necessary oncoplastic surgery or breast reconstruction skills.

Systemic therapy in mutation carriers

Retrospective series do not support inferior survival benefit for *BRCA* mutation carriers treated with standard anthracycline/taxane (neo)adjuvant chemotherapy compared with non-carriers (Bakyraktar et al., 2011); indeed, following neoadjuvant therapy *BRCA1* carrier status appears to be independently associated with higher pathological complete response (pCR) rates (Arun et al., 2011). Small studies suggest the potential for even greater pCR rates following neoadjuvant platinum therapy in carriers (Gronwald et al., 2009), but this strategy requires prospective evaluation within the context of a randomised controlled trial before adoption as standard of care in early disease. Although *BRCA* carrier status does not currently affect (neo)adjuvant agent selection outside the clinical trial setting, it seems likely that this will have a greater influence on therapy selection in the future as understanding of the underlying biology permits more rational selection of agents. Pre-clinical data suggest relatively greater efficacy for DNA-damaging approaches in context of impaired DNA double-strand break repair due to underlying *BRCA1/2* mutation (Farmer et al., 2005; McCabe et al., 2006), and in the metastatic setting a retrospective case–control study suggests that patients with *BRCA1*-associated oestrogen receptor (ER)-negative metastatic disease may derive relatively less benefit from taxane than their sporadic counterparts (Kriege et al., 2012). In advanced disease, questions regarding the relative efficacy of taxane versus platinum will be further addressed by the UK-wide randomised Phase III TNT trial (carboplatin versus docetaxel) which is recruiting in *BRCA1/BRCA2* mutation-associated breast cancer (of all phenotypes) as well as sporadic TNBC patients. In the early phase research setting, confirmed *BRCA* carrier status has a positive impact on trial eligibility compared, for example, with trials testing novel agents such as poly-ADP-ribose polymerase inhibitors which take advantage of differential sensitivity between cancerous and normal tissues in carriers to the inhibition of base excision repair. It is anticipated that selection of systemic therapy will be refined for carriers as the data from these studies are reported.

As in non-carriers, the use of endocrine therapy is driven by hormone receptor status and the data confirm adjuvant benefit in ER-positive *BRCA*-associated breast cancer as well as reduced risk of contralateral cancer in those with who have not undergone risk-reducing oophorectomy (Gronwald et al., 2006).

Management of the contralateral breast

BRCA mutation carriers are at a significantly increased risk of developing contralateral breast cancer, having 10- and 15-year estimates of 26% and 39%, respectively, compared with only 3% and 7% in non-carrier controls (hazard ratio 10.43, $P < 0.001$) (Pierce et al., 2006). Contralateral RRM reduces the risk of a new primary by up to 95% (McDonnell et al., 2001; Herrinton et al., 2005). Alternative strategies include the use of endocrine therapy or salpingo-oophorectomy, which approximately halve both ipsilateral and contralateral risk in both *BRCA1*- and *BRCA2*-associated disease (Gronwald et al., 2006; Pierce et al., 2006). The optimal length of endocrine risk-reducing manipulation is difficult to extrapolate from existing data but would usually be guided by the adjuvant recommendation for the index breast. The least intrusive option is annual breast imaging surveillance, usually by MRI or mammography according to age and the presence of *TP53* mutation, but patients need to understand that although this approach confers the benefits associated with early detection it does not prevent contralateral breast cancer (NICE, 2013).

Several tumour and patient factors need to be carefully considered, preferably by a multidisciplinary team, before any recommendations for the management of the contralateral breast are communicated to the patient. The existing stage-matched risk of distant relapse for the primary tumour (and the stage of any other existing cancers), patient perception and anxiety all need to be taken into account and the patient counselled appropriately. Other factors that need to be considered for reconstruction include existing comorbidities, body and breast habitus, previous chest radiotherapy, smoking and patient choice of post-reconstruction breast volume.

Prior to a decision to undergo risk-reducing surgery, with attendant impacts on cosmesis and body image, it is important to consider unspent residual risk from an individual's primary cancer which may far exceed the risk of new primary, at least in the first 5 years, and which is not affected by bilateral mastectomy. Where risk of metastatic relapse in the short term is high, surveillance strategies in a preserved breast may be initially more appropriate while residual distant recurrence risks dissipate. In evaluating an individual's unspent risk, online tools for predicting future distant recurrence risks such as Adjuvant!Online or PREDICT can be of value, providing 10-year estimates of risk based on clinico-pathological features including age, stage, grade and ER status. Molecular tools such as OncotypeDX for ER-positive cancer may also be informative as these become more routinely available in the clinic. The relapse-free interval provides additional information particularly, in TNBC where risk of distant recurrence and death peaks within the first 5 years after diagnosis but rapidly tails off thereafter (Dent et al., 2007). In those who received neoadjuvant chemotherapy, the magnitude of the pathological response provides further prognostic insight, and in all phenotypes complete pathological response at definitive surgery is associated with an excellent long-term prognosis that would support early consideration of risk-reducing surgery to address the risk of new primary breast or ovarian cancer (Symmans et al., 2007).

The support needs of women with hereditary breast cancer

The psychological and social impacts of a breast cancer diagnosis on a woman and her family are well documented. Common concerns include fear of recurrence and mortality and the impact of treatments on body image and physical and psychological functioning. Studies show that the period immediately following diagnosis is particularly stressful for women (Scwartz et al., 2008). These findings are even more pertinent in the context of a woman who is also facing a positive carrier result at, or shortly following, diagnosis. Women in this situation are faced with added concerns about the influence of a positive carrier result on their immediate decisions about treatment, in particular sequencing of treatment and the extent of surgery and the impact on other family members. They also have to cope with their emotions about the potential impact of a positive carrier result on their children or their plans to have a family in the future. The specific support needs of these women is an under-researched area, but close liaison between the breast, genetics and psychological support teams is essential to ensure that women are given the time they need to consider their results and to make informed choices about treatment options. Prospective evaluation of quality of life 2 years following contralateral risk-reducing mastectomy (CRRM) found levels of anxiety, depression and sexuality that were unchanged from before surgery, but more than 50% of women reported at least one concern about body image (Unukovych et al., 2012). Clear communication and discussion of results, their implications and the spectrum of treatment options is necessary to inform patient decision-making at this time and those who are considering CPM need sufficient time and support to make decisions about removal of a healthy breast (Kenen et al., 2006). Several appointments with different members of the multidisciplinary team may be necessary to ensure that women feel they have a full understanding of their situation, and it is important to ensure those wishing to consider risk-reducing surgery receive appropriate genetic and psychological counselling before surgery (NICE, 2013).

Carriers diagnosed at a relatively young age may not have completed their family at the time of first presentation. In this context fertility preservation strategies need to be recognised and addressed prior to cytotoxic exposure. Although women indicate that they can feel pressured to make decisions about fertility within the time restraints dictated by the need to start treatment, failure to address fertility preservation can have a detrimental impact on survivorship outcomes (Canada and Schover, 2012). Some women may consider risk-reducing oophorectomy to optimise future risk reduction, and clinical nurse specialists play a pivotal role in the coordination of ongoing care and provision of tailored information and support.

In the last decade there has been increasing interest in survivorship issues following cancer treatment. Many concerns are generic with fear of recurrence and prolonged side effects or consequences of treatment being common. Additional specific issues pertinent to women who are carriers include risk-reduction strategies and their impact on relationships with family and friends (Crotser and Boehmke, 2009). The communication of carrier status to partners and family members can leave women feeling vulnerable and they may find it difficult to cope with the implications of their carrier diagnosis on relatives, particularly when other family members have died from the disease (Kenen et al., 2006). This highlights the importance of ongoing psychological support from the multidisciplinary team. Lifestyle changes in relation to diet, exercise and alcohol should also be discussed.

Case studies to illustrate key issues

Carrier status detection based on risk assessment guided by age and phenotype risk factor rather than significant family history

A 39-year-old woman without any family history of malignancy was diagnosed with a 60 mm × 30 mm Grade III invasive cancer (no special type, NST) that was node negative (pre-chemotherapy sentinel lymph node negative, 0/3). The tumour was triple negative and in this context her eligibility for genetic screening was recognised due to her young age at diagnosis despite the absence of significant family history. She elected for neoadjuvant chemotherapy which allowed time to obtain the results of testing and consider the implications of this for the surgical approach without incurring a delay in treatment. *BRCA1* carrier status was subsequently confirmed while she was receiving chemotherapy.

In view of the T3 stage at presentation the requirement for adjuvant radiotherapy in her case was recognised and discussed from the outset. Following a very good radiological response to neoadjuvant sequential anthracycline–taxane-based chemotherapy she elected for bilateral mastectomy and autologous reconstruction. The final histology showed residual 10 mm × 12 mm × 5 mm, NST, and she subsequently went on to have risk-reducing salpingo-oophorectomy.

Importance of residual disease as a predictor of significant persisting risk: an example where contralateral mastectomy was advised against/delayed

A 34-year-old woman was diagnosed with Grade III invasive cancer (NST), triple negative but clinically node positive. She underwent *BRCA* testing based on her age at diagnosis and hormone receptor status and was treated with primary chemotherapy to allow time for the results of genetic testing. Interval imaging demonstrated a good response and as the patient was keen to avoid mastectomy she underwent BCS with axillary clearance. The histology showed 45 mm of residual invasive cancer incompletely excised (present at all margins) and 14 out 16 nodes were positive. These results were discussed with the patient and therapeutic mastectomy advised. At this consultation the patient raised the issue of CRRM, but following discussion about weighing the residual risk of local or distant relapse against the future risk of new contralateral breast cancer agreed to consider delayed CRRM

Definitive surgical approach: impact on reconstruction options of preceding therapy/surgical choices

A 38-year-old woman was diagnosed with Grade III NST invasive triple-negative cancer, with associated ductal carcinoma *in situ* and widespread microcalcification on imaging, rendering her unsuitable for BCS. Her family history was notable for breast cancer, which had affected her mother and maternal grandmother.

Multidisciplinary team review confirmed her eligibility for *BRCA* testing and she was referred for rapid testing after indicating her preference for simultaneous CRRM and immediate bilateral reconstruction in the event of a positive result. Following discussion regarding the available surgical reconstruction options, she indicated a preference for autologous reconstruction and DIEP microvascular reconstruction was recommended.

In this situation a fast track result was essential as DIEP is a once only procedure and cannot be repeated for the contralateral side if the patient undergoes this procedure as part of her cancer treatment and subsequently opts for a delayed CRRM and reconstruction.

Summary

The possibility of an underlying genetic susceptibility should be considered in the initial assessment of all patients presenting with a new breast cancer diagnosis. Where the 10%

threshold for genetic testing is exceeded, referral to the genetics team should take place and consideration be given to the most appropriate sequencing of cytotoxic and surgical interventions, with the aim of providing patients with a time frame that provides the greatest information on both genetic status and anticipated recurrence risk from their present cancer while optimising their involvement in decisions regarding management of the index breast and risk-reducing interventions without compromise to their oncological care. The additional decision burden faced by carriers requires effective support and communication from all members of the multidisciplinary team. This should be provided from an early stage in the diagnostic pathway, and close liaison between the breast, genetics and psychological support teams is essential in providing women with the time required to both understand their results and to make informed choices about the available treatment and risk-reducing therapy options.

References

Arun B, Bayraktar S, Liu DD, et al. 2011. Response to neoadjuvant systemic therapy for breast cancer in *BRCA* mutation carriers and noncarriers: a single-institution experience. *J Clin Oncol* **29**: 3739–3746.

Bakyraktar S, Gutierrez-Barrera AM, Liu D, et al. 2011. Outcome of triple-negative breast cancer in patients with or without deleterious *BRCA* mutations. *Breast Cancer Res Treat* **130**: 145–153.

Canada AL and Schover LR 2012. The psychosocial impact of interrupted childbearing in long-term female cancer survivors. *Psycho-Oncology* **21**: 134–143.

Crotser CB and Boehmke M 2009. Survivorship considerations in adults with hereditary breast and ovarian cancer syndrome: state of the science. *J Cancer Surv* **3**: 21–42.

Dent RA, Trudeau M, Pritchard KI, et al. 2007. Triple-negative breast cancer: clinical features and patterns of recurrence. *Clin Cancer Res* **13**: 4429–4434.

Farmer H, McCabe N, Lord C, et al. 2005. Targeting the DNA repair defect in *BRCA* mutant cells as a therapeutic strategy. *Nature* **434**: 917–921.

Gonzalez-Angulo AM, Timms KM, Liu S, et al. 2011. Incidence and outcome of *BRCA* mutations in unselected patients with triple receptor-negative breast cancer. *Clin Cancer Res* **17**: 1082–1089.

Gonzalez KD, Noltner KA, Buzin CH, et al. 2009. Beyond Li–Fraumeni syndrome: clinical characteristics of families with p53 germline mutations. *J Clin Oncol* **27**: 1250–1256.

Gronwald J, Tung N, Foulkes WD, et al. 2006. Tamoxifen and contralateral breast cancer in *BRCA1* and *BRCA2* carriers: an update. *Int J Cancer* **118**: 2281–2284.

Gronwald J, Byrski T, Huzarski T, et al. 2009. Neoadjuvant therapy with cisplatin in *BRCA1*-positive breast cancer patients [abstract]. *J Clin Oncol* **27**: 502.

Herrinton LJ, Barlow WE, Yu O, et al. 2005. Efficacy of prophylactic mastectomy in women with unilateral breast cancer: a cancer research network project. *J Clin Oncol* **23**: 4275–4286.

Heymann S, Delaloge S, Rahal A, et al. 2010. Radio-induced malignancies after breast cancer postoperative radiotherapy in patients with Li–Fraumeni syndrome. *Radiat Oncol* **5**: 104.

Kenen R, Ardern-Jones A, Eeles R 2006. 'Social separation' among women under 40 years of age diagnosed with breast cancer and carrying a *BRCA1* or *BRCA2* mutation. *J Genet Counsel* **15**: 149–162.

Kriege M, Jager A, Hooning MJ, et al. 2012. The efficacy of taxane chemotherapy for metastatic breast cancer in *BRCA1* and *BRCA2* mutation carriers. *Cancer* **118**: 899–907.

Kronowitz SJMD and Robb GLMD 2009. Radiation therapy and breast reconstruction: a critical review of the literature. *Plast Reconstruct Surg* **124**: 395–408.

McCabe N, Turner NC, Lord CJ, et al. 2006. Deficiency in the repair of DNA damage by homologous recombination and sensitivity to poly(ADP-ribose) polymerase inhibition. *Cancer Res* **66**: 8109–8115.

McDonnell SK, Schaid DJ, Myers JL, et al. 2001. Efficacy of contralateral prophylactic mastectomy in women with a personal and family history of breast cancer. *J Clin Oncol* **19**: 3938–3943.

Meiser B, Tucker K, Friedlander M, et al. 2008. Genetic counselling and testing for inherited gene mutations in newly diagnosed patients with breast cancer: a review of the existing literature and a proposed research agenda. *Breast Cancer Res* **10**: 1–14.

National Comprehensive Cancer Network 2013. *Genetic/familial high-risk assessment: breast and ovarian*, version 3.2013. Available at: <http://www.nccn.org/professionals/physician_gls/pdf/genetics_screening.pdf>.

NICE (National Institute for Health and Care Excellence) 2013. *Familial breast cancer: classification and care of people at risk of familial breast cancer and management of breast cancer and related risks in people with a family history of breast cancer*. NICE Clinical Guideline 164. London: National Institute for Health and Care Excellence.

Pierce LJ, Strawderman M, Narod SA, et al. 2000. Effect of radiotherapy after breast-conserving treatment in women with breast cancer and germline *BRCA1/2* mutations. *J Clin Oncol* **18**: 3360–3369.

Pierce LJ, Levin AM, Rebbeck TR, et al. 2006. Ten-year multi-institutional results of breast-conserving surgery and radiotherapy in *BRCA1/2*-associated stage I/II breast cancer. *J Clin Oncol* **24**: 2437–2443.

Pierce LJ, Phillips K-A, Griffith KA, et al. 2010. Local therapy in *BRCA1* and *BRCA2* mutation carriers with operable breast cancer: comparison of breast conservation and mastectomy. *Breast Cancer Res Treat* **121**: 389–398.

Robertson L, Hanson H, Seal S, et al. 2012. *BRCA1* testing should be offered to individuals with triple-negative breast cancer diagnosed below 50 years. *Br J Cancer* **106**: 1234–1238.

Scwartz R, Krauss O, Hockel M, et al. 2008. The course of anxiety and depression in patients with breast cancer and gynaecological cancer. *Breast Care (Basel)* **3**: 417–422.

Shanley S, McReynolds K, Ardern-Jones A, et al. 2006. Late toxicity is not increased in *BRCA1/BRCA2* mutation carriers undergoing breast radiotherapy in the United Kingdom. *Clin Cancer Res* **12**: 7025–7032.

Sharma P, Klemp JR, Kimler BF, et al. 2013. Prospective evaluation of *BRCA* mutation in a large triple-negative breast cancer (TNBC) registry: Implications for germline testing [abstract]. *J Clin Oncol* **31**: 1026.

Spittler C, Pallikathayil L, Bott M 2012. Exploration of how women make treatment decisions after a breast cancer diagnosis. *Oncol Nurs Forum* **39**: E425–E433.

Symmans WF, Peintinger F, Hatzis C, et al. 2007. Measurement of residual breast cancer burden to predict survival after neoadjuvant chemotherapy. *J Clin Oncol* **25**: 4414–4422.

Unukovych D, Sandelin K, Liljegren A, et al. 2012. Contralateral prophylactic mastectomy in breast cancer patients with a family history: a prospective 2-years follow-up study of health related quality of life, sexuality and body image. *Eur J Cancer* **48**: 3150–3156.

Zilliacus E, Meiser B, Gleeson M, et al. 2012. Are we being overly cautious? A qualitative inquiry into the experiences and perceptions of treatment-focused germline *BRCA* genetic testing amongst women recently diagnosed with breast cancer. *Support Care Cancer* **20**: 2949–2958.

Chapter 29

Managing hereditary colorectal and gastric cancer

Kiruthikah Thillai, Claire Coughlan, Mahmoud Ali
Zohree Ali and Paul Ross

Introduction to managing hereditary colorectal and gastric cancer

Colorectal cancer (CRC) is one of the commonest cancers, with an incidence of around 40 000 cases per year in the UK. Although less prevalent, gastric cancer is associated with a higher mortality as patients often present with advanced disease. Whilst the majority of cases of CRC are sporadic, approximately 5% are related to an inherited predisposition and a further 10–25% are familial (Vasen, 2000; Lindor, 2009). Genetic links to a small percentage of gastric cancers have also been reported. Early identification of such patients is essential as it has implications for their future oncology management. Familial links to cancers of the gastrointestinal (GI) tract include syndromes such as Lynch syndrome (LS), familial adenomatous polyposis (FAP), Li–Fraumeni syndrome and hereditary diffuse gastric cancer (HDGC) or via chronic atrophic gastritis or clusters of *Helicobacter pylori* infection in family groups.

This chapter will discuss the impact that hereditary links for CRC and gastric cancer have on oncology management and the differences between these and sporadic cases. The learning objectives for Chapter 29 are:

- to be able to discuss the benefits and challenges of offering genetic testing at CRC and gastric cancer diagnosis;
- to be able to discuss the impact of a cancer-predisposing gene mutation on the management of CRC and gastric cancer;
- to be able to discuss the current status of targeted therapies for the treatment of hereditary CRC and gastric cancer and be aware that this is a developing area.

Diagnosis

Following a diagnosis of CRC, an extensive medical history must be sought, including a three-generational family history. The challenges of identifying LS in cancer patients led to the development of the Amsterdam criteria and the Bethesda Guidelines in 1990 and 1997, respectively, to guide the selection of high-risk patients who require genetic testing. However, up to a third of patients who present with CRC before the age of 30 may be from undiagnosed LS families and so these guidelines may not highlight such cases. Therefore in this patient group early referral for genetic assessment should be considered regardless of LS family history. All newly diagnosed cases of cancer are discussed within a multidisciplinary setting to formalise a management plan. At this stage, if the patient has features suggesting that an underlying hereditary condition may be present this can be highlighted prior to clinical review. A member of the oncology or surgical team can then counsel the patient as appropriate and with their consent refer them to a genetic counsellor for consideration of testing. Whilst the benefits of collecting a detailed family history from new oncology patients to enable accurate risk assessments are clear, various studies have shown that many patients' medical records lack clear documentation of family history, suggesting that there is a greater need to correctly identify at-risk populations.

For younger patients with CRC and a background of a hereditary syndrome, the impact on fertility must be noted and patients counselled appropriately. Not only can future oncology treatment affect fertility but the implications of a diagnosed familial syndrome must also be discussed. Referral to an assisted conception unit (ACU) may be requested by patients as cytotoxic systemic chemotherapy can affect fertility in both men and women; therefore patients cannot commence chemotherapy until all procedures are completed at the ACU. Patients should therefore be counselled about the potential delays to their treatment with chemotherapy. For patients with advanced cancer, treatment is started as soon as possible, and for patients requiring adjuvant chemotherapy, treatment should ideally be started within 8 to 12 weeks of surgery.

For patients with advanced GI cancers, all treatment is with palliative intent. Referral for genetic testing, based on high clinical suspicion at presentation, remains important and should be offered where appropriate. Although it may not affect future oncology treatment for that individual, it can allow for screening of family members. As always, the patient must receive appropriate genetic counselling prior to testing. This needs to be handled sensitively, with the needs of the newly diagnosed cancer patient always being carefully considered with support from the multidisciplinary team.

Surgical resection

The only curative treatment for CRC is surgical resection (Nelson et al., 2001). When possible, the primary tumour, localised lymph nodes and adjacent vessels are removed to ensure the best outcome. Recent surgical advances have seen an increase in the use of minimally invasive surgery, which allows for a faster post-operative recovery and reduced morbidity. Several clinical trials have confirmed there is no negative impact on overall survival (OS) compared with open surgery (Bonjer et al., 2007). All patients with a new diagnosis of a colorectal tumour require a full colonoscopy to ensure that a further distal tumour is not missed. In patients with CRC secondary to an abundance of polyps, such as in FAP, there is an increased risk of synchronous tumours; for this reason, direct inspection of the full colon is important. Ideally, this should take place prior to elective surgery and the extent of polyposis needs to be assessed prior to resection where relevant as this may influence the extent of surgery. Patients with FAP are offered prophylactic colectomies at diagnosis, as there is a near 100% risk of developing CRC. Patients who have not had surgery and then develop an early CRC are offered a pan-proctocolectomy or a total colectomy with regular surveillance of the rectum. Some experts advocate extended prophylactic colectomies for patients with LS, but this remains controversial (Dunlop, 2002; Parry et al., 2011). Patients who have a total proctocolectomy remain at risk of developing an adenoma in the pouch and therefore still require regular surveillance with direct inspection of this area. Critics argue that many extended colectomies for LS are unnecessary as there are a percentage of patients that have incomplete genetic penetration. There is also the risk of extracolonic recurrence or rectal primaries that are not prevented by such surgery. Patients with *MUTYH* polyposis are offered surgery, the extent of which, after careful discussion with the patient, is dependent on the extent of polyposis.

The current standard of care for patients presenting with early gastric or oesophageal cancers includes perioperative chemotherapy combined with surgical resection (Cunningham et al., 2006). Although diagnosis of inherited genetic mutations does not alter the management of a diagnosed cancer it has implications for family members, and therefore patients who present with gastric cancer at a young age should be referred for genetic testing and family members need to be counselled to discuss genetic testing and subsequent screening. Surgery is of no benefit for patients with advanced disease that has metastatic spread from either a colorectal or gastric primary, unless for palliative symptomatic control.

Chemotherapy

For patients with resected CRC, systemic adjuvant chemotherapy is offered depending on the pathological stage of the primary combined with risk factors (Porschen et al., 2001). There is the potential for occult micrometastatic disease that can later cause recurrence. It is these cells that chemotherapy targets and there is evidence that 5-fluorouracil (5FU), with or without oxaliplatin, can reduce the risk of recurrence when given after resection for Stage III disease. However, the evidence for its use following Stage II disease is less clear (Figueredo et al., 2004). Oncologists offer patients surveillance alone or single-agent fluoropyrimidine (5FU or an oral prodrug of 5FU, capecitabine) depending on the presence of high-risk features such as a T4 lesion, obstruction, lymphovascular invasion, perineural invasion, perforation, positive margins or small lymph node harvest. Several studies have assessed OS in patients with Stage II disease on a background of LS. There is evidence that surgical resection alone offers this population a better OS compared with sporadic groups. However, studies have demonstrated no benefit in administering adjuvant 5FU to patients with Stage II disease with high microsatellite instability (MSI-high) (Ribic et al., 2003). This does not extend to Stage III disease, as there appears to be no difference between microsatellite stable and MSI-high disease. There have been some reports suggesting that irinotecan may be of benefit in patients with MSI-high disease, but as irinotecan has not been shown to have benefit in the adjuvant setting it is not currently used (Fallik et al., 2003). Immunohistochemistry of the tumour block takes places prior to any anti-cancer management, and this guides the medical team in assessing risk and in some cases affects the use of anti-cancer treatment. It is likely that management of the cancer will begin prior to complete genetics assessment, but the initial management can be determined using immunohistochemical testing.

The treatment for early gastric cancer includes resection with perioperative combination chemotherapy. Standard of care includes the combined use of epirubicin, cisplatin and capecitabine. There is no evidence to suggest that patients with a hereditary aetiology for their cancer have different responses to this regimen. Therefore, regardless of their genetic profile, patients undergo the same treatment.

In patients with advanced CRC in whom curative resection is no longer possible, treatment is with palliative intent to prolong survival and improve symptoms. Metastatic CRC is treated with combination chemotherapy with or without a targeted agent depending on performance status. Patients are managed with the same chemotherapy regimens regardless of aetiology, as there is currently no evidence to suggest different responses across subgroups. There is no globally accepted chemotherapy regimen for advanced gastric cancer, but recommended cytotoxic treatments include 5FU and a platinum agent with or without epirubicin or docetaxel.

Targeted agents

There have been recent advances in the development of targeted agents that have led to their increased use in the field of oncology. In many cancers, targeted agents are used alone or in combination with cytotoxic chemotherapy. However, at present there are no targeted agents that have shown benefit in progression-free survival when used in the adjuvant setting for CRC. A few agents such as the vascular endothelial growth factor (VEGF) antibody bevacizumab and the monoclonal antibody cetxuimab have shown an improvement in OS when used in the palliative setting. There has been no evidence to suggest differing efficacy of these treatments when used in patients with hereditary syndromes compared with sporadic cases. Recent studies conducted in patients with advanced gastric cancer have demonstrated an improvement in OS when using trastuzumab in combination with cytotoxic chemotherapy in patients whose gastric cancers over-express the protein Her-2 (Bang et al., 2010). Her-2 amplification is more commonly seen in intestinal-type than diffuse-type gastric cancer and is associated with a poorer prognosis (Hochwald et al., 2000). Studies have shown that Her-2 over-expression demonstrates an inverse association with E-cadherin (*CDH1*) mutations (Becker et al., 2000). As germline *CDH1* mutations are responsible for HDGC, these patients are unlikely to have Her-2 overexpression and thus unlikely to benefit from trastuzumab. The use of targeted treatments in patients with rare genetic syndromes such as Li–Fraumeni syndrome has not been investigated.

Surveillance

Following curative resection in patients with LS, regular surveillance is paramount due to the high risk of metachronous tumours. This has been estimated at 40% at 10 years and 72% at 40 years depending on the length of colon remaining. Following surgery, patients should be reviewed annually every 12 years with sigmoidoscopy following subtotal colectomy and with colonoscopy following subtotal partial colectomy. Surveillance for patients with FAP is dependent on the extent of prophylactic surgery that has been performed and all patients should be regularly assessed for extracolonic cancers. Patients should have surveillance CT scans and biochemistry including carcinoembryonic antigen (CEA) testing as per standard of care for all patients with CRC. If the tumour is found to be MSI-high, the options of a specialist referral to a genetic counsellor should be discussed with the patient. The patient may decline a genetics referral for a variety of reasons. A new presentation of malignancy can be an incredibly difficult time for patients who are not only coming to terms with their diagnosis of cancer but also face the prospect of surgery or chemotherapy. Therefore patients may wish to delay a referral to the genetics team. The priority of the managing physician remains the needs of their patient and the treatment of their primary cancer.

Survivorship

All cancer patients require information that is tailored to them, and for patients with hereditary syndromes this includes genetic counselling for patients and their families. For cancer survivors, completion of treatment is a very important milestone, with anxiety about recurrence amongst survivors being well documented. Patients must be advised regarding the benefits of extended routine surveillance and the importance of reporting new symptoms early. Patient education via a knowledgeable healthcare professional and genetic counsellor is of significant benefit in patient care and surveillance. In addition to the concerns that cancer survivors express, those diagnosed with familial syndromes may also have concerns regarding cancer risks in family members, especially children. It is generally accepted that communication about genetic risk information within families is largely the responsibility of family members themselves. Patients who may have already undergone lengthy treatment for an inherited cancer themselves may find this especially difficult and need the support of a knowledgeable genetic counsellor or clinical nurse specialist. The possibility of genetic testing should be discussed with the patient prior to their treatment or as soon as they are sufficiently recovered after treatment has commenced. Patients may have concerns about the psychological or physical impact on their families or financial concerns about insurance and employment. It is important that all these issues are addressed and that patients are made aware of the potential benefits of testing, and in particular of the preventative nature of regular colonoscopy and polypectomy. The existing dynamics within a family may influence the patient's decision and may lead to them declining genetic testing. The psychological impact of a potentially inherited cancer must be assessed. Healthcare professionals should offer counselling that can be accessed via referral to a psychologist or to a counsellor via the patient's GP. It is unlikely that the full psychological impact of diagnosis of an inherited cancer will become evident immediately, and any clinician responsible for the long-term follow-up of this patient group must assess the need for onward referral for psychological support at each follow-up appointment alongside the need for routine surveillance.

Summary

Early identification of familial syndromes in patients with a diagnosis of CRC or gastric cancer is important as it has implications for the overall management of the patient. For early CRC, this management may include prophylactic extended colectomy to prevent the development of metachronous cancers for high-risk patients. The choice of adjuvant chemotherapy can differ depending on aetiology of the CRC, as seen in patients with Stage II MSI disease. For gastric cancers, there are few data to support differing treatments between patients with sporadic disease or hereditary tumours, and systemic anti-cancer treatment is the same for patients with advanced GI cancers regardless of aetiology as per standard of care. However, the identification of hereditary cases will allow for early screening and surveillance of family members. With regard to targeted agents, further research needs to be undertaken to assess the efficacy in this select population. Management of all new diagnoses of CRC and gastric cancer should include multidisciplinary care. Early genetic referral facilitates patient care and allows teams to provide personalised management for patients with cancer.

References

Bang YJ, Van Cutsem E, Feyereislova A, et al. 2010. Trastuzumab in combination with chemotherapy versus chemotherapy alone for treatment of *HER2*-positive advanced gastric or gastro-oesophageal junction cancer (ToGA): a phase 3, open-label, randomised controlled trial. *Lancet* **376**: 687–697.

Becker KF, Keller G, Hoefler H 2000. The use of molecular biology in diagnosis and prognosis of gastric cancer. *Surg Oncol* **9**: 5–11.

Bonjer HJ, Hop WC, Nelson H, et al. 2007. Laparoscopically assisted vs open colectomy for colon cancer: a meta-analysis. *Arch Surg* **142**: 298–303.

Cunningham D, Allum WH, Stenning SP, et al. 2006. Perioperative chemotherapy versus surgery alone for resectable gastroesophageal cancer. *N Engl J Med* **355**: 11–20.

Dunlop MG 2002. Guidance on gastrointestinal surveillance for hereditary non-polyposis colorectal cancer, familial adenomatous polyposis, juvenile polyposis, and Peutz–Jeghers syndrome. *Gut* **51** (Suppl. 5): V21–V27.

Fallik D, Borrini F, Boige V, et al. 2003. Microsatellite instability is a predictive factor of the tumor response to irinotecan in patients with advanced colorectal cancer. *Cancer Res* **63**: 5738–5744.

Figueredo A, Charette ML, Maroun J, et al. 2004. Adjuvant therapy for stage II colon cancer: a systematic review from the Cancer Care Ontario Program in evidence-based care's gastrointestinal cancer disease site group. *J Clin Oncol* **22**: 3395–3407.

Hochwald SN, Kim S, Klimstra DS, et al. 2000. Analysis of 154 actual five-year survivors of gastric cancer. *J Gastrointest Surg* **4**: 520–525.

Lindor NM 2009. Familial colorectal cancer type X: the other half of hereditary nonpolyposis colon cancer syndrome. *Surg Oncol Clin N Am* **18**: 637–645.

Nelson H, Petrelli N, Carlin A, et al. 2001. Guidelines 2000 for colon and rectal cancer surgery. *J Natl Cancer Inst* **93**: 583–596.

Parry S, Win AK, Parry B, et al. 2011. Metachronous colorectal cancer risk for mismatch repair gene mutation carriers: the advantage of more extensive colon surgery. *Gut* **60**: 950–957.

Porschen R, Bermann A, Loffler T, et al. 2001. Fluorouracil plus leucovorin as effective adjuvant chemotherapy in curatively resected stage III colon cancer: results of the trial adjCCA-01. *J Clin Oncol* **19**: 1787–1794.

Ribic CM, Sargent DJ, Moore MJ, et al. 2003. Tumor microsatellite-instability status as a predictor of benefit from fluorouracil-based adjuvant chemotherapy for colon cancer. *N Engl J Med* **349**: 247–257.

Vasen, HF. 2000. Clinical diagnosis and management of hereditary colorectal cancer syndromes. *J Clin Oncol* **18**: 81S–92S.

Chapter 30

Managing hereditary gynaecological cancers

Charlotte Moss, Emma Crosbie and Ana Montes

Introduction to managing hereditary gynaecological cancer

As oncologists treating gynaecological malignancies, we encounter patients with hereditary cancers either when a patient with a known family predisposition is diagnosed with gynaecological cancer or when a patient with a diagnosis of gynaecological cancer has a family history or clinical features suggestive of hereditary cancer. This chapter will review the current management of patients with hereditary ovarian cancer (OC) and endometrial cancer (EC)—the commonest gynaecological malignancies with a well-recognised inherited predisposition. This is an evolving field and we will try to suggest areas where new developments are likely to arise. The learning objectives for Chapter 30 are:

+ to be able to recognise patients with a hereditary predisposition to OC and EC;
+ to be able to understand how hereditary cancers behave;
+ to be able to discuss the way in which the management of hereditary OC and EC differs from sporadic cancer.

Hereditary OC

Treatment of OC requires a multidisciplinary approach. The clinical and pathological characteristics as well as the surgical and chemotherapeutic treatment of *BRCA*-related OC and Lynch syndrome-related OC will be addressed.

BRCA-related OC

Clinical and pathological characteristics of *BRCA*-related OC

+ Age: typically, *BRCA1* carriers are diagnosed at a younger age (average 52 years) compared with *BRCA2* mutation carriers (age 62) and sporadic cases (age 63) (Boyd, 2003).
+ Histology: *BRCA1* and *BRCA2* germline mutations are almost exclusively associated with high-grade serous carcinomas (HGSC). These are rapidly growing, highly aggressive neoplasms with no well-defined precursor lesions because they are usually discovered at an advanced stage. In one large series, 22% of patients with HGSC were carriers of a *BRCA* mutation (Alsop et al., 2012).

- ◆ Primary tumour site: evaluation of risk-reducing salpingo-oophorectomies in women with *BRCA* mutations found that 10% of asymptomatic carriers have early serous cancers and that 50–100% of these are localised to the fallopian tube (Callahan et al., 2007).

- ◆ Metastases: *BRCA1/2* mutation carriers have a higher proportion of visceral metastases (30%) compared with sporadic epithelial OC (22%) (Alsop et al., 2012). In another smaller series, the incidence was 74% compared with 16% for matched non-carriers (Gourley et al., 2010).

Management of *BRCA*-related OC

Response to treatment/prognosis *BRCA* carriers typically present with advanced disease (Stage IIIC or IV), but multiple studies have demonstrated that prognosis is better than for sporadic OC: in multivariate analysis, *BRCA1/2* mutation status was an independent predictor of better overall survival (OS) and progression-free survival (PFS), after adjusting for age, stage and debulking. Compared with sporadic epithelial OC, patients with *BRCA*-related OC were less likely to have disease progression within 6 months of the end of primary treatment compared with those not carrying mutations (14.9% compared with 31.7%) (Alsop et al., 2012). A pooled analysis of 26 observational studies with 1213 *BRCA* carriers and 2666 non-carriers demonstrated a 5-year OS of 36% for non-carriers, 44% for *BRCA1* and 52% for *BRCA2* mutation carriers (Bolton et al., 2012).

Surgery *BRCA*-related OC typically presents late with advanced disease. An elevated level of cancer antigen 125 (CA125) with bilateral complex cystic/solid adnexal masses, ascites and omental disease on computed tomography (CT) scan favours a diagnosis of advanced OC. The standard of care is primary surgical staging and debulking of the tumour, with the aim of achieving complete cytoreduction. For mutation-positive women, late tumour stage and suboptimal tumour debulking were significantly associated with reduced survival in univariate analysis (Alsop et al., 2012).

Where OC is picked up early, surgical cure is much more likely. Patients who present with an isolated ovarian mass have their risk of malignancy index (RMI) calculated. This score is based on ultrasound scan features, CA125 level and the woman's menopausal status (Jacobs et al., 1990). Women with a RMI > 250 are generally considered to have OC until histological assessment proves otherwise. A high index of suspicion is key to the management of young women with a strong family history or known hereditary predisposition to OC. Even in the presence of a low or intermediate RMI, it is appropriate to consider these patients as high risk.

Surgery is conducted through a midline vertical abdominal incision (laparotomy): (1) for adequate exposure of the pelvic and abdominal contents; (2) so that adnexal masses can be removed intact, without spillage of their contents into the abdominal cavity; and (3) to facilitate resection of supracolic omental or other upper abdominal (e.g. diaphragmatic or splenic) disease. Surgical staging implies careful inspection and palpation of all peritoneal and bowel serosal surfaces, excision of suspicious nodules or tumour deposits, as well as random biopsies and peritoneal washings. A total hysterectomy, removal of both tubes and ovaries and infracolic omentectomy are completed as a minimum. The aim is to remove all macroscopically visible tumour since residual disease of 1 cm or more is associated with a poorer outcome (Elattar et al., 2011).

Some young patients who are at intermediate or high risk of OC based on their RMI may not have completed their families at the time of presentation. Total hysterectomy and bilateral salpingo-oophorectomy will render these women infertile. Counselling will be important for these patients, faced with two devastating diagnoses simultaneously (OC and infertility). If disease appears restricted to one ovary, it may be appropriate to carry out modified surgical staging (midline laparotomy, unilateral salpingo-oophorectomy, biopsy of the contralateral ovary, omental biopsy, peritoneal washings and biopsies) and await histological assessment. Where the histology is benign, the patient is still able to complete her family. Where borderline or malignant, completion surgery may be conducted immediately (if disease is advanced or aggressive) or after a short delay (if disease is early stage, borderline or low risk) to enable the patient to complete her family. The need for two operations rather than one may be acceptable for some women if there is a chance that their fertility can be spared for a time. Women with a strong family history or known hereditary predisposition must be regarded as high risk and a two-stage surgical procedure may not be appropriate for them.

Neoadjuvant chemotherapy Two Phase III studies, EORT-NCIC and CHORUS, explored the use of induction, or neoadjuvant chemotherapy in advanced OC. Both found that induction chemotherapy followed by delayed primary surgery was equally effective but carried less surgical morbidity (Kehoe et al., 2013). Patients treated with neoadjuvant chemotherapy are assessed after three cycles at a gynaecological oncology multidisciplinary team meeting (comprising gynaecological oncologists, medical oncologists and radiologists) to decide whether surgery is likely to achieve complete cytoreduction, based on the CT scan images. Occasionally, a laparoscopic assessment of operability may be necessary. If the disease is still not operable, six cycles of chemotherapy are given. A final attempt to incorporate surgical debulking of the tumour is made after the six cycles. Surgery at this time is not evidence-based, but most surgeons would consider it with sufficient response to chemotherapy. Patients who progress through chemotherapy are unlikely to undergo surgery because it is extremely doubtful that it will achieve optimal cytoreduction.

Choice of first-line chemotherapy The improved prognosis seen in women with *BRCA*-related OC seems to be linked to the exquisite sensitivity of *BRCA*-mutated cancer cells to platinum-based chemotherapy, demonstrated in both clinical and pre-clinical studies. *BRCA1* and *BRCA2* play an important role in DNA repair, specifically in the repair of double-strand breaks (DSBs) by homologous recombination (HR). While normal cells can repair DSBs via the error-free gene conversion subpathway of HR, loss of BRCA function forces cells to repair DSBs via non-homologous end-joining or the single-strand annealing subpathway of HR, both of which are error-prone mechanisms leading to genomic instability. BRCA-deficient cells die as a consequence of numerous aberrations or survive accumulating DNA mutations with an increased risk of cancer.

Conventional agents used in the adjuvant and neoadjuvant setting include carboplatin and the combination of carboplatin and paclitaxel given 3-weekly for six cycles. Most guidelines recommend the use of combination chemotherapy, but in patients for whom toxicity or poor performance status prevents the use of combination therapy, single-agent carboplatin is recommended. The results of the ICON 3 study support this recommendation (ICON Group, 2002). A retrospective analysis comparing the outcome of *BRCA*-related OC patients with sporadic OC found improved outcomes for the *BRCA*-related cohort. There was no apparent difference in outcome between first-line treatment with paclitaxel and platinum or single-agent platinum (Vencken et al., 2011).

Follow-up of *BRCA*-related OC

Patients are routinely monitored with clinical review and measurement of serum CA125. Imaging is performed mainly to investigate symptoms or persistent maker elevation. Routine imaging is not advised in the absence of symptoms or marker progression.

In *BRCA1/2* mutation carriers there is evidence of increased sensitivity to diagnostic radiation, therefore the use of imaging techniques involving non-ionising radiation, such as MRI, for abdominal surveillance in young women with *BRCA1/2* mutations seems reasonable (Pijpe et al., 2012).

Treatment of recurrent disease in *BRCA*-related OC

Chemotherapy *BRCA*-related OC responds better to chemotherapy treatment than sporadic epithelial OC (response rates to second-line platinum-based chemotherapy were 64.6% versus 58.6% ($P = 0.07$) in a prospective, population-based observational study). Higher response rates to second-line non-platinum-based treatment were also seen in patients with mutations versus non-carriers (52.9% versus 21.7%; $P = 0.05$) (Alsop et al., 2012).

The choice of agents should be based on the platinum-free interval, patient fitness and toxicity from previous regimens. In the absence of clear progression during platinum treatment, it is reasonable to use platinum alone or in combination in *BRCA* carriers. The only prospective data suggest that patients with *BRCA*-related OC are likely to undertake more lines of chemotherapy than those with sporadic epithelial OC: 30/134 (22%) of patients with *BRCA*-related OC had third-line chemotherapy compared with 98/700 (14%) mutation-negative women. *BRCA*-related OC remains more responsive to platinum agents with repeated exposure: 20/30 (66%) of *BRCA*-related OC patients had a CA125 response to third-line platinum chemotherapy while 37/98 (37%) of patients with sporadic epithelial OC responded (Alsop et al., 2012).

Synthetic lethality/PARP inhibition Poly ADP-ribose polymerase (PARP) plays an essential role in the repair of single-stranded DNA breaks, through the base excision repair pathway. PARP inhibition leads to the formation of DSBs that cannot be accurately repaired in tumours with homologous recombination deficiency, a concept known as synthetic lethality (Ashworth, 2008). PARP inhibitors were originally tested as chemosensitisers in combination with chemotherapy and more recently in BRCA-deficient cancers. Although PARP inhibitors have shown some encouraging results in recent trials in patients with *BRCA*-related OC (Audeh et al., 2010), they are still investigational agents and are not routinely available in the clinic.

The first study of olaparib in a *BRCA*-enriched population was conducted as a Phase I study, initially in unselected solid tumours and subsequently enriched for *BRCA*-mutated cancers. Sixty patients were treated; the maximum tolerated dose was 400 mg twice daily. Objective anti-tumour activity was noted only in patients with *BRCA1/2* mutations and in one patient with a strong family history of *BRCA* mutation (Fong, 2009). The promising activity of olaparib in patients with *BRCA1*- and *BRCA2*-related OC was confirmed in a Phase II study: 57 assessable patients with *BRCA1* and *BRCA2* mutations, treated at two dose levels (400 and 100 mg twice daily), showed response rates of 33% and 12.5%, respectively. Toxicity was mild; the only reported grade 3 toxic effects were nausea (7%) and leucopenia (5%) (Audeh et al., 2010).

Another Phase II study compared olaparib with liposomal doxorubicin in patients with platinum-resistant *BRCA*-related OC. Although the activity of a PARP inhibitor was confirmed, no difference was seen in progression free survival (PFS) (Kaye et al., 2012).

Exploiting 'BRCA-ness' It is thought that up to 50% of women with high-grade serous OC are deficient in HR as a result of germline or somatically acquired *BRCA1/2* mutations, epigenetic inactivation of *BRCA1* or defects in the HR pathway independent of *BRCA1/2*. The resultant phenotype is described as '*BRCA*-ness' and has similarities to that seen in patients with germline mutations in *BRCA1/2* (i.e. high morphological grade, aggressive clinical behaviour, platinum sensitivity retained through multiple relapses). Microarray studies in serous epithelial OC have identified a *BRCA*-ness gene expression profile which demonstrates responsiveness to both platinum-based chemotherapy and PARP inhibitors (Rigakos and Razis, 2012).

The largest study to date of PARP inhibitors in OC used a population enriched for *BRCA*-ness. In a placebo-controlled Phase II study evaluating maintenance treatment with olaparib in patients with platinum-sensitive, high-grade serous ovarian cancer, 136 were assigned to olaparib and 129 to placebo; median PFS was significantly longer with olaparib with a median of 8.4 versus 4.8 months (Ledermann et al., 2012).

A recent study assessed response to third-line chemotherapy in patients without a germline *BRCA* mutation: 25% of patients who responded to third-line chemotherapy had detectable somatic *BRCA* mutations, compared with 6% of unselected HGSC (Alsop et al., 2012).

The concepts of synthetic lethality and *BRCA*-ness have led to numerous clinical trials: because of the higher prevalence of *BRCA*-ness it is hoped the results may apply to the wider population. Several PARP inhibitors are under investigation (veliparib, rucaparib, niraparib, etc.) in addition to trabectedin, a DNA-binding agent which binds the minor groove of DNA, slowing progression of cells through the cell cycle; pre-clinical studies demonstrate that its cytotoxic effect is greatly enhanced by loss of BRCA (D'Incalci et al., 2003). It is important to appreciate that this is an evolving area and new data are emerging constantly.

BRCA genetic testing for women with high-grade serous OC

The significant activity of PARP inhibitors in *BRCA* mutation carriers has focused attention on *BRCA1/2* testing early in disease management, though this is not performed routinely at present. Once these agents are licensed and available for general clinical use, there will be a clear indication for *BRCA* mutation testing. However, as discussed, *BRCA* positivity affects an individual's prognosis, may provide access to additional therapeutic agents via clinical trials, may guide treatment choice and imaging modality for follow-up and has implications for cancer risk in family members. We therefore propose that women are routinely referred for genetic counselling and genetic testing, either during or soon after their primary systemic therapy is completed, so that this information is available in a timely fashion for inclusion in decisions about subsequent treatment strategies in the event of a relapse.

Lynch syndrome-related OC

Clinical and pathological characteristics of LS-related OC

The following characteristics are typical:

◆ Age: up to 10% of all OC in patients aged 50 or younger may be associated with LS (Ketabi et al., 2011). Approximately 30% of LS-associated OC is diagnosed before the age of 35 (Watson et al., 2008). Ovarian clear cell carcinoma (CCC), particularly in younger patients, appears to be associated most strongly with LS.

◆ Histology: the majority of OCs in LS patients are of non-serous histology; most are endometrioid, CCC or undifferentiated carcinomas (Ketabi et al., 2011). Borderline ovarian tumours do not seem to be associated with LS (Watson, 2001). Studies to date indicate that high levels of Microsatellite Instability (MSI) and associated loss of mismatch repair (MMR) gene expression are found more frequently in OC with non-serous ovarian histology, particularly endometrioid and related clear cell types, than in serous carcinomas, which are more common in the general population (Pal et al., 2008; Murphy and Wentzensen, 2011). Atypical endometriosis is the precursor lesion of endometrioid and CCC of the ovary, and a direct transition from ovarian atypical endometriosis to endometrioid or CCC has been described in 15–32% of cases. In cases of endometrioid carcinoma associated with endometriosis, common genetic alterations have been encountered in the adjacent endometriosis, atypical endometriosis and adenocarcinoma (Fuseya et al., 2012).

◆ Stage at presentation: patients with LS are diagnosed at an early stage, with approximately 75% presenting in Stage I. Similarly, 75% are unilateral (Grindedal et al., 2010).

◆ Association with other cancers: in 25% of cases of OC there is synchronous EC, often at an early stage (Kim et al., 2011).

Management of LS-related OC

Treatment of OC associated with LS is similar to that for sporadic disease. Most patients present with a large unilateral ovarian mass; the most important prognostic factor is complete surgical debulking. As these cancers tend to be less chemosensitive, than sporadic OC, it is of utmost importance to achieve complete surgical clearance.

Patients with LS-related OC tend to present at an earlier stage with non-serous histology. A European retrospective study of 11 centres which examined survival in patients with a pathogenic MMR mutation who had a diagnosis of OC suggested that OC in LS had a better prognosis than *BRCA*-related OC or OC in the general population (Grindedal et al., 2010). A small study showed no difference in outcome between LS-related OC and controls with sporadic OC (Crijnen et al., 2005).

When a new OC is diagnosed in a LS family, genetic testing is indicated. In addition, patients fulfilling the Amsterdam II criteria should be tested (described in Chapter 9). We would suggest that patients with OC with either endometrioid or clear cell histology presenting at a young age (under 50) are questioned thoroughly for a family history. Genetic counselling, screening and risk-reducing treatment should be offered to patients with histology suggestive of a MMR mutation.

Hereditary EC

This can be classified in two types:

1 Familial site-specific EC. The clustering of EC alone may constitute a separate entity. Eight per cent of this group have been reported to have germline MMR mutations. This mutation rate is lower than that of patients with LS-associated with EC, of whom 15% show MMR mutations. The difference in MMR mutation rate therefore suggests the existence of different genetic alteration pathways in familial site-specific EC.

2 LS-related EC. More than half of LS patients present with a gynaecological malignancy, usually EC, as the sentinel cancer (Lu et al., 2005). The risk for subsequent EC in women with LS presenting first with colorectal cancer (CRC) has been estimated at 26% within 10 years of the initial CRC diagnosis (Obermair, 2010). The frequency of LS-associated germline mutations in EC has been estimated at 1.8–2.1%, which is similar to that in CRC.

Lynch syndrome-related EC

Clinical and pathological characteristics of LS-related EC

The following characteristics are typical:

◆ Age at diagnosis: initial studies performed in high-risk families found an average age of diagnosis of approximately 48 years; in population-based studies, a later age of diagnosis (62 years) has been found (Hampel et al., 2005).

◆ Body mass index (BMI): most endometrioid adenocarcinomas in young patients are associated with oestrogen excess and patients are often obese or overweight. However,

LS patients with EC tend to have a low BMI (Shih et al., 2011). Recent studies in women aged under 50 have not confirmed this observation; therefore the strength of this association is unclear (Ring et al., 2013).

- Synchronous cancers: several studies have reported an association between LS and synchronous endometrioid carcinomas of the ovary and endometrium. There are a small number of reported cases of synchronous uterine endometrioid carcinoma and ovarian CCC in women with MMR protein defects (Kim et al., 2011).
- Histology: EC show a wide spectrum of histological subtypes. Endometrioid carcinomas are the most common, but non-endometrioid carcinomas also occur; including serous carcinoma, CCC and carcinosarcoma (Broaddus et al., 2006).

Management of LS-related EC

Response to treatment/prognosis The endometrioid carcinomas associated with LS are usually well to moderately differentiated, present at an early stage and have favourable clinical outcomes. A survival advantage similar to that in LS-related CRC has been reported in LS-related EC (Maxwell et al., 2001). There are no large studies investigating the effect of chemotherapy and radiotherapy in patients with LS. Pre-clinical data and limited observational studies suggest that deficient DNA MMR can modify the responses to chemotherapy and radiation (Resnick et al., 2010).

Surgery EC usually presents at an early stage following the onset of post-menopausal bleeding. The mainstay of treatment for early stage disease is hysterectomy and bilateral salpingo-oophorectomy. Traditionally this was via a midline laparotomy or transverse lower abdominal incision, but open surgery has now been largely superseded by the laparoscopic approach. Compared with open surgery, laparoscopic hysterectomy is associated with a faster post-operative recovery, reduced length of hospital stay and an earlier return to normal activities (Galaal et al., 2012). Intra-operative complications and post-operative morbidity rates are similar in open and laparoscopic approaches. Laparoscopic surgery is challenging for women with extensive adhesions from previous pelvic surgery, reduced vaginal access and/or a bulky uterus and in the presence of extreme obesity (Crosbie et al., 2010). It may be appropriate to perform a laparoscopic assessment before embarking on definitive surgical treatment. Newer surgical techniques, including robot-assisted laparoscopic hysterectomy, are undergoing evaluation but there is insufficient evidence at present to recommend robotic surgery over standard 'straight stick' laparoscopy.

When the disease is confined to the uterus, surgery for EC is generally curative. This is reflected in the excellent overall 5-year survival rate (85%) for EC. In the presence of advanced disease, or when histological parameters indicate a biologically aggressive tumour, adjuvant treatment with radiotherapy and/or chemotherapy may be recommended. Histological hallmarks of intermediate- or high-risk disease include non-endometrioid histology (Type 2 tumours, e.g. clear cell or serous subtypes), moderate or poorly differentiated disease (Grade 2 or 3) and evidence of tumour spread within vascular and/or lymphatic channels (lymphovascular space invasion). In this setting, adjuvant radiotherapy has been shown to reduce the risk of central pelvic recurrence but overall survival is not improved (Kong et al., 2012).

References

Alsop K, Fereday S, Meldrum C, et al. 2012. *BRCA* mutation frequency and patterns of treatment response in *BRCA* mutation-positive women with ovarian cancer: a report from the Australian Ovarian Cancer Study Group. *J Clin Oncol* **31**: 2654–2663.

Ashworth A 2008. A synthetic lethal therapeutic approach: poly(ADP) ribose polymerase inhibitors for the treatment of cancers deficient in DNA double-strand break repair. *J Clin Oncol* **26**: 3785–3790.

Audeh MW, Carmichael J, Penson RT, et al. 2010. Oral poly(ADP-ribose) polymerase inhibitor olaparib in patients with *BRCA1* or *BRCA2* mutations and recurrent ovarian cancer: a proof-of-concept trial. *Lancet* **376**: 245–251.

Bolton KL, Chevenix-Trench G, Goh C, et al. 2012. Association between *BRCA1* and *BRCA2* mutations and survival in women with invasive epithelial ovarian cancer. *J Am Med Assoc* **307**: 382–389.

Boyd J 2003. Specific keynote: hereditary ovarian cancer: what we know. *Gynecol Oncol* **88**: S8–S10 (discussion S11–S13).

Broaddus RR, Lynch HT, Chen L-M, et al. 2006. Pathologic features of endometrial carcinoma associated with HNPCC. *Cancer* **106**: 87–94.

Callahan MJ, Crum CP, Medeiros F, et al. 2007. Primary fallopian tube malignancies in *BRCA*-positive women undergoing surgery for ovarian cancer risk reduction. *J Clin Oncol* **25**: 3985–3990.

Crijnen TE, Janssen-Heijnen ML, Gelderblom H, et al. 2005. Survival of patients with ovarian cancer due to a mismatch repair defect. *Fam Cancer* **4**: 301–305.

Crosbie EJ, Zwahlen M, Kitchener HC, et al. 2010. Body mass index, hormone replacement therapy, and endometrial cancer risk: a meta-analysis. *Cancer Epidemiol Biomarkers Prev* **19**: 3119–3130.

D'Incalci M, Colombo T, Ubezio P, et al. 2003. The combination of yondelis and cisplatin is synergistic against human tumor xenografts. *Eur J Cancer* **39**: 1920–1926.

Elattar A, Bryant A, Winter-Roach BA, et al. 2011. Optimal primary surgical treatment for advanced epithelial ovarian cancer. *Cochrane Database Syst Rev* **8**: CD007565.

Fong PC, Boss DS, Yap TA, et al. 2009. Inhibition of poly(ADP-ribose) polymerase in tumours from *BRCA* mutation carriers. *N Engl J Med* **361**: 123–134.

Fuseya C, Horiuchi A, Hayashi A, et al. 2012. Involvement of pelvic inflammation—related mismatch repair abnormalities and microsatellite instability in the malignant transformation of ovarian endometriosis. *Hum Pathol* **43**: 1964–1972.

Galaal K, Bryant A, Fisher AD, et al. 2012. Laparoscopy versus laparotomy for the management of early stage endometrial cancer. *Cochrane Database Syst Rev* **9**: CD006655.

Grindedal EM, Renkonen-Sinisalo L, Vasen H, et al. 2010. Survival in women with MMR mutations and ovarian cancer: a multicentre study in Lynch syndrome kindreds. *J Med Genet* **47**: 99–102.

Gourley C, Michie CO, Roxburgh P, et al. 2010. Increased incidence of visceral metastases in Scottish patients with *BRCA1/2*-defective ovarian cancer: an extension of the ovarian *BRCA*ness phenotype. *J Clin Oncol* **28**: 2505–2511.

Hampel H, Stephens JA, Pukkala E, et al. 2005. Cancer risk in hereditary nonpolyposis colorectal cancer syndrome: later age of onset. *Gastroenterology* **129**: 415–421.

International Collaborative Ovarian Neoplasm Group 2002. Paclitaxel plus carboplatin versus standard chemotherapy with either single-agent carboplatin or cyclophosphamide, doxorubicin, and cisplatin in women with ovarian cancer: the ICON3 randomised trial. *Lancet* **360**: 505–515.

Jacobs I, Oram D, Fairbanks J, et al. 1990. A risk of malignancy index incorporating CA 125, ultrasound and menopausal status for the accurate preoperative diagnosis of ovarian cancer. *Br J Obstet Gynaecol* **97**: 922–929.

Kaye SB, Lubinski J, Matulonis U, et al. 2012. Phase II, open-label, randomized, multicenter study comparing the efficacy and safety of olaparib, a poly (ADP—ribose) polymerase inhibitor, and pegylated liposomal doxorubicin in patients with *BRCA1* or *BRCA2* mutations and recurrent ovarian cancer. *J Clin Oncol* **30**: 372–379.

Kehoe S, Hook J, Nankivell M, et al. 2013. Chemotherapy or upfront surgery for newly diagnosed advanced ovarian cancer: results for MRC CHORUS trial. *J Clin Oncol* **31** (Suppl.): abstract 5500.

Ketabi Z, Bartuma K, Bernstein I, et al. 2011. Ovarian cancer linked to Lynch syndrome typically presents as early-onset, non-serous epithelial tumors. *Gynecol Oncol* **121**: 462–465.

Kim MK, Song SY, Do IG, et al. 2011. Synchronous gynecologic malignancy and preliminary results of Lynch syndrome. *J Gynecol Oncol* **22**: 233–238.

Kong A, Johnson N, Kitchener HC, et al. 2012. Adjuvant radiotherapy for stage I endometrial cancer: an updated Cochrane systematic review and meta-analysis. *J Natl Cancer Inst* **104**: 1625–1634.

Ledermann J, Harter P, Gourley C, et al. 2012. Olaparib maintenance therapy in platinum-sensitive relapsed ovarian cancer. *N Engl J Med* **366**: 1382–1392.

Lu KH, Dinh M, Kohlmann W, et al. 2005. Gynecologic cancer as a 'sentinel cancer' for women with hereditary nonpolyposis colorectal cancer syndrome. *Obstet Gynecol* **105**: 569–574.

Maxwell GL, Risinger JI, Alvarez AA, et al. 2001. Favorable survival associated with microsatellite instability in endometrioid endometrial cancers. *Obstet Gynecol* **97**: 417–422.

Murphy MA and Wentzensen N 2011. Frequency of mismatch repair deficiency in ovarian cancer: a systematic review. *Int J Cancer* **129**: 1914–1922.

Obermair A, Youlden DR, Young JP, et al. 2010. Risk of endometrial cancer for women diagnosed with HNPCC-related colorectal carcinoma. *Int J Cancer* **127**: 2678–2684.

Pal T, Permuth-Wey J, Sellers TA, et al. 2008. A review of the clinical relevance of mismatch-repair deficiency in ovarian cancer. *Cancer* **113**: 733–772.

Pijpe A, Andrieu N, Easton DF, et al. 2012. Exposure to diagnostic radiation and risk of breast cancer among carriers of *BRCA1/2* mutations: retrospective cohort study (GENE-RAD-RISK). *Br Med J* **345**: e5660.

Resnick KE, Frankel WL, Morrison CD, et al. 2010. Mismatch repair status and outcomes after adjuvant therapy in patients with surgically staged endometrial cancer. *Gynecol Oncol* **117**: 234–238.

Rigakos G and Razis E 2012. *BRCA*ness: finding the Achilles heel in ovarian cancer. *Oncologist* **17**: 956–962.

Ring KL, Connor EV, Atkins KA, et al. 2013. Women 50 years or younger with endometrial cancer: the argument for universal mismatch repair screening and potential for targeted therapeutics. *Int J Gynecol Cancer* **23**: 853–860.

Shih KK, Garg K, Levine DA, et al. 2011. Clinicopathologic significance of DNA mismatch repair protein defects and endometrial cancer in women 40 years of age and younger. *Gynecol Oncol* **123**: 88–94.

Vencken PM, Kriege M, Hoogwerf D, et al. 2011. Chemosensitivity and outcome of *BRCA1*- and *BRCA2*-associated ovarian cancer patients after first-line chemotherapy compared with sporadic ovarian cancer patients. *Ann Oncol* **22**: 1346–1352.

Watson P and Lynch HT, 2001. Cancer in mismatch repair gene mutation carriers. *Fam Cancer* **1**: 57–60.

Watson P, Vasen HF, Mecklin JP, et al. 2008. The risk of extra-colonic, extra-endometrial cancer in the Lynch syndrome. *Int J Cancer* **123**: 444–449.

Chapter 31

Managing hereditary cancer. Summary

Patricia Webb and Lorraine Robinson

Introduction to section 7 summary

Section 7 discusses the difference that identifying a cancer-predisposing gene mutation can make to the management of patients with a diagnosis of hereditary cancer, highlighting the importance of identifying cancer patients who may benefit from genetic assessment and considering the benefits, disadvantages and challenges of this for patients and health professionals.

Until recently patients with cancer have tended to be referred for genetics assessment after completing cancer treatment. Advances in genetic technology and cancer management have resulted in the involvement of genetics services much closer to diagnosis, affecting decision-making both about cancer treatment and the management of future cancer risks. Although only 5–10% of cancer is due to a high-risk single gene mutation, identifying those who might carry a mutation is important for the patient with cancer as well as for 'at-risk' relatives.

It is important that health professionals specialising in cancer care are able to identify patients who may be at risk of hereditary cancer; that they have sufficient knowledge of the genes that may be involved and the potential impact of a gene mutation on cancer treatment and future cancer risks; and that they are able to facilitate decision-making about whether or not to undergo a genetics assessment and know how to refer cancer patients for a genetics opinion. Understanding the possibility that an individual with breast cancer may exceed the 10% risk threshold, therefore qualifying for genetic testing (without a family history), is one of the key learning objectives of this section.

Chapter 27. Managing hereditary cancer. Introduction

Chapter 27 reflects on the research into the psychological impact of genetic testing at cancer diagnosis and acknowledges the practical challenges for patients and health professionals in genetics and cancer care of managing genetic risk assessment and testing at diagnosis. The importance of close collaboration, multidisciplinary working and robust pathways between genetics and cancer care are emphasised.

Guided activities for Chapter 27

- Select a patient and family for whom identification of carrier status is likely or confirmed. Produce a plan of care and support with some idea of timelines and how they interact with strategic parts of the patient journey, from diagnosis, through treatments and to the possibilities for the future. Support includes information-giving and eliciting information through history-taking. Advanced communication skills are required for this. Further help with this may be found in the Further resources (in particular <http://www.sageandthymetraining.org.uk>). If you do not have direct access to patients in this category, talk to colleagues who may be willing to share unidentified/anonymised patient histories for you to work on. If possible discuss your plan with someone working regularly in the field.

◆ Do you routinely speak to your cancer patients about family history? Consider how you might approach this and work with a colleague to make sure you are able to raise and discuss this issue in a sensitive and informed way.

◆ If you are unsure about how to refer a patient with cancer for a genetics assessment, contact your local genetics centre to find out.

Chapters 28–30. Managing hereditary cancer

Chapters 28–30 discuss the management of patients with specific cancers once a cancer-predisposing mutation has been identified.

Confirmed carrier status already affects early decisions regarding the choice and extent of surgery for patients with breast cancer. Extra time for confirmatory testing for carrier status is offered by cytotoxic sequencing. Decisions at this stage are important; and patients and families need time and may feel bombarded by new information of a somewhat technical nature. The psychological impact of confirmation of carrier status on individuals may be under-reported. Support strategies for patients need to be explored at this stage. Details of therapy sequencing strategies in breast cancer treatment are provided in Chapter 27. Examples of the impact of carrier status on treatment decisions include eligibility for novel target agents used in trials and for metastatic relapse.

Guided activities for Chapters 28–30

◆ Produce a grid of the differences between the various mutations and their implications for patients with cancer. This will provide you with a quick reminder of key features for future patients.

◆ With a colleague consider the benefits and challenges of offering genetic testing at cancer diagnosis, relating this to your own area of specialty.

◆ Write a narrative of how you would explain the impact that a genetic mutation might have on cancer treatment in your own area of specialty—draw a diagram to help with this. Produce your own pack of visual aids to help explanations in the future.

◆ Oncology treatment and the diagnosis of a hereditary syndrome can have an impact on fertility. Patients may need information regarding assisted conception units and referrals made as appropriate. Potential delays in commencement of treatment may be considered. Consider how you might discuss this sensitive situation in young, fertile individuals.

Further resources for Chapters 28–30

Alsop K, Fereday S, Meldrum C, et al. 2012. *BRCA* mutation frequency and patterns of treatment response in BRCA mutation—positive women with ovarian cancer: a report from the Australian Ovarian Cancer Study Group. *J Clin Oncol* 31: 2654–2663.

Lalloo F, Kerr B, Friedman J, Evans G 2005. *Risk assessment and management in cancer genetics.* Oxford: Oxford University Press.

NICE (National Institute for Health and Care Excellence) 2013. *Familial breast cancer: classification and care of people at risk of familial breast cancer and management of breast cancer and related risks in people with a family history of breast cancer.* NICE Clinical Guideline 164. London: National Institute for Health and Care Excellence.

Parry S, Win AK, Parry B, et al. 2011. Metachronous colorectal cancer risk for mismatch repair gene mutation carriers: the advantage of more extensive colon surgery. *Gut* 60: 950–957.

Sclich-Bakker KJ, ten Kroode HH, Ausems MG 2006. A literature review of the psychological impact of genetic testing on breast cancer patients. *Patient Educ Counsel* 62: 13–20.

University of Hospital of South Manchester. *Sage and Thyme training: how to listen to patients/dealing with patients in distress.* Details at: <http://sageandthymetraining. org.uk> (last accessed 24 August 2013).

Genetic counselling and supporting individuals with a family history of cancer

Chapter 32

Genetic counselling and supporting individuals with a family history of cancer. Introduction

Chris Jacobs

Introduction to genetic counselling and supporting individuals with a family history of cancer

Once a patient has been identified as being at high risk of cancer, either through assessment of their family history or by genetic testing, many challenging issues can be raised for the individual themselves and for their family. Coming to terms with the feeling of increased risk can affect decisions about risk management and information that is communicated to the wider family. It is helpful for health professionals in primary and secondary care to be aware of the psychosocial, ethical and cultural issues and information and support needs of individuals and families at high risk in order to help them to prepare for their genetic counselling appointment and to provide ongoing support. The learning objectives for Chapter 32 are:

+ to become aware of the principles underpinning genetic counselling for a genetic predisposition to cancer;

+ to consider the implications of a genetic predisposition to cancer and/or a cancer family history on the wider family;

+ to be able to discuss the information and support needs for patients with a genetic predisposition to cancer and/or a cancer family history.

The process of genetic counselling

Genetic counselling is a relatively new area of expertise, first introduced by Sheldon Reed in 1974 (Resta, 2006). Much of the early genetic counselling work involved diagnosing chromosome disorders and children with dysmorphic syndromes and counselling individuals with a family history of hereditary disorders based on empirical evidence.

The identification of specific genes predisposing to conditions, such as Huntington's disease (HD), in the early 1990s heralded a new era for healthcare, enabling pre-symptomatic testing of unaffected individuals for known genetic conditions. The availability of genetic testing necessitated changes to the way in which genetic counselling was approached and a protocol was drawn up for the genetic counselling of patients considering pre-symptomatic testing for HD (Craufurd and Tyler, 1992). This ensured that healthy individuals were provided with full information, an opportunity to explore their motivation for and implications of testing, an extended period of reflection and informed consent. Although modified over time, the HD protocol has formed the basis of current practice in the genetic counselling of affected and unaffected patients about hereditary cancer and other genetic conditions.

The concept of non-directiveness (i.e. not recommending a course of action and leaving the decision and responsibility to the counsellee) has been the central ethos of genetic counselling for over 30 years. However, there has been debate about whether non-directiveness continues to be relevant to genetic counselling, particularly in cancer where measures to reduce risk are available, and whether in fact addressing psychosocial issues should replace non-directiveness as the central ethos (Biesecker, 2003; Weil, 2003). The US National Society of Genetic Counselors defines genetic counselling as: 'the process of helping people understand and adapt to the medical, psychological and familial implications of genetic contributions to disease'. The definition goes onto explain that the process 'integrates interpretation of family histories to assess the chance of disease occurrence or recurrence, education about inheritance, resources and research and counselling to promote informed choices and adaptation to the risk of the condition' (Resta et al., 2006).

The provision of genetic counselling in the UK and Europe

Genetic counselling in the UK and the Netherlands (and North America and Australasia) is provided by medical and non-medical health professionals. Clinical geneticists are medical doctors who have trained and specialised in medical genetics and may have subspecialty expertise. Genetic counsellors are health professionals with training and expertise in clinical genetics and genetic counselling. In the UK genetic counsellors are registered by the Genetic Counsellor Registration Board (GCRB) (<http://www.gcrb.org.uk>). There are two routes to entry into the profession: attainment of an accredited master of science degree in genetic counselling, or a first or masters degree plus a professional qualification as a registered nurse or midwife with training in counselling skills and human genetics. To become a registered genetic counsellor requires employment within a clinical genetics service, evidence of counselling supervision and submission of a portfolio. Re-registration is required every 5 years.

The European Board of Medical Genetics (EBMG) (<https://www.eshg.org/471.0.html>) has recently been established under the auspices of the European Society of Human Genetics (ESHG) with responsibility for developing systems of certification and recertification for health professionals working in genetics within Europe. A code of professional practice has been agreed and competencies developed for genetic nurses and counsellors, clinical geneticists and clinical laboratory geneticists (Skirton et al., 2010). A European register for genetic nurses and counsellors is now in place.

Evaluating the effectiveness of genetic counselling

Evaluating the effectiveness of healthcare is vitally important for service users, commissioners and policy-makers. Although there are a number of validated outcome measures to evaluate a range of different aspects within clinical genetics services, such as understanding, satisfaction, anxiety and depression, quality of life and risk perception (Hilgart et al., 2012), there is no single measure of the benefits of genetic counselling to patients.

The measure of 'perceived personal control' (Berkenstadt et al., 1999) captures the ability to make decisions about family life, but only for the patient themselves. Yet the family is central to genetic counselling. It has been suggested that the concept of perceived personal control could be further developed to include a new construct of 'empowerment', enabling an individual from a family with a genetic condition to make informed decisions, have sufficient information, make use of health and social care services, and have hope for the future for themselves, their family and their future descendants (McAllister et al., 2011).

The concept of family in relation to genetics

Identifying cancer susceptibility inevitably involves the wider family. For health professionals working in primary and secondary care, the focus tends to be on the individual rather than the family and so the concept of family in relation to genetics and family history may not be familiar. Within western culture the term 'family' has many different meanings (Richards, 1996). In the context of genetics, the family refers to biological relatives connected by 'blood line'. Yet the western concept of family is complex and fluid in nature, relying less on biological or traditional legal ties and more on non-traditional legal ties, interpersonal commitments and medical advances in reproduction (Bylund et al., 2010). These changes in family structure and culture inevitably impact on family dynamics and communication, leading to challenges for patients and health professionals, both in gathering confidential medical information about family members and in communicating genetic information to those at risk.

Family communication about hereditary cancer

Sharing information within a family once a cancer-predisposing gene mutation has been identified generally falls to the individual with cancer who receives the initial genetic test result (Hayat Roshanai et al., 2010). In general, families prefer information to be communicated to relatives by the patient than by the clinician (Forrest et al., 2003) and most families do share this information (Hayat Roshanai et al., 2010).

There are several well-documented barriers to family communication (Gaff et al., 2007; Chivers Seymour et al., 2010). Barriers include lack of close relationship (Forrest et al., 2003), family culture (Dancyger et al., 2011), reluctance to upset relatives (Hughes et al., 2002), youth or emotional readiness of relatives (Dancyger et al., 2010) lack of understanding (Forrest et al., 2007) or perceived risks and benefits of the information (Gallo et al., 2009) and personal beliefs about the causes of genetic illness (Michie et al., 2003). Several studies have shown that genetic information is more commonly shared with first- and second-degree relatives, in particular with sisters (Armstrong et al., 2012) or with siblings and children (Claes et al., 2003).

If a gene mutation is identified, the patient may be provided with a copy of the genetic test result and/or a letter for relatives explaining how to access genetic counselling, testing and screening. It can be helpful to include a copy of this information if the relative is subsequently referred for genetic counselling.

Information and support

Access to sound, reliable and evidence-based information is extremely important for people with a genetic predisposition and/or a family history of cancer. The need to provide this information for women at risk of breast cancer has been identified in several studies (Iredale et al., 2003; Werner-Lin, 2008) and highlighted by the National Institute for Health and Care Excellence (NICE) guidelines for familial breast cancer (NICE, 2013). These guidelines emphasise that in addition to individualised tailored information, patients need access to standard information that should not contradict messages from other service providers and is commonly agreed across localities. The need for robust patient information applies across all types of hereditary cancer. In response to this evidence, online story banks have been established and standardised patient information has been developed by several of the cancer charities with input from genetics health professionals.

In addition, patients require access to professional and peer support in identifying a family history of cancer, coming to terms with the outcome of genetic testing and decision-making about genetic testing and risk management. Some genetics services may provide access to therapeutic counselling or peer support. In addition, professional and peer support is provided for patients and families by the voluntary sector in the form of telephone helplines, online chat rooms and patient support groups.

Summary

Genetics health professionals have an important role in the provision of genetic counselling, support and information to patients and families with a genetic predisposition and/or a cancer family history. The issues raised by genetic testing for cancer susceptibility are discussed in Chapter 33. In Chapter 34, the psychosocial and support needs of individuals with a cancer family history are addressed in more detail. Ethical and cultural issues surrounding decision-making and risk management of patients and families with a genetic predisposition to cancer and/or a cancer family history are addressed in Chapter 35.

References

Armstrong K, Putt M, Halbert CH, et al. 2012. The influence of health care policies and health care system distrust on willingness to undergo genetic testing. *Med Care* **50**: 381–387.

Barsevick AM 2008. Intention to communicate *BRCA1/BRCA2* genetic test results to the family. *J Fam Psychol* **22**: 303–312.

Berkenstadt M, Shiloh S, Barkai G, et al. 1999. Perceived personal control (PPC): a new concept in measuring outcome of genetic counseling. *Am J Med Genet* **82**: 53–59.

Biesecker B 2003. Back to the future of genetic counseling: commentary of 'Psychosocial genetic counseling in the post–non directive era'. *J Genet Counsel* **12**: 213–217.

Bylund CL, Galvin KM, Gaff CL 2010. Principles of family communication. In: *Family communication about genetics. Theory and practice* (ed. CL Gaff and CL Bylund), pp. 3–17. Oxford: Oxford University Press.

Chivers Seymour K, Addington-Hall J, Lucassen AM, Foster CL 2010. What facilitates or impedes family communication following genetic testing for cancer risk? A systematic review and meta-synthesis of primary qualitative research. *J Genet Counsel* **19**: 330–342.

Claes E, Evers-Kiebooms G, Boogaerts A, et al. 2003. Communication with close and distant relatives in the context of genetic testing for hereditary breast and ovarian cancer in cancer patients. *Am J Med Genet A* **116A**: 11–19.

Craufurd D and Tyler A 1992. Predictive testing for Huntington's disease: protocol of the UK Huntington's Prediction Consortium. *J Med Genet* **29**: 915–918.

Dancyger C, Smith JA, Jacobs C, et al. 2010. Comparing family members' motivations and attitudes towards genetic testing for hereditary breast and ovarian cancer: a qualitative analysis. *Eur J Hum Genet* **18**: 1289–1295.

Dancyger C, Wiseman M, Jacobs C, et al. 2011. Communicating *BRCA1/2* genetic test results within the family: a qualitative analysis. *Psychol Health* **26**: 1018–1035.

Forrest K, Simpson SA, Wilson BJ, et al. 2003. To tell or not to tell: barriers and facilitators in family communication about genetic risk. *Clin Genet* **64**: 317–326.

Forrest LE, Delatycki MB, Skene L, Aitken M 2007. Communicating genetic information in families—a review of guidelines and position papers. *Eur J Hum Genet* **15**: 612–618.

Gaff CL, Clarke AJ, Atkinson P, et al. 2007. Process and outcome in communication of genetic information within families: a systematic review. *Eur J Hum Genet*, **15**: 999–1011.

Gallo AM, Angst DB, Knafl KA 2009. Disclosure of genetic information within families. *Am J Nurs* **109**: 65–69.

Hayat Roshanai A, Lampic C, Rosenquist R, Nordin K 2010. Disclosing cancer genetic information within families: perspectives of counselees and their at-risk relatives. *Fam Cancer* **9**: 669–679.

Hilgart JS, Coles B, Iredale R 2012. Cancer genetic risk assessment for individuals at risk of familial breast cancer. *Cochrane Database Syst Rev* **2**: CD003721.

Hughes C, Lerman C, Schwartz M, et al. 2002. All in the family: evaluation of the process and content of sisters' communication about *BRCA1* and *BRCA2* genetic test results. *Am J Med Genet* **107**: 143–150.

Iredale R, Brain K, Gray J, France E 2003. The information and support needs of women at high risk of familial breast and ovarian cancer: how can cancer genetic services give patients what they want? *Fam Cancer* **2**: 119–121.

Landsbergen K, Verhaak C, Kraaimaat F, Hoogerbrugge N 2005. Genetic uptake in *BRCA*-mutation families is related to emotional and behavioral communication characteristics of index patients. *Fam Cancer* **4**: 115–119.

McAllister M, Dunn G, Todd C 2011. Empowerment: qualitative underpinning of a new clinical genetics-specific patient-reported outcome. *Eur J Hum Genet* **19**: 125–130.

Michie S, Smith JA, Senior V, Marteau TM 2003. Understanding why negative genetic test results sometimes fail to reassure. *Am J Med Genet A* **119A**: 340–347.

NICE (National Institute for Health and Care Excellence) 2013. *Familial breast cancer: classification and care of people at risk of familial breast cancer and management of breast cancer and related risks in people with a family history of breast cancer.* NICE Clinical Guideline 164. London: National Institute for Health and Care Excellence.

Resta RG 2006. Defining and redefining the scope and goals of genetic counseling. *Am J Med Genet C* **142C**: 269–275.

Resta R, Biesecker BB, Bennett RL, et al. 2006. A new definition of genetic counseling: National Society of Genetic Counselors' Task Force report. *J Genet Counsel* **15**: 77–83.

Richards M 1996. Families, kinship and genetics. In: *The troubled helix: social and psychological implications of the new human genetics* (ed. T Marteau and M Richards), pp. 249–273. Cambridge: Cambridge University Press.

Skirton H, Lewis C, Kent A, and Coviello DA 2010. Genetic education and the challenge of genomic medicine: development of core competences to support preparation of health professionals in Europe. *Eur J Hum Genet* **18**: 972–977.

Weil J 2003. Psychosocial genetic counseling in the post-nondirective era: a point of view. *J Genet Counsel* **12**: 199–211.

Werner-Lin A 2008. Formal and informal support needs of young women with *BRCA* mutations. *J Psychosoc Oncol* **26**: 111–133.

Chapter 33

Genetic counselling about cancer predisposition

Chris Jacobs, Eshika Haque and Gillian Scott

Introduction to genetic counselling about cancer predisposition

Individuals from families with a known cancer-predisposing gene mutation and those who are assessed to be at high risk of cancer or who have complex cancer family histories may be referred to a genetics clinic where, for some, genetic testing may become a possibility. Genetic testing for cancer predisposition raises many complex and challenging issues for the individual seen in the clinic and for their relatives. The learning objectives for Chapter 33 are:

- to become aware of the process of genetic counselling for cancer predisposition;
- to be able to discuss the psychological impact of genetic testing for individuals with and at risk of cancer;
- to be able to consider the guidelines and implications of genetic testing in childhood and the reproductive choices available for individuals with a cancer-predisposing gene mutation.

The initial genetic counselling consultation

Once a referral is accepted, the patient is offered an appointment for genetic counselling with a genetics health professional. Prior to the appointment, patients are usually asked to provide details about their family history.

The initial consultation lasts for approximately 45 minutes. The health professional obtains personal and family history information over at least three generations, identifying any cancer diagnoses and other major health issues and documenting this information on a pedigree. The patient's perception of risk and his or her expectations of the consultation are explored, enabling the health professional to tailor the communication to the individual. A risk assessment is calculated and explained along with any other information regarding lifestyle or screening recommendations for the patient and other family members. In many cases, before risk and screening advice can be provided, the family history will be verified. This may involve asking the patient to provide copies of medical letters or death certificates pertaining to deceased family members or obtaining consent to access medical records of living relatives in order to confirm the diagnosis via the cancer registry or the histopathology department of the hospital where the relative was treated.

Pre-test genetic counselling

Genetic testing may be available at the first appointment, for example if the patient has had cancer, is able to give informed consent and wishes to have a test or if there is a known cancer-predisposing gene in the family, the laboratory report has been verified and the patient is ready to give informed consent to testing. However, for many patients the first consultation does not result in genetic testing because the family history does not meet the genetic testing criteria, the patient is not ready for testing or analysis of a sample from a relative with cancer is required before genetic testing can be offered to unaffected individuals.

Where genetic testing is possible, pre-test genetic counselling aims to enable people to understand the risk and empower them to make informed decisions about risk management. Addressing the psychological issues is essential for effective genetic counselling (Weil, 2003). Pre-test genetic counselling includes discussion of the likelihood of carrying a cancer-predisposing gene mutation, the inheritance pattern of the disease, the possible genes involved, penetrance, possible outcomes and the benefits, risks and limitations of genetic testing. The genetics health professional explores with the patient their understanding, their thoughts and feelings about their family history, the risks associated with a genetic predisposition to cancer and how they might feel if they have/have not inherited the mutation. Preparation for the possible outcome of the test is extremely important and the genetic counselling includes anticipated reaction to the result, identification of support networks and coping strategies. Failure to anticipate reactions to the result can lead to increased emotional distress which can persist for many months afterwards (Dorval et al., 2000). During the consultation, issues such as bereavement, guilt, blame, fear, anxiety and specific cancer worry may be addressed. Before genetic testing, important issues are discussed, such as: sharing the result; the possibility of genetic discrimination, including telling employers and issues surrounding mortgages and insurance; the impact of testing on the family and coping with a positive or negative result, especially when other family members may receive different results; the timing of the test, especially if they are undergoing testing before a screening test is available; thoughts and feelings about risk management; feelings about the possibility of passing the mutation on to children and reproductive options. For individuals with cancer, the discussion may also include feelings about coping with a current cancer diagnosis, the risks of developing further cancers and facing further treatments. The genetics health professional helps the patient to prepare for the result and discusses the timescale and arrangements for how the result will be communicated. For patients undergoing cancer treatment and waiting for the result in order to plan surgery, for example, this may involve liaison with other members of the multidisciplinary team in order to ensure that the result is available in time for the patient to process and reflect on the result before any planned surgery (see Chapter 27). Once the patient is ready and able to give informed consent, a consent form is signed and the blood sample drawn.

Sometimes the genetics health professional may make the assessment that the patient is not able to give informed consent, for example because they do not have the mental capacity, they have not fully thought through the implications or do not understand the issues, they are not psychologically ready for the test or they are under the age of 18 and the test is for an adult-onset cancer. The genetics health professional may seek advice from the multidisciplinary team or other agencies, arrange a further genetic counselling appointment, suggest a period of reflection about the reasons for testing and how they will cope with the result, suggest talking to family members or their partner or refer them for supportive counselling.

Post-test genetic counselling and management of mutation carriers

Delivery of the result of the genetic test varies between genetics centres and between patients. Some services communicate all genetic test results in a face-to-face appointment, others give the patient a choice of how they wish to be informed. There is limited evidence of the optimal way to deliver genetic test results, although the studies that have compared the delivery of results by telephone and in clinic have found no difference in satisfaction (Baumanis et al., 2009; Doughty Rice et al., 2010).

Individuals who do not carry a cancer-predisposing gene mutation may require a further follow-up appointment or telephone discussion in order to help them to adjust to the result or clarify the meaning of the result and establish the screening recommendations for themselves and other family members.

Mutation carriers are generally offered at least one further genetic counselling appointment in order to help them to understand the result and to come to terms with the change in their personal health circumstances. This consultation also enables further discussion and contextualisation of the risks and risk management options, implications for other family members, an opportunity to explore when and how to share the information and even to rehearse telling relatives. Post-test genetic counselling involves the provision of psychosocial support and onward referral to other specialists to discuss risk management. Some centres provide one-stop carrier clinics, enabling the patient to consult with various members of the multidisciplinary team in a coordinated way (Bancroft et al., 2010; Pichert et al., 2010).

The psychological impact of genetic counselling and genetic testing

A review of the literature evaluating the psychological impact of genetic testing for cancer susceptibility amongst unaffected mutation carriers (Meiser, 2005) found that most studies reported no change in psychological outcomes compared with baseline at any time point after receiving the genetic test result. However, several studies (Meiser et al., 2002; van Roosmalen et al., 2004; Watson et al., 2004) reported a short-term increase in breast cancer-related anxiety and/or depression requiring increased professional support among a small subset of individuals. In those at risk of Lynch syndrome and familial adenomatous polyposis (FAP) no adverse long-term effects on carriers were seen, changes in distress following disclosure of the result appeared to be temporary (Aktan-Collan et al., 2001) and increases in general anxiety were followed by decreases in depression (Meiser et al., 2004). A short- and long-term decrease in anxiety relating to colorectal cancer, generalised anxiety and depression was seen in those who received a negative predictive test result (Meiser, 2005). Studies that have examined the psychological impact on children with an *APC* mutation and their parents found no evidence of a negative impact and a review of the divergent findings of the impact of genetic testing for other cancers led to the conclusion that testing for each type of familial cancer raises unique issues (Meiser, 2005).

Despite the fact that the genetic testing process usually begins with the affected family member, fewer studies have examined the psychological impact of genetic counselling and testing on patients with cancer who undergo genetic testing at some time after completion of their cancer treatment. These studies are mainly focused on women with breast cancer. Dorval et al. (2000) found that women with breast cancer underestimated the level of sadness, anger and worry that they would feel after a positive *BRCA1* result and suggested that the result rekindled distress relating to the cancer diagnosis and treatment. The review by Meiser (2005) showed no change in psychological distress following testing amongst individuals with cancer, but concluded that the psychological response to genetic testing amongst women with breast cancer is mediated by their personal experience of cancer (Hallowell et al., 2004). Similar conclusions were drawn in a systematic review of the psychological effects of genetic testing in symptomatic patients with a variety of genetic conditions, including patients with cancer (Vansenne et al., 2009).

Case study 1: genetic counselling of individuals with and without cancer

John's brother died from colorectal cancer at the age of 43 and his mother died from the disease aged 54. His aunt Sylvia, the only surviving member of his mother's family, had been diagnosed three years earlier with endometrial cancer at the age of 62. Sylvia had two sons, aged 40 and 42, both of whom had young daughters.

At his genetic counselling appointment John learned that he was at high risk of Lynch syndrome and was recommended to have 2-yearly colonoscopies. The genetic counsellor explained that genetic testing would only be possible for John if a mutation were to be identified in his aunt. John was concerned about approaching her as they were not close. After some months he felt able to contact her and several months later Sylvia was referred to the genetics clinic.

Sylvia was accompanied by her youngest son who was anxious about his mother. His brother was worried about the insurance implications and angry with John for raising the issues. Sylvia was upset to discover that her children and grandchildren could be at risk and anxious about the possibility of developing colorectal cancer. She did, however, consent to tumour block testing and DNA analysis and was later informed that a mutation had been identified in the *MSH2* gene. John tested negative for the mutation.

Issues raised in case study 1: genetic counselling of individuals with and without cancer

1 Approaching relatives to request their help is difficult, particularly when relationships are not close. The genetics health professional will not contact relatives directly in this situation but may provide information for the patient to pass on to relatives. Affected relatives may feel obliged to be tested (Dancyger et al., 2010).

2 Attending a genetics appointment for the purpose of helping another relative may reveal unexpected information about the risk of further cancers for the affected individual and their offspring. If Sylvia's oncology team had identified the family history earlier in her treatment, this may have been helpful for the whole family.

3 Genetic discrimination is a valid concern, although there is currently a moratorium on insurance companies asking clients about genetic testing for cancer predisposition which extends until 2017 (HM Government/Association of British Insurers, 2011).

Genetic testing in childhood

Genetic testing in childhood is based on the principle of balancing the loss of the child's future autonomy and privacy against the wishes and anxiety of the parent in the best interests of the child (Clarke, 2010). Comprehensive guidance is provided for health professionals on the genetic testing of children (British Society for Human Genetics, 2010) but parental requests for genetic testing in childhood are rarely straightforward and multidisciplinary discussion of the case in the context of the guidelines and the principles of biomedical ethics is often required (see Chapter 34).

Diagnostic genetic testing may be appropriate in circumstances where a genetic test will enable a diagnosis and reduce the need for multiple invasive tests, make treatment available or relieve family anxiety (British Society for Human Genetics, 2010). However, even in a symptomatic child, the decision to undertake testing in childhood needs to be made with a caution and consideration of whether the timing of the test is in the child's best interests.

Predictive genetic testing is not available in childhood when a child is healthy but at risk of an adult-onset genetic condition (British Society for Human Genetics, 2010). The Gillick decision in 1985 identified the importance of children's rights of autonomy and established that children with sufficient understanding of the matter being decided have the legal authority to give consent to treatment. Similar rights apply in Scotland (The Age of Legal Capacity Act 1991). Requests from Gillick-competent children or 16- or 17-year-olds who are mature enough to make a decision may be upheld provided the young person is fully engaged in discussion about the pros and cons, and is able to understand and reflect on the issues involved.

In genetic conditions which arise in childhood, such as multiple endocrine neoplasia or FAP, predictive testing is often appropriate before the age of 18 as early surveillance and risk-reducing treatments can mitigate the risk. Understandably parents are often extremely anxious and may request testing at a very young age in the hope that the child does not carry the mutation. There are good arguments for deferring testing until the age at which screening or treatment would be offered. For example, a request to test a 5-year-old in a family with FAP is best deferred until the child is 11; at that age, screening will become available and the child is more likely to be able to be involved in the decision and therefore better placed to take on the responsibility for managing their cancer risk as they develop into adulthood. Labelling a child from a young age as being at risk of a genetic condition may be harmful, leading the child to be treated differently in subtle ways (Clarke and Gaff, 2008). However, if the child is too young to be involved and testing at a young age is indicated, parents are encouraged to talk with their child about their family history in order to enable understanding and adjustment as the child grows up.

Reproductive options for genetic testing

Reproductive issues are relevant and appropriate for young carriers who have not started or completed their families, yet this is an option about which women may have limited awareness (Ormondroyd et al., 2012). Decisions about whether to have children at all, to adopt or to embark on invasive testing during pregnancy are challenging. For many, there is a belief that medical science will lead to the availability of improved prevention and treatment options for the next generation. For some, however, the risk of passing on a mutation is too great to take a chance. Although testing for adult-onset conditions is not available during childhood, prenatal genetic diagnosis (PND) and pre-implantation genetic diagnosis (PGD) are options that parents may consider.

Prenatal diagnosis

PND followed by termination of an affected pregnancy is an option for couples wanting a biological child who has not inherited the mutation. Two invasive tests are offered during pregnancy enabling predictive genetic testing of the foetus. Chorionic villous sampling (CVS) is offered between 10 and 13 weeks of pregnancy and involves taking a sample of cells from the placenta. Complications include a 2% risk of miscarriage. Amniocentesis involves taking a sample of amniotic fluid and is offered between 15 and 20 weeks of pregnancy. The risk of miscarriage associated with amniocentesis is 1%. Genetic counselling about reproductive options involves balancing the risks to the pregnancy, the ethical implications of the loss of autonomy for the child should the couple decide not to terminate the pregnancy, the psychological impact on the parents and other members of the family, the cancer risks and the available risk management options.

In families where there is a *BRCA1* or *BRCA2* mutation, some couples might be less worried should a male child inherit the gene mutation. By testing foetal DNA in the maternal circulation, known as free foetal DNA (ffDNA), the sex of the foetus can be determined

(Wright and Chitty, 2009). Although this procedure does not pose the risk of miscarriage, the reliability and accuracy of ffDNA sex testing is currently being assessed. For couples wishing to pursue CVS or amniocentesis, ffDNA testing may minimise the risk of miscarriage by limiting prenatal tests to female foetuses.

Pre-implantation genetic diagnosis

PGD is an option for some couples at risk of having a child with a serious genetic condition. PGD aims to limit the chance of transmission of the gene while avoiding termination of pregnancy. PGD involves using *in vitro* fertilisation (IVF) to produce embryos cultured in the laboratory from the eggs and sperm of that couple. The embryo is then biopsied at the eight-cell stage and a cell removed and tested for the mutation. One or two embryos unaffected by the genetic condition may then be transferred into the womb, in the hope that a viable pregnancy will occur. The chance of a live birth is around 30% per IVF cycle (Human Fertilisation and Embryology Authority, 2013) and the procedure is costly, although NHS funding may be available.

PGD is available for highly penetrant cancer-predisposition syndromes, including several where screening and treatment options are available, such as FAP, Von Hippel–Lindau disease, *BRCA1* and *BRCA2* and Lynch syndrome. For some people, PGD poses religious, moral or ethical concerns. For others, PGD offers the potential to avoid termination of pregnancy for conditions where treatments are available, but where these treatments are of limited acceptability.

Case study 2: genetic counselling about PND for a BRCA2 mutation

Carla underwent predictive genetic testing for a *BRCA2* mutation when she was 34 weeks' pregnant. She already had two children, aged 4 and 2, and felt able to cope with the result during pregnancy. She was informed about the possibility of PND should she consider further children and understood that PND was not possible in her current pregnancy.

Eighteen months later Carla got in touch to say that she was 13 weeks' pregnant and wanted to have PND. Carla attended the appointment alone and was anxious and distracted. It emerged that her partner was reluctant to consider PND and that her heightened anxiety stemmed from feelings of guilt about having a baby while knowing her own genetic status. She acknowledged that she was seeking testing for her peace of mind and that a positive gene test would make her feel overwhelmingly guilty. She could not contemplate terminating the pregnancy. The issue of the child's autonomy was discussed, at which point Carla said that she would not tell the child but would allow him/her to find out the outcome of testing for him/herself in adulthood.

Carla was encouraged to reflect on the issues with her partner. A further appointment was arranged for them both to attend a few days later. In the meantime the case was discussed at the genetics clinical meeting where it was agreed that the loss of autonomy for the child and the potential impact on the family meant that on balance PND would not be in the best interests of the child, the family or the parents.

Carla called before the next appointment to say that, on reflection, she and her partner had decided against testing.

Issues raised in case study 2: genetic counselling about PND for a BRCA2 mutation

1 Carla presented at 13 weeks of pregnancy although she knew CVS would not be possible. This, together with her partner's response and the inconsistency in her arguments suggested that the request for PND was symptomatic of her feelings of guilt and anxiety. Helping her to recognise this may have helped her to resolve the issue and to reach a joint decision with her partner.

2 Her suggested solution to protect the autonomy of the child could have led to further problems for the child and for her relationship with the child. Encouraging Carla to consider how this might feel from the child's perspective and posing alternative scenarios (Smith et al., 2013) was a helpful strategy in genetic counselling in this circumstance.

3 Helping Carla to consider whether knowing the status of one child might have led to that child being treated differently and the potential impact of that on the whole family may have affected on her final decision. If she had gone ahead with PND it is possible that she would have requested genetic testing for the other children at a later date.

Summary

Living with a genetic predisposition to cancer and/or a strong family history of the disease raises complex and challenging issues. Genetic counselling aims to help individuals and families to understand, adjust to and make decisions about how to manage their cancer risks.

References

Aktan-Collan K, Haukkala A, Mecklin JP, et al. 2001. Comprehension of cancer risk one and 12 months after predictive genetic testing for hereditary non-polyposis colorectal cancer. *J Med Genet* **38**: 787–792

Bancroft EK, Locke I, Ardern-Jones A, et al. 2010. The carrier clinic: an evaluation of a novel clinic dedicated to the follow-up of *BRCA1* and *BRCA2* carriers—implications for oncogenetics practice. *J Med Genet* **47**: 486–491.

Baumanis L, Evans JP, Callanan N, Susswein LR 2009. Telephoned *BRCA1/2* genetic test results: prevalence, practice, and patient satisfaction. *J Genet Counsel* **18**: 447–463.

British Society for Human Genetics 2010. *Report on the genetic testing of children 2010*. Birmingham: British Society for Human Genetics.

Clarke A 2010. What is at stake in the predictive genetic testing of children? *Fam Cancer* **9**: 19–22.

Clarke AJ and Gaff C 2008. Challenges in the genetic testing of children for familial cancers. *Arch Dis Child* **93**: 911–914.

Dancyger C, Smith JA, Jacobs C, et al. 2010. Comparing family members' motivations and attitudes towards genetic testing for hereditary breast and ovarian cancer: a qualitative analysis. *Eur J Hum Genet* **18**: 1289–1295.

Dorval M, Patenaude AF, Schneider KA, et al. 2000. Anticipated versus actual emotional reactions to disclosure of results of genetic tests for cancer susceptibility: findings from *p53* and *BRCA1* testing programs. *J Clin Oncol* **18**: 2135–2142.

Doughty Rice C, Ruschman JG, Martin LJ, et al. 2010. Retrospective comparison of patient outcomes after in-person and telephone results disclosure counseling for *BRCA1/2* genetic testing. *Fam Cancer* **9**: 203–212.

Hallowell N, Foster C, Eeles R. et al. 2004. Accommodating risk: responses to *BRCA1/2* genetic testing of women who have had cancer. *Soc Sci Med* **59**: 553–565.

HM Government/Association of British Insurers 2011. *Concordat and moratorium on genetics and insurance*. London: Department of Health/Association of British Insurers.

Human Fertilisation and Embryology Authority 2013. *Pre-implantation genetic diagnosis* [online]. Available at: <http://www.hfea.gov.uk/preimplantation-genetic-diagnosis.html> (last accessed 21 July 2013).

Meiser B 2005. Psychological impact of genetic testing for cancer susceptibility: an update of the literature. *Psycho-Oncology* **14**: 1060–1074.

Meiser B, Butow P, Friedlander M, et al. 2002. Psychological impact of genetic testing in women from high-risk breast cancer families. *Eur J Cancer* **38**: 2025–2031.

Meiser B, Collins V, Warren R, et al. 2004. Psychological impact of genetic testing for hereditary non-polyposis colorectal cancer. *Clin Genet* **66**: 502–511.

Ormondroyd E, Donnelly L, Moynihan C, et al. 2012. Attitudes to reproductive genetic testing in women who had a positive *BRCA* test before having children: a qualitative analysis. *Eur J Hum Genet* **20**: 4–10.

Pichert G, Jacobs C, Jacobs I, et al. 2010. Novel one-stop multidisciplinary follow-up clinic significantly improves cancer risk management in *BRCA1/2* carriers. *Fam Cancer* **9**: 313–319.

Smith JA, Stephenson M, Jacobs C, Quarrell O 2013. Doing the right thing for one's children: deciding whether to take the genetic test for Huntington's disease as a moral dilemma. *Clin Genet* **83**: 417–421.

Van Roosmalen MS, Stalmeier PFM, Verhoef LCG, et al. 2004. Impact of *BRCA1/2* testing and disclosure of a positive test result on women affected and unaffected with breast or ovarian cancer. *Am J Med Genet A* **124A**: 346–355.

Vansenne F, Bossuyt PM, De Borgie CA 2009. Evaluating the psychological effects of genetic testing in symptomatic patients: a systematic review. *Genet Test Mol Biomarkers* **13**: 555–563.

Watson M, Foster C, Eeles R, et al. 2004. Psychosocial impact of breast/ovarian (*BRCA1/2*) cancer-predictive genetic testing in a UK multi-centre clinical cohort. *Br J Cancer* **91**: 1787–1794.

Weil J 2003. Psychosocial genetic counseling in the post-nondirective era: a point of view. *J Genet Counsel* **12**: 199–211.

Wright CF and Chitty LS 2009. Cell-free fetal DNA and RNA in maternal blood: implications for safer antenatal testing. *Br Med J* **339**: b2451.

Chapter 34

Psychosocial issues and supporting individuals with a family history of cancer

Clare Firth

Introduction to psychosocial issues and supporting individuals with a family history of cancer

Individuals with a family history of cancer face multiple challenges and a range of psychosocial issues. Attention to psychological needs is a key component of satisfaction with cancer services and genetic counselling services (Holloway et al., 2004). This chapter describes some of the main psychosocial issues faced by individuals at high risk of hereditary cancer and with a known genetic mutation. It is intended to apply to a range of genetic cancer disorders and draws from research and the author's clinical experience, highlighting the particular issues of risk management and information on management of psychological issues and the role of counselling services and peer support. The learning objectives for Chapter 34 are:

- to be able to understand the psychological and social impact of hereditary cancer on the individual and the family;
- to be aware of the psychosocial issues surrounding decision-making about risk management options;
- to be able to describe the role of psychological and counselling services in the provision of support.

Psychosocial issues involved in living with a cancer family history

Patients who have been diagnosed with a cancer genetic condition have already faced several challenges leading up to the diagnosis. They may have already experienced the loss of several close family members or have been diagnosed with cancer themselves. They may have experienced difficulty in deciding whether to have a genetic test and in telling family members, friends and partners about the possibility of an inherited condition.

After being diagnosed with a cancer genetic condition there are a mixed range of emotions that patients encounter—ranging from numbness, anxiety and guilt to grief and uncertainty, some patients experience acceptance and hope as they move through the process.

The diagnosis of a genetic risk of cancer for some individuals is a traumatic event which can challenge fundamental beliefs about life, themselves and their future, and leave them feeling numb, overwhelmed and powerless. It can also raise huge decisions about risk management. For some it can also lead to information about risks for a variety of other cancers that they had not anticipated.

Understandably, many patients report a strong rise in cancer anxiety in the days and weeks following a genetic diagnosis and a strong sense of uncertainty about the future and their life expectancy. Some patients report a sense that the genetic diagnosis is synonymous with a cancer diagnosis or a feeling that they are a 'ticking time bomb'. This can manifest itself in panic attacks, intrusive thoughts, worries about death and illness, preoccupation with a foreshortened future and hypervigilance about bodily symptoms and sensations. Some patients report a sense of disengagement, loss of motivation and hopelessness and an inability to move on and to plan for the future. Research on large samples of patients supports this; for example, Watson et al. (2004) found that cancer worry increased in the month following a positive *BRCA1/2* genetic test result.

Themes of loss and unresolved grief are common in people at high risk of cancer, due to the many potential causes of loss, for example losing parents at a young age, loss of health security or of multiple family members (Hopwood et al., 1998). Processing the loss is especially difficult when there may be other ongoing issues such as immediate health concerns or dealing with young children.

A large proportion of patients experience feelings of guilt relating to the possibility of passing the mutation on to their children. There may also be guilt regarding the negative consequences of risk management strategies for partners and children or about informing family members.

Health-related problems can leave patients feeling out of control and with a sense of increased vulnerability, which may lead to low self-esteem and an inability to cope with day to day problems (Burns, 2005). Some individuals may feel that their concerns are unique to themselves and/or may hold a sense of shame about their condition which can lead to difficulty in talking about their situation.

What and how to tell children about the genetic condition can be a major issue for patients who find the prospect of talking to their children about the genetic diagnosis difficult and distressing, particularly as a parent's first instinct is to protect their child. There may be difficulties in knowing what or how to communicate to children, and a sense that disclosing any information may raise children's anxieties to uncontrollable levels. Providing information, checking understanding and explaining and managing the emotional feelings that arise are integral to helping children cope with genetic risk information (Metcalfe et al., 2008).

Patients with a diagnosis of cancer who are undergoing genetic testing often experience multiple challenges such as accepting the diagnosis, coping with the side effects of treatment, maintaining independence and activity, adjusting to loss and change, seeking support and understanding medical information.

Having a genetic test in the midst of treatment might be seen as an extra burden for patients (Ardern-Jones et al., 2005). However, other studies have found no difference in distress between cancer patients who are found to have a breast cancer-predisposing gene mutation and those in whom no mutation is identified (Croyle et al., 1997). Some patients cite the benefit that genetic knowledge can inform their cancer management.

As patients adjust to the genetic diagnosis, some report a sense of relief at discovering an answer to why so many family members and/or themselves have developed cancer. Many patients report that difficult feelings start to improve as they come to terms with the diagnosis and begin to make a plan for risk management. This is related to feeling empowered by the options for risk management which might not have been available had they not tested positive for the mutation.

These issues are not exhaustive or mutually exclusive, rather they are a set of interrelated challenges to be considered within the person's familial, cultural and spiritual circumstances. As with any challenges, the psychological issues will vary according to many different factors, such as age, experience of cancer within the family, previous psychological issues and/or stage of diagnosis.

Psychosocial issues involved in decisions about risk management

Major psychological and social issues can arise when making decisions about risk management, such as whether to have risk-reducing surgery or screening. Screening can be a highly anxiety-provoking and traumatic experience that can feel intolerable. Risk-reducing surgery can feel like a big step and can elicit many different emotions both for the patient and the people they discuss it with.

Risk-reducing mastectomy is a major operation and there may be additional considerations such as whether or not to have breast reconstruction. Some patients are concerned about the impact on relationships and the effects on family members, like being able to care for young children, or have concerns about the views of friends and family. There may also be issues in terms of the impact of the loss of shape and sensation of the breasts, and the subsequent effect of both on feelings of femininity and body image. There may be work-related issues, such as the ability to take time off work and financial considerations.

The majority of patients are satisfied with their decision and are relieved that they no longer face the worry of cancer (Patenaude, 2012). Some also feel improvements in their emotional stability and self-esteem (Frost et al., 2000). Surgery may be less traumatic and painful than patients expect (Rolnick et al., 2007). However, difficulties have been reported for a minority of patients involving impact on body image and attractiveness, with minor levels of psychological problems (Hopwood et al., 2000). This is related to low levels of social support, unresolved grief issues, past psychiatric illness, stressful life events, low levels of self-esteem and levels of surgical complications. Patients have also reported wishing that they had more information to prepare for their expectations with regard to recovery, complications and the impact on their femininity (Rolnik et al., 2007).

Although risk-reducing salpingo-oophorectomy offers a significant reduction in worry about the risk of developing ovarian cancer, there are psychosocial issues to consider relating to the side effects of early menopause and the resulting issues such as coping with a loss of libido. Some women may mourn the loss of reproductive ability and their sense of femininity (Hallowell, 2004).

Assessment of psychological issues

Psychological assessment and support for patients with a high risk of cancer and their carers may be required at any point in the patient care pathway and may be undertaken by a variety of health professionals, depending on the nature of the intervention required. Since genetic issues can affect many family members, individuals may be eager for help outside the family if they prefer to discuss feelings and decisions that may have implications for their relatives. Support for partners and carers should also be considered.

There are many ways to assess a patient's psychological status, depending upon the clinician's experience, preference, the needs of the patient and the preferences of local services. At the early stages in a patient's pathway, for example in a family history clinic, it is important to be aware of any psychological distress during the consultation. Some patients may naturally volunteer information about their emotional well-being, but others may require prompting, for example by asking 'How are you feeling about the information we have covered so far?'. It can also be helpful to ask about a patient's sense of their ability to cope in the future. Listening in a permissive and non-judgemental manner establishes a sense of trust which can help to elicit worries and other difficult feelings.

Screening questionnaires can be a useful way to find out more about how a patient is feeling, particularly if they are reluctant to openly disclose their distress. Validated tools are available and preference will vary between practices. The Distress Thermometer (National Comprehensive Cancer Network, 2014) is a single-item question screen that can identify distress from any source and has been developed specifically for use in cancer care. The scale asks: "Please circle the number (0–10) that best describes how much distress you have been experiencing in the past week including today." Scores of 4 or more indicate a significant level of distress that should be investigated further (Jacobsen et al., 2005). Supplementary questions covering various areas of distress (such as family problems and physical problems) can then be covered. The Distress Thermometer has been adapted for use with patients with a *BRCA1/2* mutation in the *BRCA* clinic at Guy's Hospital (Fig. 34.1). A number of other assessment tools might also potentially be useful, as recommended in the National Institute for Health and Care Excellence (NICE) depression guideline (NICE, 2009).

Onward referral for further assessment and/or intervention may be appropriate if initial screening indicates a need for input from a specialist mental health practitioner such as a counsellor, clinical/health psychologist, liaison psychiatrist or social worker. The decision about when to refer on, and for what type of treatment, should be made in partnership with the patient and health professionals. Different mental health services may favour different methods of assessment and treatment and so it is important to link up with local teams, consult about referrals where necessary and develop joint approaches.

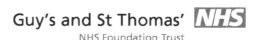

Guy's and St Thomas'

NHS Foundation Trust

Name: Reference Number:

___

Questionnaire to help us help you at your clinic appointment

We would be grateful if you would complete this questionnaire so that we can help you to get the most from your clinic visit.

This questionnaire will help us to see how you are doing physically and emotionally. If you have specific problems, it will help us to make sure we address these with you at your appointment. Your answers will be confidential and only shared with the clinic team.

Please complete both sides of the questionnaire and return it in the SAE provided together with the form telling us which specialists you wish to see in the clinic.

If you have any further questions or concerns about the questionnaire or the clinic before your appointment please call the clinic coordinator.

Thank you very much for your help.

___

Please tell us how you have been feeling about the following statements during the past week, including today.

Please circle one number between 1 (not at all) and 5 (all the time) for each statement:

		Not at all			All the time	
1.	I have felt anxious or worried about cancer	1	2	3	4	5
2.	I have been experiencing guilt related to the result of my genetic test	1	2	3	4	5
3.	I have been experiencing anger related to the result of my genetic test	1	2	3	4	5
4.	I have been experiencing stress related to communicating my genetic test result to others	1	2	3	4	5
5.	I have been experiencing stress concerning future decisions related to my genetic test	1	2	3	4	5
6.	I have been experiencing stress related to loss/bereavement Issues	1	2	3	4	5
7.	I have been experiencing stress related to other issues	1	2	3	4	5

If other issues are causing you distress it would be helpful if you can explain what these are:

....

....

....

....

Please turn the page over

Figure 34.1 The Distress Thermometer adapted for use with patients with a *BRCA1/2* mutation.

Reproduced and adapted with permission from the NCCN Clinical Practice Guidelines in Oncology (NCCN Guidelines®) for Distress Management (V.2.2013). © 2013 National Comprehensive Cancer Network, Inc. All rights reserved. The NCCN Guidelines® and illustrations herein may not be reproduced in any form for any purpose without the express written permission of the NCCN. To view the most recent and complete version of the NCCN Guidelines®, go online to NCCN.org. NATIONAL COMPREHENSIVE CANCER NETWORK®, NCCN®, NCCN GUIDELINES®, and all other NCCN Content are trademarks owned by the National Comprehensive Cancer Network, Inc. This adaptation is courtesy of the Department of Clinical Genetics, Guy's and St Thomas' Hospital, United Kingdom.

Guy's and St Thomas' NHS
NHS Foundation Trust

Please circle the number between 0 (no distress) to 10 (extreme distress) on the thermometer opposite that best describes how much distress you have been experiencing over the past week

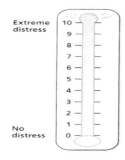

In particular, WHICH of the following is a cause of distress? (please tick, you may tick more than one):

Practical Problems
Childcare
Housing
Insurance/Finance
Transport
Work/School

Family Problems
Dealing with partner
Dealing with children

Emotional Problems
Depression
Fears
Nervousness
Sadness
Worry
Anger
Guilt

Spiritual/ Religious Concerns

Physical Problems
Appearance
Bathing/ Dressing
Breathing
Changes in urination
Constipation
Diarrhoea
Eating
Feeling swollen
Fevers
Getting around
Hot flushes
Indigestion
Memory/concentration
Mouth sores
Nausea
Nose dry/ congested
Pain
Sexual
Skin dry/ itchy
Sleep
Tingling in hands/ feet
Lymphoedema
Shoulder limitation
Menopausal symptoms

Figure 34.1 *(continued)*

Sometimes the health professional might receive information about a history of previous mental health difficulties, and if the patient is already receiving psychological care it is important to consult with the mental health practitioner or team and plan care accordingly. Although rare, if the patient presents during the consultation as a considerable and immediate risk to themselves or others, urgent referral to emergency services or specialist mental health services is indicated and/or advice must be sought from another health professional as soon as possible. The National Comprehensive Cancer Network® (NCCN®) (2014) has developed useful guidelines for assessing and managing distress in cancer patients which might be helpful for patients at high risk of hereditary cancer.

Management of psychosocial issues

When faced with a patient who is particularly anxious or distressed, it will be therapeutic if the health professional is aware of their issues, is able to deal with them in a sensitive manner, gives the patient a chance to express and explore their feelings with empathy and provides useful information. The use of additional listening skills can help a patient feel that their concerns are being heard and understood, for example empathising with a patient's feelings in way that affirms them and paraphrasing and summarising what they are saying to ensure they feel listened to.

It can also be useful to 'listen with a constructive ear' (Lipchik, 2002); this involves looking out for the strengths that the patient brings and methods they have already developed to deal with adversity and reflecting these back to the patient in a way that reinforces their self-efficacy. Coping questions (George et al., 1990) can also help a patient feel empowered to deal with their problems, for example 'How are you managing such a difficult situation?' and 'How have you coped so far?'.

If further input is required it may be helpful to refer a patient for specific psychological interventions delivered according to an explicit theoretical framework. Some of the most common approaches are cognitive behavioural therapy (CBT), solution-focused therapy (SFT) and systemic or family therapy.

Cognitive behavioural therapy

CBT is a talking therapy that helps people to manage their problems by addressing the way they think and behave (see, for example, Moorey and Greer, 2002). It is based on the idea that people sometimes develop maladaptive thought (cognitive) processes which affect their feelings and behaviour. Treatment works by identifying negative spirals of thoughts and interrupting these cycles by replacing them with more realistic and helpful thoughts and encouraging people to behave in different ways according to these new thoughts. Common issues relevant to a person with a family history of cancer that might benefit from CBT include dealing with cancer anxiety or guilty thoughts about passing the gene on to their children.

Solution focused therapy

This is a type of talking therapy that focuses on what the patient wants to achieve through therapy rather than on the problems that made them seek help (see, for example, George et al., 1990). The patient is asked to envision their preferred future. This helps to gain a concrete vision of what that person would like to see being different and in this way provides a sense of hope and empowerment. The therapist helps the client to identify times in their life that are closer to this future and any small successes that helped to achieve them. Patients are more likely to repeat these successes when they need to. The approach assumes that the patient has the necessary skills and resources to cope and to deal with their problems and the therapist's role is to help uncover them.

SFT can be useful for patients and families at high risk of cancer, for example when discussing how best to tell the family about test results, making decisions for risk-reducing surgery or Moving forward from bereavement.

Systemic or family therapy

Some patients may benefit from family therapy, sometimes called systemic therapy or family counselling. This is a branch of psychotherapy that emphasises family relationships as an important factor in psychological health (Hills, 2012). There are a number of branches including narrative therapy, structural therapy and MRI brief therapy (developed at the Mental Research Institute in California). For patients with a family history of cancer the issues involved may bring to the surface difficult family dynamics or couple relationship problems which may benefit from this therapy.

Other approaches

Other useful models include person-centred counselling as developed by Carl Rogers (1961), who introduced the 'core conditions' for a positive counselling relationship—genuineness, empathy and warmth. There is also, psychodynamic psychotherapy which involves analysis of how unconscious thoughts and past experiences shape current behaviour (Cabaniss, 2010). It can be helpful, for example, with a patient who identifies problems from their childhood which they feel are adding to the sense of burden of having a family history of cancer.

The role of peer support

Some individuals find it useful to connect with others who are in a similar situation. Some genetic services may hold a list of clients who are willing to speak to others or run local support groups. Telephone access to patients with similar issues or an online support group may be more practical. Timing can be important; Kausemeyer et al. (2006) noted that there may be a limited time frame during which patients with an inherited genetic predisposition find support groups relevant to their needs.

Case study: example of support for a patient diagnosed with a family history of breast cancer

SB, a 34-year-old woman with a family history of breast cancer, was referred to the family history clinic due to concerns about having a *BRCA* gene mutation as her sister had recently been diagnosed with breast cancer and found to have a *BRCA1* gene mutation.

She was seen by a nurse in the breast cancer family history clinic. During the consultation the nurse noticed the patient become visibly upset when asked about her family history of cancer. When asked what was making her feel upset, SB said that her mother had passed away from breast cancer when SB was 18 years old. On further prompting, SB revealed that the questions about her family history were bringing back difficult memories of her mother's cancer and also causing high anxiety about having the *BRCA* gene mutation and how to manage the risk if she was diagnosed with it. SB also explained about her sister's recent diagnosis of cancer and that she was currently doing a lot to support her sister. SB had two young children and was worried about their future.

The nurse decided to ask SB to complete a Distress Thermometer, which gave a distress score of 5 and indicated that work-related issues were causing her additional stress. The nurse reflected back SB's concerns and empathised with how she was feeling. The nurse asked SB how she felt she was coping and how she felt she would cope in the future were she to undergo genetic testing. SB said that she had a supportive husband and friends and was managing to cope by talking to them about things and keeping herself busy, which usually worked for her. On further discussion SB felt that she would like to be referred to the genetics centre as her sister wanted her to find out if she carried the gene mutation so she could manage her risk. She also wanted to find out for the sake of her children.

The nurse discussed with SB her support needs during the upcoming genetics referral and raised the possibility of being referred for more specialist help. SB said that if she were found to carry the gene fault she would welcome some additional support. At the end of the appointment the nurse highlighted SB's coping skills as well as her strength in supporting her sister.

SB was referred to the local clinical genetics service where she underwent genetic counselling prior to testing positive for the *BRCA1* gene mutation. Upon disclosure of the result SB became very tearful and expressed her concerns about future risk management with the genetic counsellor. She also talked about the ongoing issues with her sister's cancer and her work stress. She did, however, express that knowing about the mutation would help her to be able to gain some control over the cancer in her family and make informed choices about risk management. The genetic counsellor and SB discussed referral to local specialist counselling services for help with making a decision about whether to have risk-reducing surgery and to help support her with the external issues. SB and her husband agreed that she would benefit from further help and, as he also wanted to be involved in decisions about risk management, he attended further counselling with her.

Summary

Individuals and their families living with a cancer family history and a known genetic risk may be experiencing a range of different emotions that will vary from person to person and family to family. Decisions around risk management are often complex and involve the consideration of multiple issues for both individuals and their families and may require support from external sources. Treatment needs can be assessed in a variety of ways ranging from clinical judgement to formal screening tools depending on patient, clinician and local service preference. The support needs of an individual will vary, and may include input from general counselling, information provision, peer support or specific interventions by a trained counsellor. Patients will often have their own range of resources and coping skills that it may be useful to highlight during consultations.

References

Arden Jones A, Keenen R, Eeles R 2005. Too much, too soon? Patients and health professionals' views concerning the impact of genetic testing at the time of breast cancer diagnosis in women under the age of 40. *Eur J Cancer Care* **14**: 272–281.

Burns K 2005. *Focus on solutions: a health professional's guide*. London: Whurr Publishers Ltd.

Cabaniss D, Cherry S, Douglas CJ, et al. 2010. *Psychodynamic psychotherapy: a clinical manual*. Chichester: John Wiley and Sons.

Croyle RT, Smith KR, Botkin JR, et al. 1997. Psychological responses to *BRCA1* mutation testing: preliminary findings. *Health Psychol* **16**: 63–72.

Frost MH, Schaid DJ, Sellers TA, et al. 2000. Long-term satisfaction and psychological and social function following bilateral prophylactic mastectomy. *J Am Med Assoc* **284**: 319–324.

George E, Iveson C, Ratner H 1990. *Problem to solution: brief therapy with individuals and families*. London: BT Press.

Hallowell N, Mackay J, Richards M, et al. 2004. High-risk premenopausal women's experiences of undergoing prophylactic oophorectomy: a descriptive study. *Genet Test* **8**: 148–156.

Hills J 2012. *Introduction to systemic and family therapy: a user's guide*. Basingstoke: Palgrave Macmillan.

Holloway S, Porteous M, Cetnarskyj R, et al. 2004. Patient satisfaction with two different models of cancer genetic services in south-east Scotland. *Br J Cancer* **90**: 582–589.

Hopwood P, Keeling F, Long A, et al. 1998. Psychological support needs for women at high genetic risk of breast cancer: some preliminary indicators. *Psycho-Oncology* **7**: 402–412.

Hopwood P, Lee A, Shenton A, et al. 2000. Clinical follow-up after bilateral risk reducing ('prophylactic') mastectomy: mental health and body image outcomes. *Psycho-Oncology* **9**: 462–472.

Jacobsen PB, Donovan KA, Trask PC, et al. 2005. Screening for psychologic distress in ambulatory cancer patients. *Cancer* **103**: 1494–1502.

Kausmeyer DT, Lengerich EJ, Kluhsman BC, et al. 2006. A survey of patients' experiences with the cancer genetic counselling process: recommendations for cancer genetics programs. *J Genet Counsel* **15**: 409–431.

Lipchik E 2002. *Beyond technique in solution focused therapy*. New York: Guilford Press.

Metcalfe A, Coad J, Plumridge GM, et al. 2008. Family communication between children and their parents about inherited genetic conditions: a meta-synthesis of the research. *Eur J Hum Genet* **16**: 1193–1200.

Moorey S and Greer S 2002. *Cognitive behaviour therapy for people with cancer*. Oxford: Oxford University Press.

NICE (National Institute for Health and Care Excellence) 2009. *Depression in adults. The treatment and management of depression in adults*. NICE Clinical Guideline 90. London: National Institute for Health and Care Excellence. Available at: <http://www.nice.org.uk/nicemedia/live/12329/45888/45888.pdf> (last accessed 8 January 2014).

National Comprehensive Cancer Network 2014. Referenced with permission from the NCCN Clinical Practice Guidelines in Oncology (NCCN Guidelines®) for Distress Management V.1.2014. © National Comprehensive Cancer Network, Inc. 2014. All rights reserved. Accessed 6 June 2014. To view the most recent and complete version of the guideline, go online to NCCN.org. NATIONAL COMPREHENSIVE CANCER NETWORK®, NCCN®, NCCN GUIDELINES®, and all other NCCN content are trademarks owned by the National Comprehensive Cancer Network, Inc.

Patenaude AF 2012. Prophylactic mastectomy: insights from women who chose to reduce their risk. Westport, CT: Praeger Publishers.

Rogers CR 1961. *On becoming a person*. London: Constable and Co. Ltd.

Rolnick SJ, Altschuler A, Nekhlyudov L, et al. 2007. What women wish they knew before prophylactic mastectomy. *Cancer Nurs* **30**: 285–291.

Watson M, Foster C, Eeles R, et al. 2004. Psychosocial impact of breast/ovarian (*BRCA1/2*) cancer-predictive genetic testing in a UK multicentre clinical cohort. *Br J Cancer* **91**: 1787–1794.

Chapter 35

Ethical and cultural issues

Athalie Melville and Sally Watts

Introduction to ethical and cultural issues

Genetic counselling within cancer genetics almost always involves the wider family. The families encountered during genetic counselling come from various parts of the world and comprise a wide range of ethnicities, religions and languages. Even families who share a common language may have different uses for particular words. They will have developed practices that combine many aspects of their cultural background. Some practices will be common but others may be more specific to a family or even one individual within a family. Life experience will vary. Each family will have developed their own 'culture'. Ethical issues arise when there are differences in opinion, values and beliefs within families or between individuals and their healthcare providers.

The focus of this chapter is to explore the impact that ethical issues and culture may have on individuals and families undergoing genetic assessment and testing for cancer conditions, and the practical implications of this for healthcare professionals. One of the competencies for nurses from the National Genetics and Genomics Education Centre is to develop an understanding and awareness of the need to tailor genetic/genomic information and services according to a client's culture, knowledge, language ability and developmental stage (Kirk et al., 2011). This is also applicable to any health professional working with families with an inherited condition. The learning outcomes for Chapter 35 are:

- to consider the impact that 'culture' may have on decision-making about managing a family history of cancer;
- to be able to discuss the biomedical ethical principles in the context of cancer genetics.
- to be able to apply these biomedical ethical principles to a clinical scenario within cancer genetics.

Culture

Culture is defined by the *Oxford English dictionary* as 'the distinctive ideas, customs, social behaviour, products, or way of life of a particular nation, society, people or period'. Different aspects of a person's culture may influence their knowledge, values and beliefs about genetic disease and the impact this will have on their family. Genetic information and services need to be 'tailored' to the individual (Middleton et al., 2005). It is impossible to consider all possible aspects of culture in this chapter; however, we would stress that good communication is key to understanding the culture of an individual and/or a family. Open discussion can lead to shared understanding, recognition and respect for similarities and differences. For example, some families do not to discuss medical problems with relatives; other families have an open style of communication whereby information is passed freely between relatives. Sometimes there is a definite desire not to disclose information (active non-disclosure), but a more subtle form of withholding information is passive non-disclosure, whereby an individual does not share information with relatives but does not explicitly reveal that that is their intention (Hodgson and Gaff, 2013). It may be possible to resolve these issues by establishing at the outset any concerns the patient may have about sharing information. Baile et al. (2000) produced a guide for healthcare professionals on how to break bad news in the form of a six-stage model, and that model could also be used to help patients share information with their relatives.

To compound the possible burden of caring for relatives with cancer, there can be significant implications for other family members. For some families the identification of a genetic mutation which explains the family history of cancer is empowering, enabling other members to access screening or risk-reducing treatment; for others, it is a devastating outcome and increases the worry and concern within the family. The knowledge of a cancer predisposition within the family and the responsibility that individuals feel to share this information with relatives can be a huge burden (Hallowell, 1999).

Genetic testing may be offered in different ways depending on local practice or ethnicity. For example, *BRCA* gene testing is available in Poland as part of local workplace screening programmes. There is evidence that individuals from minority ethnic groups with a family history of cancer are less likely to access clinical genetics services (Genetic Alliance UK, 2012).

From our practice as genetic counsellors we have learnt that not all families function or communicate as one might imagine based on our own culture and experience of family life. It is important not to make assumptions, and to be aware that the unexpected can occur. We have experience of parents withholding their cancer diagnosis from their adult children, relatives not passing on a genetic test result because of a long-standing feud within the family and genetic test results from an estranged parent being delivered via someone in a pub or a social networking site. There are no right or wrong answers in many ethical or family scenarios, but the skills to assess each situation and help individuals explore different viewpoints are essential.

A value is defined by the *Oxford English dictionary* as the 'worth or desirability or utility, or qualities on which these depend'. During the genetic assessment and testing process there are a number of different stakeholders, including the patient, the wider family, local cancer clinic staff, genetics healthcare professionals, general practitioners and laboratory staff. All will have different values from a personal, professional, cultural or ethical viewpoint. Many ethical dilemmas arise due to a conflict in values and the challenge is to explore how to resolve the conflicts that result (Parker and Lucassen, 2003).

Ethical principles

The biomedical ethical framework that is most commonly used in clinical genetics is that of Beauchamp and Childress (1979). They suggest four main principles of biomedical ethics, namely:

- respect for autonomy
- justice
- non-maleficence
- beneficence.

This framework is suited to genetic scenarios as the principles can be applied to more than one individual and therefore the rights, limits and concerns for a family can be considered.

Case study

To demonstrate the use of these ethical principles from the viewpoint of clinical genetics we will apply them to a case study. The aim is to provide readers with a framework to facilitate decision-making in clinical practice. We have used hereditary breast and ovarian cancer as an example but other cancer predispositions can be considered in a similar way.

Susan, who is 45 years old and has two daughters, was referred to the genetics clinic to discuss her family history of breast and ovarian cancer. Her mother, Christine, is 73 years old and suffers with dementia. Christine has two sisters, Pamela who was diagnosed with breast cancer aged 45 years and Denise who was reported to have been diagnosed with ovarian cancer at 46 years and died 2 years later (Fig. 35.1). Pamela had previously undergone diagnostic genetic testing and was found to carry a *BRCA2* gene mutation. Predictive testing was therefore available to other family members.

The principle of respect for *autonomy* is underpinned by the moral and political tradition of the importance of individual freedom and choice, whereby an individual can act without controlling influences to make their own decisions, and make a reasoned informed choice (Beauchamp, 2007).

Susan wants to know if she is at an increased risk of developing breast and ovarian cancer so she can access early screening if necessary. However, her mother Christine has refused to have a blood test. If we test Susan and she carries the familial mutation we will know, by default, that Christine is a *BRCA2* mutation carrier. Both family members have the right to autonomy but the two decisions are not compatible. Does one family member have more right to autonomy?

Consideration of the remaining three principles may help with further reflection on the scenario.

Beneficence is the 'duty to do good' (Beauchamp, 2007). If beneficence outweighs the risk of maleficence in any given situation, the particular action could be justified. We could ask who would benefit more from the genetic testing, Susan or Christine? As Susan is younger, a positive test result would enable her to access early screening and risk-reducing surgery which could prolong her life expectancy. It would also provide risk information for her children.

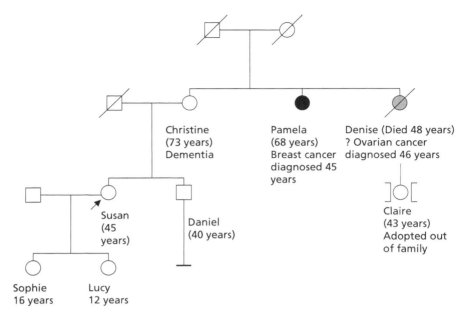

Figure 35.1 Pedigree of the family in our case study. The black shading represents a diagnosis of breast cancer and the grey shading represents a diagnosis of ovarian cancer.

The principle of *non-maleficence* is to avoid causing harm (Beauchamp, 2007). Would testing Susan first cause significant harm to her mother? It may be beneficial to involve the health professionals looking after Christine in the discussion. As Christine has a diagnosis of dementia, guidance from the Mental Capacity Act (2005) could be used. Christine's age, medical condition and mental capacity will influence any decisions.

Justice relates to doing what is fair, due or owed and to equity of care (Beauchamp, 2007). What is right for Susan may be wrong for Christine or other family members but a balance of care needs to be reached. What is motivating each person to make their decision? The outcome for this family may be different from that for another family as each case needs to be resolved separately. Appropriate care needs to be given to individuals and families but it must also be as fair and equitable as possible for the wider population within the NHS.

Use of the above four principles of biomedical ethics can facilitate communication between a genetics health professional and the family. It can enable family members to see the 'other side' of a scenario if each point is discussed and can help health professionals to identify specific issues, evaluate facts, consider alternative actions and facilitate decision-making. These factors will also need consideration within a cultural context.

We can now consider how this information can be applied to individual family members in the case study. The possible applications of the ethical principles to Christine's situation are:

♦ Autonomy—we have a responsibility to support Christine's decision not to have a genetic test.

+ Justice—protecting Christine's autonomy is fair. Christine has the right not to know her genetic status. However, we also have a responsibility to Susan and the two are not compatible.

+ Beneficence—where we support Christine's decision not to be tested.

+ Non-maleficence—where we do not insist that Christine has a genetic test and offer her breast screening instead due to increased cancer risks.

The possible applications of the ethical principles to Susan's situation are:

+ Autonomy—we support Susan's decision by offering her a genetic test.

+ Justice—Susan has the right to know her genetic status. It is her DNA sample and she is entitled to know any results. It would be unfair to refuse to test Susan. We could consider the possible unnecessary cost of extra breast screening if Susan does not carry the *BRCA2* gene mutation.

+ Beneficence—where we support Susan's decision to be tested.

+ Non-maleficence—if Susan is found to carry the *BRCA2* gene mutation, this will reveal Christine's genetic status. We need to consider the implications of this for Christine in terms of emotional well-being and her relationship with her daughter.

Informed consent

Informed consent is when an individual is aware of all the relevant information and has the competence and capacity to make an informed decision. Sometimes an individual's competence or capacity to give informed consent may be impaired, such as with Christine in the case study. Other situations may involve a child who is not of sufficient intellectual maturity to appreciate all the implications of a test or an adult with significant learning difficulties. Sometimes it is difficult to assess whether an individual is able to give informed consent. Whenever there is doubt, it is important to seek advice. Genetic testing in childhood can be a contentious issue, particularly where the wishes and views of the parents are in conflict with the views of the healthcare professional about the child's best interest (Parker, 2009). The British Society for Human Genetics (2010) (now renamed the British Society for Genetic Medicine) has published a useful guide to childhood testing.

Susan, from our case study, said that if she was found to carry the *BRCA2* gene mutation she would also want her daughters to undergo testing. She felt that her 16-year-old daughter could cope with a result which showed that she carried the mutation but is unsure how her 12-year-old daughter, Lucy, would react. She asked if we could test Lucy without revealing what the blood test was for.

+ How would you feel about this request?

+ What are the implications for Lucy?

When a parent or relative signs a consent form on behalf of a child or relative, it is important to ensure that the individual being tested is giving *informed* consent.

- Does the individual understand why a test is being offered, and the limitations of the test?
- Do they know and understand all the possible test outcomes and implications for them and/or their relatives?
- Should children be offered genetic testing for adult-onset disorders?
- When is a child competent to be involved in the decision-making process (i.e. are they Gillick competent; Wheeler, 2006)?

Confidentiality and disclosure

In genetics, confidentiality is paramount in order to protect individuals. Some questions that arise are: who owns genetic or family information and who should have access to this information? In genetics we are careful not to disclose information about other relatives unless it is necessary and then only if we have written or explicit consent to do so.

We often ask patients and relatives to disclose information to others, such as sharing information about their cancer diagnosis in order to accurately assess cancer risk in the family or asking individuals to share genetic test results with at-risk relatives. Individuals may have difficulty obtaining information about or sharing information with their relatives, particularly if relatives are dead or they do not live locally. Non-disclosure can occur in the case of adopted people or those who do not know their biological family history. Are there occasions where a clinician may pass on this information?

In our case study family Pamela's genetic counsellor wrote a 'to whom it may concern' letter for Pamela to pass on to her relatives to share the genetic information. But what if a number of relatives remain uniformed, such as Claire (see Fig. 35.1) who was adopted out of the case study family after birth? Consideration of the four ethical principles can be helpful in this situation.

Non-disclosure often comes about through fear. In some cases, patients need a clinician to give them 'permission' to share information. In our experience family members who feel supported are empowered to be proactive about contacting and sharing information with relatives. Partial or inaccurate disclosure can occur. For example, patients are sometimes informed that a *BRCA* mutation has been identified in an estranged family member. It is difficult to offer predictive testing to family members without knowing the specific mutation due to the large number of different mutations known to occur within these genes. If an estranged family member is reluctant to give such full and personal information, as they think it unnecessary, accurate predictive testing cannot be offered. This denies their relative(s) the right to know their genetic status.

Is knowing that there is a *BRCA* mutation in the family different from knowing the exact mutation within the *BRCA1* or *BRCA2* gene? Although the patient may not see the importance of this information, from the laboratory and clinical viewpoint it makes the difference between being able to offer an accurate genetic test or not.

Other questions to be considered are:

+ If the patient had a positive predictive test, and therefore the mutation was revealed, could the estranged relative view this as a breach of confidentiality?

+ How does a genetic counsellor best support the needs of their patient and where do the limits of his or her responsibility lie?

Guidance on genetic testing and sharing information has been published by the Royal College of Physicians, Royal College of Pathologists and British Society for Human Genetics (RCP, 2011). Many families take part in research programmes associated with cancer predisposition and it is important that there is a clear distinction between clinical and research care offered to patients (Hallowell, 2010).

Cases of non-paternity are less likely to be identified in cancer families than in other cases involving genetics, but this situation could arise. A degree of diplomacy and tact may need to be applied. It would be important to consider whether such information needs to be disclosed and the effect that this may have on family dynamics.

The right to know versus the right not to know

Once an individual has been told that there is a family history of a genetic condition, their right not to know about it has been removed. It is almost impossible to find out in advance whether or not someone would want to have specific genetic information. By asking them, we are removing their right not to know. Some individuals may be aware that they have a risk of carrying a particular genetic condition, such as Lynch syndrome, but may choose not to go ahead with predictive genetic testing.

A typical problem that could be encountered is if a child or an identical twin wants to find out their genetic status for a known *MSH2* gene mutation within their family, but their test result will reveal the result to another relative who does not wish to know.

Ethical dilemmas in cancer genetics and how these are managed

The advantage of improved technology is that it allows us to target testing and screening more specifically to high-risk individuals and their families but, as with all advances, this leads to challenges for the healthcare professional. It is now possible to offer prenatal testing or pre-implantation genetic diagnosis (PGD) for some cancer-predisposition syndromes (see Chapter 34), but this can also involve ethical dilemmas (Clancy, 2010): for example,

+ Is it ethical to offer prenatal testing/PGD for an adult-onset disorder?

+ Does it make a difference if the foetus is male or female?

+ If we can offer PGD, should we test children?

The laboratory techniques used for genetic testing are rapidly evolving with advances in technology and knowledge. These are going to bring new clinical challenges for health professionals. An example of this is where a child is offered a genetic test to try to establish why they may have developmental delay and/or dysmorphic features. These new technologies may reveal a number of unexpected results, for example that the child also carries a previously unidentified *APC* gene mutation. The dilemma can come when deciding what information to disclose to the family. In this situation it is important to highlight to the family the possibility that unexpected results may be revealed. Clinicians may have access to local NHS hospital trust clinical ethics committees (which are different from research ethics committees). These multidisciplinary groups, which consist of a mixture of health professionals, law and ethics experts and lay members including patients, can discuss ethical dilemmas from any specialty. It is particularly helpful to have an 'outside' perspective on a scenario. A similar forum specific to genetics is available at the national Genethics Club (<http://www.ethox.org.uk/copy_of_ethics-support/the-genethics-club>)—the website offers further examples of ethical dilemmas in genetics and relevant documentation. It is essential to share good practice and gain views from other health, law and ethics experts to provide a comprehensive approach to ethical dilemmas and clinical challenges. Sharing clinical cases could also be useful because other genetic centres may be caring for different branches of the family. In some cases centres may be able to facilitate communication or share information on behalf of a family which informs day-to-day clinical practice.

Summary

We hope that this chapter has raised awareness of some possible ethical issues and pitfalls that can arise in clinical practice. By pre-empting issues, major ethical dilemmas may be avoided. Use of the biomedical ethical framework can enable health professionals to explore situations in more detail from their own viewpoint or those of a patient and/or their family members, and facilitate discussion and debate so that issues are resolved.

References

Baile WF, Buckman R, Lenzi R, et al. 2000. SPIKES—a six-step protocol for delivering bad news: application to the patient with cancer. *Oncologist* **5**: 302–311.

Beauchamp TL 2007. The 'four principles' approach to health care ethics. In: *Principles of healthcare ethics*, 2nd edn (ed. R Ashcroft, A Dawson, H Draper and JR McMillan), pp. 3–10. Chichester: John Wiley and Sons.

Beauchamp TL and Childress JF 1979. *Principles of biomedical ethics*. New York: Oxford University Press.

British Society for Human Genetics 2010. *Report on the genetic testing of children*. Birmingham: British Society for Human Genetics. Available at: <http://www.bsgm.org.uk/media/678741/gtoc_booklet_final_new.pdf> (last accessed 7 June 2013).

Clancy T 2010. A clinical perspective on ethical arguments around prenatal diagnosis and preimplantation genetic diagnosis for later onset inherited cancer. *Fam Cancer* **9**: 9–14.

Genetic Alliance UK 2012. *Identifying families at risk of cancer: why is this more difficult for ethnic minority communities and what would help?* London: Genetic Alliance UK.

Hallowell N 1999. Doing the right thing: genetic risk and responsibility. *Sociol Health Illness* **21**: 597–621.

Hallowell N, Cooke S, Crawford G, et al. 2010. An investigation of patients motivations for their participation in genetics-related research. *J Med Ethics* **36**: 37–45.

Hodgson J and Gaff C 2013. Enhancing family communication about genetics: ethical and professional dilemmas. *J Genet Counsel* **22**: 16–21.

Kirk M, Tonkin E, Skirton H 2011. *Fit for practice in the genetics/genomics era: a revised competence based framework with learning outcomes and practice indicators. A guide for nurse education and training.* Birmingham: National Genetics Education and Development Centre.

Mental Capacity Act 2005. London: Her Majesty's Stationery Office. Available at: <http://www.legislation.gov.uk/ukpga/2005/9/contents> (last accessed 9 January 2014).

Middleton A, Ahmed M, Levene S 2005. Tailoring genetic information and services to clients culture, knowledge and language level. *Nurs Stand* **20**(2): 52–56.

Parker M 2009. Genetic testing in children and young people. *Fam Cancer* **9**: 15–18.

Parker M and Lucassen A 2003. Concern for families and individuals in clinical genetics. *J Med Ethics* **29**: 70–73.

RCP (Royal College of Physicians, Royal College of Pathologists and British Society for Human Genetics) 2011. *Consent and confidentiality in clinical genetic practice: guidance on genetic testing and sharing genetic information*, 2nd edn. Report of the Joint Committee on Medical Genetics. London: RCP, RCPath.

Wheeler R 2006. Gillick or Fraser? A plea for consistency over competence in children. *Br Med J* **332**: 7545.

Chapter 36

Genetic counselling and supporting individuals with a family history of cancer. Summary

Patricia Webb and Lorraine Robinson

Introduction to section 8 summary

Section 8 focuses on the key issues and support needs of patients and families who undergo genetic counselling and testing for hereditary cancer. A sound understanding of the issues discussed in Sections 2–4 is important in order to become familiar with the principles underpinning genetic counselling for hereditary cancer.

Once an individual has been identified as being at risk of cancer they face immediate and ongoing challenges. At all times the implications for the wider family need to be considered. Health professionals need to be aware of the psychosocial, ethical and cultural issues in order to help patients to prepare for genetic counselling and to come to terms with knowledge of their genetic status.

Chapter 32. Genetic counselling and supporting individuals with a family history of cancer. Introduction

Pre-symptomatic testing for disease can be seen in the most positive of lights if treatment can prevent a serious condition developing. However, learning about a genetic predisposition without the tangible certainty of having a disease is not easy to cope with. Decisions are left to individuals as to what action they take, if any, with health professionals providing the necessary information and support. As a general rule, health professionals have avoided giving advice. However, although that has been the case for 30 years or so, there now appears to be the beginning of a trend to offer guidance in decision-making.

Yet how do we know genetic counselling helps? There is currently no single measure of the benefits or risks of genetic counselling. A useful tool is the perceived personal control measure developed by Berkenstadt et al. (1999). This captures decisions regarding family life, but only from the individual's point of view. Further developments to the tool to include the family are being considered.

Guided activity for Chapter 32

◆ Read or listen to personal experiences of hereditary cancer at <http://www.tellingstories. nhs.uk>. What were the support and information needs of the participants? How might the cancer health professionals have helped to support and inform these individuals and families?

Further resource for Chapter 32

Bryan E 2008. *Singing the life: the story of a family living in the shadow of cancer*. London: Vermilion.

Chapter 33. Genetic counselling about cancer predisposition

This chapter highlights many of the issues surrounding genetic testing, such as non-directive counselling, relationships within families, testing in childhood, prenatal testing and pre-implantation genetic diagnosis.

Guided activity for Chapter 33

◆ Drawing on Case study 1 in Chapter 33, consider how the oncology team might have managed Sylvia's family history differently and the challenges this might have raised.

Further resources for Chapter 33

British Society for Human Genetics 2010. *Report on the genetic testing of children 2010*. Birmingham: British Society for Human Genetics.
Harper P 2010. *Practical genetic counselling*, 7th edn. London: Edward Arnold.
Riley BD, Culver JO, Skrzynia C, et al. 2012. Essential elements of genetic cancer risk assessment, counseling and testing: updated recommendations of the National Society of Genetic Counselors. *J Genet Counsel* 21: 151–161.

Chapter 34. Psychosocial issues and supporting individuals with a family history of cancer

The psychological issues raised by a cancer family history are addressed throughout the book but this chapter draws together the research in the area and the strategies for helping individuals to come to terms with these difficult issues.

Guided activity for Chapter 34

◆ Reflect on the information and support about cancer family history and/or genetics that is provided by the cancer charities in your specialist area. How accessible is each website? Is the information clear, comprehensible and accurate? Is there professional/ peer input? What support is provided for individuals or families concerned about family history? Is a helpline or chat room provided? When was the website last updated? Would you direct your patients to the website? If not, why not?

Further resources for Chapter 34

Meiser B 2005. Psychological impact of genetic testing for cancer susceptibility: an update of the literature. *Psycho-Oncology* 14: 1060–1074.

Patenaude AF 2005. *Genetic testing for cancer. Psychological approaches for helping patients and families.* Washington, DC: American Psychological Association.

Chapter 35. Ethical and cultural issues

Ethical and cultural issues can arise in any area of clinical practice, but these may be particularly complex in clinical genetics because they often concern the wider family as well as the individual.

It is important to be aware of the possible ethical and cultural issues that may arise in your practice so that you are prepared for difficult situations. Sometimes it is impossible to predict a particular issue. When difficult issues arise it is useful to share your concerns with a colleague or your team or seek external support. This can help to resolve some of the conflict in your own mind and help you to communicate with the patient or family. Sharing your concerns with the patient and family may enable you to work together to resolve issues.

Guided activity for Chapter 35

◆ Reflect on the issues raised by the case study presented in this chapter.

Further resources for Chapter 35

Parker M 2012. *Ethical problems and genetics practice.* Cambridge: Cambridge University Press.

Parker M and Lucassen A 2003. Concern for families and individuals in cancer genetics. *J Med Ethics* 29: 70–73.

References

Berkenstadt M, Shiloh S, Barkai G, et al. 1999. Perceived personal control (PCC): a new concept in measuring outcome of genetic counseling. *Am J Med Genet* 82: 53–59.

Managing cancer family history in primary, secondary and palliative care

Managing cancer family history in primary, secondary and palliative care. Introduction

Chris Jacobs

Introduction to managing cancer family history in primary, secondary and palliative care

Managing a cancer family history appropriately involves knowledge, skills and time. The competencies and training strategy set out by the NHS National Genetics and Genomics Education Centre aim to address the deficiency in knowledge and skills about genetics that has been reported amongst health professionals. However, appropriate management of cancer family history requires more time than is available in the average general practitioner (GP) consultation or symptomatic clinic visit. A qualitative study of women's views of GP consultations about family history of breast cancer concluded that women were not reassured by the explanation provided by GPs (Grande et al., 2002). This is unsurprising given that the average length of a GP consultation is 11.7 minutes (HSCIC, 2007). Without a systematic approach to assessing family history, there is a danger that at-risk patients may be missed in a busy cancer clinic (Dudley-Brown and Freivogel, 2009; Foo et al., 2009).

This chapter presents various different approaches to managing cancer family history in primary and secondary care and considers the implications of cancer family history in palliative care. The learning objectives for Chapter 37 are:

- to be able to identify at least two models for managing a cancer family history;
- to be able to discuss the benefits and limitations of the different models.

Background

In 2001, the average GP saw approximately one patient a month with concerns about a family history of breast or ovarian cancer (Rose, 2001) and approximately one patient in 14 with a positive family history seen in primary care needed to be referred to a regional genetics centre (RGC) (DoH, 2004; Wallace et al., 2004). At that time there was insufficient demand for GPs to be required to gain the knowledge needed to assess and explain cancer risk, and consequently patients were generally referred to genetics services or to symptomatic clinics for family history follow-up. Within symptomatic clinics there was little time for investigation into family history and little or no consistency of screening for family history risk.

In 1998 a Department of Health report for the Chief Medical Officer (DoH, 1998) recommended a 'filtered' system of referrals using a 'hub and spoke' model with the 'spokes' being secondary care clinics and the 'hubs' RGCs. Various different models of risk assessment clinic were set up but there was no consistency about how risk should be assessed or recommendations for screening,

In 2004, following the government White Paper 'Our inheritance, our future' (DoH, 2004), a number of pilot projects were set up in an attempt to establish a single model for managing cancer family history within primary and secondary care. Although no single model emerged as the ideal for all areas and all populations, several key elements were identified as important for successful implementation, including: working with specialist genetics services; understanding the working practices of all specialties involved; identifying key stakeholders and involving them at an early stage; demonstrating the importance of genetics in healthcare; and improving the genetic literacy of health professionals, patients and the public in order to improve the use of services (Bennett et al., 2010).

The importance of cancer family history is referred to in several sets of National Institute for Health and Care Excellence (NICE) guidelines (NICE, 2004, 2011, 2013). The competences set out by the NHS National Genetics and Genomics Education Centre requires health professionals to identify individuals who might benefit from genetic services. Health professionals in primary and secondary care are not required to make a genetic diagnosis or to explain the implications of genetic testing and this discussion is often best undertaken by genetics health professionals who have training and expertise in this area.

As discussed in Chapter 1, growing awareness of the importance of family history for health and a shift in the organisation and delivery of genetic healthcare means that identifying ways to manage cancer family history in primary, secondary and palliative care is important for all health professionals.

Managing cancer family history within genetics services

The overwhelming demand for cancer genetics services means that many RGCs in the UK triage referrals using cancer family history questionnaires (FHQs). This involves the patient being sent a FHQ requesting details of family members such as name and date of birth, type of cancer and treatment details. FHQs are sometimes used in combination with other models. Following risk assessment, patients at average/near population or moderate cancer risk may be sent a letter; only those at high risk or with a complex family history are usually offered a genetic counselling appointment.

The standard model of delivery of genetic counselling is in an individual face-to-face appointment. Although genetics services are regionally based with many patients attending outpatients clinics at the RGC, many services offer genetic counselling in outreach clinics. Other models of delivering cancer genetic counselling have been described, such as the use of videoconferencing technology (telemedicine) for patients in rural areas and group genetic counselling (Cohen et al., 2013). Genetic counselling within primary care has also been reported. A project targeting a 'hard to reach' minority ethnic group through the provision of genetic services in primary care showed only a small increase in referrals from the target community despite the huge amount of effort involved in promoting the service (Srinivasa et al., 2007). A cluster randomised factorial trial of a genetic counselling service based within primary care showed an improvement in the appropriateness of referrals from better-educated GPs and higher rates of attendance than usual (Westwood et al., 2012).

Managing cancer family history within primary and secondary care

Surveillance is not appropriate for all patients with a cancer family history, and cancer units do not have the capacity to manage asymptomatic patients who have concerns about their family history. In many cancer units medical teams assess cancer risk but alternative ways to manage cancer family history in primary and secondary care have been developed to cope with the demand on services.

Family history questionnaires

A study evaluating the administration of FHQs to triage patients in primary care found that although the majority of people who needed specialist referral were identified, this system was less effective at identifying those with a single gene disorder where more detailed information was often required (Qureshi et al., 2005). FHQs pose a number of potential problems for patients and health professionals. For example, obtaining family history information can be upsetting for patients, family members may be unable or unwilling to provide details and some patients may have difficulty understanding or completing the FHQ due to language problems or learning difficulties. The use of FHQs can generate an additional workload for health professionals, particularly when further information is required in order to make a risk assessment, and FHQs may not be returned, leaving the patient's risk unknown and health professionals with the problem of how to manage this (Armel et al., 2011).

Telephone clinics

A telephone-led cancer triage model was described by Shanley et al. (2007) whereby a virtual telephone clinic was offered as a first point of contact for all new genetics referrals to triage patients to discharge, screening or genetic counselling. The flexibility of this model made it convenient and acceptable for patients and led to fewer missed appointments and more focused face-to-face consultations. However, limitations included under-representation of ethnic minorities and difficulty of managing patients' distress, assessing anxiety and providing reassurance.

Nurse-led cancer family history clinics

In one model described by Brennan et al. (2007), family history referrals across the whole cancer network were triaged by RGC-based cancer nurses with specialist training in genetics risk assessment. Other nurse-led clinics have been established within cancer services (McAllister et al., 2002) and in primary care (Allen et al., 2007). The nurse-led cancer risk assessment clinic model is described in more detail in Chapters 39 and 41.

Managing cancer family history within palliative care

It can be difficult for all involved when a patient with cancer is identified as having a family history, particularly if the prognosis is poor. The few studies that have been undertaken in palliative care suggest that nurses are concerned about raising issues concerning family history at the end of life (Lillie et al., 2011) and lack confidence in their ability to provide appropriate care and support for families with inherited cancer (Metcalfe et al., 2010). Health professionals working with terminally ill cancer patients need to be aware of how to identify families at increased cancer risk and how to access genetics specialists so that advice and discussion can take place without delay and with minimal distress to the family.

Summary

The choice of model for managing cancer family history will depend on the availability of services and the needs of the local population. Implementation of each of these models presents challenges such as accessibility, involving hard to reach groups, difficulty with obtaining reliable family history information, maintaining confidentiality across families, keeping up to date with guidelines, the dynamic nature of family histories and working across organisational boundaries.

The chapters in this section aim to provide practical examples of managing cancer family history in primary, secondary and palliative care and to demonstrate how some of these challenges may be addressed.

References

Allen H, Maxwell L, Dibley N, et al. 2007. Patient perspectives on the Poole PCT cancer genetics service. *Fam Cancer* **6**: 231–239.

Armel SR, Hitchman K, Millar K, et al. 2011. The use of family history questionnaires: an examination of genetic risk estimates and genetic testing eligibility in the non-responder population. *J Genet Counsel* **20**: 355–364.

Bennett C, Burke S, Burton H, Farndon P 2010. A toolkit for incorporating genetics into mainstream medical services: learning from service development pilots in England. *BMC Health Serv Res* **10**: 125.

Brennan P, Claber O, Shaw T 2007. The Teesside cancer family history service: change management and innovation at cancer network level. *Fam Cancer* **6**: 181–187.

Cohen SA, Marvin ML, Riley BD, et al. 2013. Identification of genetic counseling service delivery models in practice: a report from the NSGC Service Delivery Model Task Force. *J Genet Counsel* **22**: 411–421.

DOH (**Department of Health**) 1998. *Genetics and cancer services*. Report of a working group for the Chief Medical Officer. London: Department of Health

DoH (**Department of Health**) 2004. *Our inheritance, our future. Realising the potential of genetics in the NHS*. London: The Stationery Office.

Dudley-Brown S and Freivogel M 2009. Hereditary colorectal cancer in the gastroenterology clinic: how common are at-risk patients and how do we find them? *Gastroenterol Nurs* **32**: 8–16.

Foo W, Young JM, Solomon MJ, Wright CM 2009. Family history? The forgotten question in high-risk colorectal cancer patients. *Colorectal Dis* **11**: 450–455.

Grande GE, Hyland F, Walter FM, Kinmonth AL 2002. Women's views of consultations about familial risk of breast cancer in primary care. *Patient Educ Counsel* **48**: 275–282.

HSCIC (**Health and Social Care Information Centre**) 2007. *GP workload survey results* [online]. Available at: <http://www.hscic.gov.uk/pubs/gpworkload> (last accessed 8 June 2013).

Lillie AK, Clifford C, Metcalfe A 2011. Caring for families with a family history of cancer: why concerns about genetic predisposition are missing from the palliative agenda. *Palliat Med* **25**: 117–124.

McAllister M, O'Malley K, Hopwood P, et al. 2002. Management of women with a family history of breast cancer in the north west region of England: training for implementing a vision of the future. *J Med Genet* **39**: 531–535.

Metcalfe A, Pumphrey R, Clifford C 2010. Hospice nurses and genetics: implications for end-of-life care. *J Clin Nurs* **19**: 192–207.

NICE (**National Institute for Health and Care Excellence**) 2004. *Improving outcomes in colorectal cancers. Manual update*. London: National Institute for Health and Care Excellence.

NICE (**National Institute for Health and Care Excellence**) 2011. *Ovarian cancer: the recognition and initial management of ovarian cancer*. NICE Clinical Guideline 122. London: National Institute for Health and Care Excellence.

NICE (**National Institute for Health and Care Excellence**) 2013. *Familial breast cancer: classification and care of people at risk of familial breast cancer and management of breast cancer and related risks in people with a family history of breast cancer*. NICE Clinical Guideline 164. London: National Institute for Health and Care Excellence.

Qureshi N, Bethea J, Modell B, et al. 2005. Collecting genetic information in primary care: evaluating a new family history tool. *Fam Pract* **22**: 663–669.

Rose PW 2001. Referral of patients with a family history of breast/ovarian cancer—GPs' knowledge and expectations. *Fam Pract* **18**: 487–490.

Shanley S, Myhill K, Doherty R, et al. 2007. Delivery of cancer genetics services: the Royal Marsden telephone clinic model. *Fam Cancer* **6**: 213–219.

Srinivasa J, Rowett E, Dharni N, et al. 2007. Improving access to cancer genetics services in primary care: socio-economic data from North Kirklees. *Fam Cancer* **6**: 197–203.

Wallace E, Hinds A, Campbell H, et al. 2004. A cross-sectional survey to estimate the prevalence of family history of colorectal, breast and ovarian cancer in a Scottish general practice population. *Br J Cancer* **91**: 1575–1579.

Westwood G, Pickering R, Latter S, et al. 2012. A primary care specialist genetics service: a cluster-randomised factorial trial. *Br J Gen Pract* **62**: e191–e197.

Chapter 38

Experiences of managing cancer family history in primary care

Belinda Lötter and Kati Harris

Introduction to experiences of managing cancer family history in primary care

The aim of managing cancer family history in primary care is to provide an accessible service for patients, targeted screening and genetic counselling and ease of referral for health professionals. However, there are many challenges to overcome. This chapter reflects on the experience of setting up and running nurse-led cancer family history clinics in primary care in an inner city area of London. The nurses running the service describe the background, organisation, benefits and challenges. The learning objectives for Chapter 38 are:

- to be able to discuss the role of the health professional in managing cancer family history in primary care;
- to consider the challenges and benefits of setting up and running cancer risk assessment clinics in primary care.

Breast cancer family history clinics in primary care

The Breast Cancer Risk Assessment Service

The nurse-led Breast Cancer Risk Assessment Service (BCRAS) was introduced in 2010 following a successful pilot project funded by Macmillan and the Department of Health (Jacobs et al., 2007). The service was established to meet the need for breast cancer risk assessment amongst the population of Lambeth, Southwark and Lewisham, three inner London boroughs, following publication of a government report (DoH, 2004) and national guidelines for familial breast cancer (McIntosh et al., 2004). These three boroughs have areas of considerable deprivation and are culturally and socially diverse, with approximately 35% of the population from minority ethnic groups (ONS, 2001). Prior to the pilot project, the proportion of patients from black and minority ethnic (BME) groups accessing the cancer genetics service was just 3% (Jacobs et al., 2007).

The BCRAS is based within Guy's Regional Genetics Centre (RGC) but all clinics take place within general practitioner (GP) clinics and community centres across the three boroughs, with the nurses attending different clinics every day in one of seven locations. The service is available to women and men who are concerned about their family history of breast and/or ovarian cancer. A unique aspect of the service is that self-referrals are accepted in order to increase access and availability.

The BCRAS is run by two full-time Band 6 nurses from a varied nursing background and supported by a half-time Band 4 administrator. In order to meet the genetics competencies (Kirk et al., 2003, 2011) training included attending the course in advanced healthcare practice in cancer genetics course run by King's College London in conjunction with St George's, University of London and the London RGCs, and one-to-one supervised clinics with genetic counsellors. The nurses have gone on to undertake the postgraduate certificate in genetic healthcare at Plymouth University.

The primary role of the nurses is to assess the risk of individuals who have a family and/or personal history of breast and/or ovarian cancer and to refer on for appropriate risk management. All patients referred to the service are offered an individual face-to-face appointment in a local clinic or, if they prefer, a telephone appointment in which a three-generation family history is taken, a pedigree is drawn, risk assessment is made and risk management information and health education are provided. Patients who meet criteria for early breast screening (NICE, 2013) are referred to the local NHS breast screening unit. Those at high risk are given the opportunity to access genetic counselling and are referred directly without the delay of going back to their GP. Patients who do not require further intervention are discharged with breast awareness information and lifestyle advice. All patients are sent a brief letter summarising the appointment, copied to the referring clinician and their GP (Harris and Lötter, 2012).

The nurses are managed, supported and supervised by the RGC, providing access to genetics clinical meetings, lectures and expert opinion. The BCRAS and breast screening service are commissioned by the local clinical commissioning groups (CCG) with a service level agreement between the South East London Breast Screening Service and the BCRAS. Governance is the responsibility of the RGC. Quarterly audit meetings are attended by the BCRAS manager, breast screening managers and breast screening commissioners. The business case is reviewed on a 2-yearly basis.

Evaluation of the BCRAS over the third year of the service

The number of referrals has steadily increased as new clinics have opened and awareness of the clinics has been raised amongst the local community. It is interesting to note that the monthly referral rate increased threefold between 1 and 30 June 2013 in response to media publicity and publication of revised familial breast cancer guidelines (NICE, 2013). The clinical outcome data from 1 June 2012 to 31 May 2013 are presented in Table 38.1 and Fig. 38.1.

Of the 478 patients referred to the service, the majority were female with a mean age of 37.6 years. Just under half of the patients seen identified themselves as being from BME groups, demonstrating that the service is reaching the target local population. The majority of patients were referred by health professionals, but 18% were self-referrals.

Over the 12-month period, 48% (228) were assessed to be at high risk, 29% (141) at moderately increased risk and 23% (109) at near population risk. Amongst the patients

Table 38.1 Demographic data from the Breast Cancer Risk Assessment Service (BCRAS) from 1 June 2012 to 31 May 2013

Total number of patients seen	478
Age range	18–81 years (mean 37.6 years)
Gender	470 (98%) female
Ethnicity	214 (45%) from BME groups
Self-referrals	84 (18%)

BME, black and minority ethnic.

Source: data from clinical activity from BCRAS from 1 June 2012 to 31 May 2013.

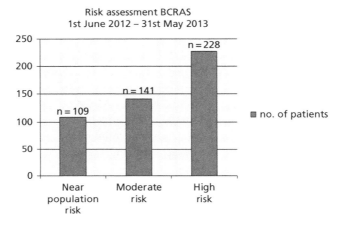

Figure 38.1 BRCAS Risk assessment between 1 June 2012 and 31 May 2013.

Source: data from clinical activity from the Breast Cancer Risk Assessment Service (BCRAS) from 1 June 2012 to 31 May 2013.

who referred themselves to the service, 71.4% (60) were assessed to be at moderate or high risk of breast cancer, in line with the patients referred by health professionals and indicating that patients triage themselves and seek risk assessment appropriately. Of those at higher than average risk, 22% (103) were referred directly into screening and 20% (96) were referred to genetics. Forty-eight per cent (229) were under the age of 40 at the time of the risk assessment and were advised to enter screening at the appropriate age where necessary.

Benefits and challenges

Location of clinics

The community-based location of the clinics enables patients to be seen close to home by a trained health professional, increasing convenience and accessibility. In order to maximise clinic attendance, the administrator contacts each patient prior to their appointment. This acts as a reminder and provides an opportunity for them to change the appointment if necessary. Patients are able to contact the clinic by post, telephone or email, with access to a staffed helpline during office hours.

Funding for the service does not include paying for clinic space. Finding suitable and affordable clinic space that has good transport links has been one of the main challenges in setting up the service. The clinic space provider can sometimes make changes to room availability at short notice, leading to disruption of the clinic. These challenges require open communication and flexibility from both parties. Because of the financial constraints on clinic room availability, there are a limited number of geographical locations where clinics can be held, requiring regular re-evaluation of the suitability and accessibility of clinics to service users.

Accessing the clinics

Robust and seamless pathways have been established to and from local GP practices, breast units and the breast screening service, reducing waiting times for patients and facilitating easy referral for clinicians. GPs, practice nurses and hospital specialists are able to refer asymptomatic patients directly to the service by letter, email, fax or telephone. Alternatively, health professionals can provide patients with the contact details of the service so that they can refer themselves. The self-referral pathway enables patients to get back in touch with the service if their family history changes and they require reassessment. Providing equitable access to all groups of the population is one of the main objectives of the service. In an area where many different languages are spoken, appointments with an interpreter present or three-way telephone interpretations are sometimes necessary.

Regular audit helps to identify areas that do not refer to the service, enabling these areas to be targeted. GPs who continue to refer asymptomatic patients inquiring about their family history to the symptomatic breast service are contacted and informed of the referral pathway.

For symptomatic women with a family history, the pathway involves onward referral by the breast unit to the BCRAS once symptoms have been managed. Seeing these women has been challenging, both in terms of the breast units referring to the service and the women attending the clinic. To overcome this, clinics are in the process of being set up within several of the local breast units.

Raising awareness and developing relationships across organisational boundaries

Excellent working relationships have been established with many of the local GP practices and specialist breast units. Gaining the trust and respect of local health professionals has been achieved by identifying key individuals, attending meetings, delivering talks about the service and responding quickly and appropriately to queries. Establishing clinics within the local breast units has the added advantage of increasing the visibility of the nurses, helping to build relationships and providing a helpful resource for the breast unit multidisciplinary team. Having a base within the RGC has enabled close integration between the BCRAS, primary care, the genetics service and the breast screening service. This has led to the development of streamlined patient pathways and improved communication, which is beneficial to all parties.

Ongoing promotion amongst local service users is necessary to maintain awareness of the service. The promotion strategy includes mail shots to local GP surgeries, community centres, community groups, libraries, children's centres and specialist units, a webpage on the trust website with links from the breast unit and RGC, development and distribution of patient information leaflets and regular attendance at local events and stands in shopping centres and hospitals. The Health and Social Care Act (2012) has resulted in enormous changes in primary care, making it difficult at times to gain access to GPs who are flooded with information.

Providing accurate risk assessment

The BCRAS has provided the local population with access to expert risk assessment and seamless referral to appropriate screening and genetic counselling. Providing a risk assessment service in primary care to such a socially and ethnically diverse population has not been without its challenges. Recognising and respecting cultural diversity and personal beliefs is extremely important as is sensitivity to the differences in the way illness and death are discussed within different cultures. Reluctance to talk about illness and death can make accurate risk assessment very difficult. This is managed by acknowledging cultural differences, explaining to patients that the risk assessment can only be as accurate as the information they provide and helping them to understand what further information would be required. In addition, patients may not be aware of the details of cancer diagnoses of relatives living abroad, meaning that confirmation of diagnosis is often impossible and access to genetic testing and screening may not be available for those relatives.

Summary

Undertaking breast cancer risk assessment within primary care has provided patients and health professionals with a local, accessible service and seamless pathways into appropriate breast cancer risk management. Although there are challenges and the outcomes and requirements of the service need to be re-evaluated on a regular basis, the experience to date the service is becoming integrated into local health services and is reaching local 'hard to reach' groups.

References

DoH (Department Of Health) 2004. *Our inheritance, our future. Realising the potential of genetics in the NHS*. London: The Stationery Office.

Harris K and Lötter B 2012. Focus on patients with a family history of cancer. *Cancer Nurs Pract* **11**: 14–19.

Jacobs C, Rawson R., Campion C, et al. 2007. Providing a community-based cancer risk assessment service for a socially and ethnically diverse population. *Fam Cancer* **6**: 189–195.

Kirk M, Macdonald K, Longley M, Anstey S 2003. *Fit for practice in the genetics era: a competence based education framework for nurses, midwives and health visitors*. Pontypridd: University of Glamorgan.

Kirk M, Calzone K, Arimori N, Tonkin E. 2011. Genetics-genomics competencies and nursing regulation. *J Nurs Scholar* **43**: 107–116.

McIntosh A, Shaw C, Evans G, et al. 2004. *Clinical guidelines for the classification and care of women at risk of familial breast cancer* [updated October 2006]. London: National Collaborating Centre for Primary Care/University of Sheffield.

NICE (National Institute for Health and Care Excellence) 2013. *Familial breast cancer: classification and care of people at risk of familial breast cancer and management of breast cancer and related risks in people with a family history of breast cancer*. NICE Clinical Guideline 164. London: National Institute for Health and Care Excellence.

ONS (Office for National Statistics). 2001. *2001 census* [online]. Available at: <http://www.ons.gov.uk/ons/guide-method/census/census-2001/index.html> (last accessed 16 May 2013).

Chapter 39

Experiences of managing cancer family history in secondary care

Gillian Bowman and Linda Dyer

Introduction to experiences of managing cancer family history in secondary care

This chapter will focus on the management within secondary care of patients with a family history (FH) of breast cancer and colorectal cancer (CRC), drawing on the experience of two nurse-led FH clinics in the southeast of England. The rationale for establishing the clinics, the way the services were delivered and the benefits, challenges and lessons learned will be discussed. The learning objectives for Chapter 39 are:

- to be able to discuss the role of the health professional in managing FH in secondary care;
- to consider the challenges and benefits of setting up and running a cancer FH clinic in the hospital setting.

Rationale for setting up the clinics

Both clinics were set up in the late 1990s, following publication of a report for the Chief Medical Officer about the organisation of cancer genetics services (DoH, 1998). The clinics aimed to improve consistency of management, triage referrals for screening and genetics assessment and move well patients out of the symptomatic clinics. National risk assessment guidelines were not available at that time so referral pathways and guidelines were developed in consultation with the regional genetics centre (RGC) based on the available evidence. Support and training for the clinical nurse specialists (CNS) running the clinics was provided by the RGC.

Prior to establishing the clinics, patients concerned about their FH were seen in the symptomatic clinic by a surgeon alongside patients undergoing cancer treatment. Screening and genetics referrals were undertaken at the patient's request or the clinician's judgment, and although patients diagnosed with cancer were generally asked if they had a FH of the disease, a thorough FH and systematic risk assessment was rarely undertaken. Clinicians were often influenced by patients' concerns or the reported frequency of screening amongst other family members, leading to a lack of consistency in the organisation of screening. Asymptomatic patients who reported a FH were often followed up on a regular basis from the age at which they were referred (with clinical breast examinations and/mammograms or ultrasound scans or colonoscopies), strengthening dependency on screening. As a consequence, many patients were exposed to unnecessary procedures and overwhelming demand was placed on symptomatic clinics and screening services.

Experience of running the clinics

The Breast Cancer Family History Clinic

Initially, monthly clinics were held but demand quickly grew, and within 9 months the CNS was seeing six to eight patients per clinic for up to 30 minutes each. Referrals were accepted from general practitioners (GPs) or the symptomatic clinic. All patients were offered a one-off appointment at which a three-generation family history was taken, a pedigree drawn, risk and further management explained and, where appropriate, screening and/or genetics referral made. Patients presented for many reasons, including seeking reassurance, requesting screening and asking about genetic testing. Often referral was requested when a close family member or friend had been diagnosed or died from cancer. As described by Watson et al. (1999), there was a tendency for patients to overestimate their risk, and those in the average- and moderate-risk groups invariably stated that they felt reassured that their risk was lower than they had originally thought (Brain et al., 2002). The referral pathway for the Breast Cancer Family History Clinic is shown in Fig. 39.1.

The Colorectal Cancer Family History Clinic

At the outset, the CNS saw eight patients a month in a face-to face appointment. However, demand quickly grew and by 2004 the clinic was receiving in excess of 50 GP referrals a

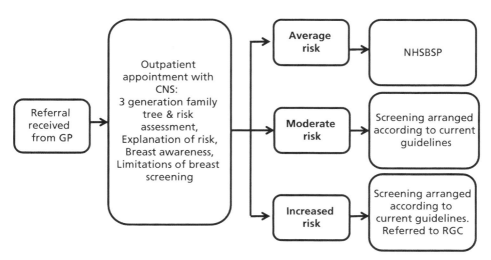

Figure 39.1 Breast Cancer Family History Clinic referral pathway (GP, general practitioner; CNS, clinical nurse specialist(s); NHSBSP, NHS Breast Screening Programme; RGC, regional genetics centre).

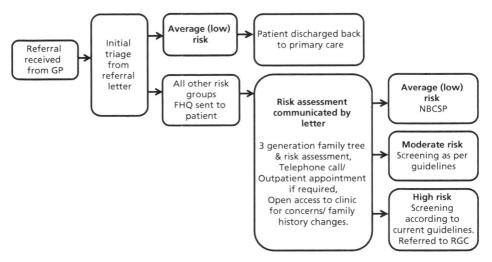

Figure 39.2 Colorectal Cancer Family History Clinic revised referral pathway (GP, general practitioner; FHQ, family history questionnaire; NBCSP, National Bowel Cancer Screening Programme; RGC, regional genetics centre).

month, in addition to referrals from local consultants. The service became the local 'hub' for referrals, monitoring outcomes and follow-up. Growing demand for the service and the publication of guidelines for CRC risk assessment (Dunlop, 2002) prompted an audit of the service. This showed that as a result of the clinic, 40% of patients were either taken out of or not entered into screening, but that although patients were asked if there was a FH of CRC they were not always asked about other cancers; consequently patients with an Amsterdam positive FH or a history of polyposis were not consistently offered referral to the RGC. The decision was made to send referral guidelines to local GPs in order to increase the appropriateness of referrals and a triage system was established so that patients at average risk were managed in primary care. Follow-up audit in 2007 showed that referrals were appropriate and demand for the service continued to increase to the point that demand exceeded capacity. Further revision of the referral pathway became necessary (Fig. 39.2).

Benefits

Over time, both clinics became integral to the local cancer services and local communities. The clinics provided accurate risk and management advice to individuals and families, improved the appropriateness of referrals and reduced demand on overstretched symptomatic and screening services (Table 39.1).

Challenges and lessons learned

Facilitating transition to the new service

Changing access to screening caused some anxiety, confusion and, at times, anger amongst patients who had previously been told that they should be having regular screening. It

Table 39.1 Summary of the benefits of the FH clinics for patients and local services

Benefits for patients	Benefits to local services
Accurate risk assessment for individuals	Coordinated centralised care
Appropriate screening organised and genetics referral made	Inappropriate demand on symptomatic clinics and screening services reduced
Implementation of evidence-based guidelines enabled consistent advice to be provided across local families	Provided a specialist resource for local services

was sometimes difficult to explain why patients no longer required early or more frequent screening. The following case is typical example:

> Jane's maternal aunt and grandmother developed breast cancer in their 60s. Jane had been advised by her aunt's GP that she should undergo screening from the age of 35. She was assessed to be at near population risk and advised to enter the NHS Breast Screening Programme at the age of 50. Jane found this difficult to accept. It was helpful to work through the pedigree and risk assessment tool with Jane so that she had a better understanding of her risk and the rationale for the advice given.

Gradual transition to the new service, introducing the changes over a 1-year period, helped to alleviate some of these difficulties. Careful explanation of the rationale for the change of advice, open access to the clinics in the event of a change to FH and reference to links with the RGC were also helpful. The RGC provided advice and support for the CNS and, where necessary, a second opinion for patients, although obtaining a response from the RGC and then getting back in touch with the patient was sometimes time-consuming.

Managing family dynamics and maintaining confidentiality

Health professionals working in cancer care generally manage the care of the individual rather than the family. Because the clinics were local, several family members were sometimes referred without the others' knowledge. This became particularly difficult when family dynamics were complex. For example:

> The father of Jason (who died from gastric cancer at the age of 26) refused permission to discuss the diagnosis or consider testing of Jason's tumour, which would have helped with risk assessment and screening advice for the whole family. Maintaining confidentiality became a huge issue, preventing other family members from accessing screening. This was resolved when, unfortunately, another female relative presented with CRC at the age of 30. This relative was referred to the FH clinic and then on to the RGC where a mutation was identified in the *MLH2* gene, enabling other family members to access genetic testing.

It is helpful in such situations to explain why it is important for relatives to be informed and to help patients find ways to discuss the FH. Respecting privacy and confidentiality, for example by seeking consent and not documenting the full names of family members on the pedigree (RCP, 2011), was also important. Training in genetics and close links with the RGC helped provide support to the CNS in these situations.

Helping patients to accept screening recommendations

It was sometimes difficult to explain to a patient why screening would commence later than the age at which a relative had been diagnosed with cancer. For example:

> Karen was aged 35. Her mother developed breast cancer at the age of 37 but there was no other cancer FH. Karen was assessed to be at moderate risk of breast cancer and advised to commence annual mammograms from the age of 40. Careful explanation about lack of evidence for the effectiveness of mammography in younger women, the potentially harmful effects of radiation and breast awareness and lifestyle factors, helped Karen to accept the screening recommendations.

Through close links with the RGC from the outset, consultation about referral pathways, consistent use of risk assessment tools and training in communicating risk were facilitated. As national guidelines became available (Dunlop, 2002; McIntosh et al., 2004; Cairns et al., 2010) explaining risk estimates to patients became less challenging.

Establishing confidence amongst local colleagues

Consultants were sometimes cautious about handing over the care of patients to the FH clinic. For example:

> Nine members of one family were all found to have a mutation in the *MSH6* gene at predictive testing. Each relative was under the care of a different consultant in the area and a range of screening arrangements were in place. The consultants were unaware of the extent of the FH or the different screening regimes. The clinic enabled the FH notes of each family member to be matched up and screening to be standardised across the family.

Gaining the trust and confidence of local colleagues in the specialist and related areas involved in the management of patients with a FH of hereditary cancers (such as gynaecology, dermatology, ophthalmology), required communication, time and diplomacy.

Changing funding and support needs

When the clinics were initially set up, funding and management support were not formalised. As the workload increased, so did the need for administrative and technical support. Although the clinics could demonstrate efficiency savings in the long term, due to targeted screening, resources for the clinic were not prioritised. As a result, clinics ran on minimal staffing with no cover for annual/sick leave:

> The Breast Cancer Family History Clinic had been running for many years when the administrative support was reduced due to staff sickness and changing priorities within the breast unit. The clinic could no longer function effectively and had to be suspended. The case was presented to the manager with the support of the RGC. After much discussion, staffing issues were resolved and the clinic was reinstated.

Careful business planning and ongoing audit help to overcome the practical and organisational challenges of setting up a new clinic.

Summary

These two dedicated FH clinics within secondary care provided a valuable local service for patients, families and local clinicians and facilitated appropriate referral to screening services and the RGC. The clinics were set up in response to a clinical need and policy changes before national guidelines had been agreed. Valuable lessons were learned from these experiences, in particular the importance of engaging all stakeholders in setting up new services, developing a business case and establishing systems for monitoring the service.

References

Brain K, Norman P, Gray J, et al. 2002. A randomized trial of specialist genetic assessment: psychological impact on women at different levels of familial breast cancer risk. *Br J Cancer* **86**: 233–238.

Cairns SR, Scholefield JH, Steele RJ, et al. 2010. Guidelines for colorectal cancer screening and surveillance in moderate and high risk groups (update from 2002). *Gut* **59**: 666–689.

DoH (Department of Health) 1998. *Genetics and cancer services*. Report of a working group for the Chief Medical Officer. London: Department of Health.

Dunlop MG 2002. Guidance on gastrointestinal surveillance for hereditary non-polyposis colorectal cancer, familial adenomatous polyposis, juvenile polyposis, and Peutz–Jeghers syndrome. *Gut* **51** (Suppl. 5): V21–V27.

McIntosh A, Shaw C, Evans G, et al. 2004. *Clinical guidelines for the classification and care of women at risk of familial breast cancer* [updated October 2006]. London: National Collaborating Centre for Primary Care/University of Sheffield.

RCP (Royal College of Physicians Royal College of Pathologists and British Society for Human Genetics) 2011. *Consent and confidentiality in clinical genetic practice: guidance on genetic testing and sharing genetic information*, 2nd edn. Report of the Joint Committee on Medical Genetics. London: RCP/RCPath.

Watson M, Lloyd S, Davidson J, et al. 1999. The impact of genetic counselling on risk perception and mental health in women with a family history of breast cancer. *Br J Cancer* **79**: 868–874.

Chapter 40

Experiences of managing cancer family history in palliative care

Sheila Goff

Introduction to experiences of managing cancer family history in palliative care

In 2010, 157 275 people in the UK died from cancer (CRUK, 2012). A large proportion of these will have come into contact with health professionals working in palliative care. It is estimated that 5–10% of people with cancer have a genetic predisposition to the condition (Offit, 1998). Health professionals in palliative care will therefore care for many people who have a family history of the disease during the end stages of their cancer illness. Despite this, evidence suggests that there is usually no discussion of family history with patients receiving palliative care at the end of life. There appears to be an assumption that by the time the patient reaches that stage of their illness, the family history will have been assessed and acted upon by other teams involved earlier on.

This chapter will look at some of the evidence that family history is not assessed in palliative care settings and consider why this may be. It will also highlight the importance of addressing this and look at the opportunities and challenges facing health professionals, patients and families when this issue is raised at the end of life. The learning objectives for Chapter 40 are:

- to be able to discuss the role of the health professional in identifying a significant cancer family history in palliative care;
- to consider the challenges and benefits of cancer risk assessment in the hospice/dying patient's home setting.

Palliative care

The World Health Organization defines palliative care as 'an approach that improves the quality of life of patients and their families facing the problems associated with life-threatening illness, through the prevention and relief of suffering by means of early identification and impeccable assessment and treatment of pain and other problems, physical, psychosocial and spiritual' (World Health Organization, 2012). This definition includes the care of the family, and indeed the biological family and all other people who are important to the patient should be given care and time by health professionals engaged in palliative care (Payne et al., 2008). Central to a holistic assessment of a patient referred for palliative care is the collection of details about their family and those close to them, but the focus of this discussion is usually to determine the nature of the support structures available to the patient in that phase of their illness and the effect of the situation on those family members or friends. Thus, health professionals working in palliative care are skilled in asking about family but research shows that taking and checking a three-generation family history for risk of a genetic predisposition to cancer often does not take place. Quillin et al. (2010) reviewed medical notes and interviewed 43 cancer patients receiving palliative care; they found that although nine (21%) had a strong genetic risk none had undergone genetic counselling. This study indicates that the prevalence of individuals with a significant risk of hereditary cancer in the palliative care population is as high as in the general population but it is not being addressed. Other studies looking at the assessment of family history in women with advanced ovarian cancer from both the United States and the UK also indicate that family history assessment is sometimes missed altogether, or if carried out is not always acted upon even when significant (Meyer et al., 2010; Lanceley et al., 2012).

Why so late?

When a patient with cancer enters the end of life phase, palliative care health professionals may assume that the family history assessment has been done at an earlier stage in the illness trajectory and that, in any case, it is not the right time or place to ask such questions (Quillin et al., 2008). The problem is that there is never a right time in the illness path to raise the issue of family history. Health professionals may believe that at cancer diagnosis it is not a good time for such discussion and assessment because patients are shocked and have so much information to take in (Ardern- Jones et al., 2005); neither is the time of a relapse or difficult treatment. Patients may be unwilling to disclose or think about a family history at certain stages of their illness, or they may overestimate the length of time they have left and feel that it is an issue that can be addressed at a later date. It may be that more significant family history emerges as estranged or out of contact family members become involved when the death of their relative approaches. For all these reasons, the health professional in palliative care may be the most appropriate person to gather all the information about the family history and to make the risk assessment (Quillin et al., 2008).

However, there is evidence of a lack of confidence and knowledge in this field amongst palliative care professionals. Metcalfe et al. (2010) carried out a large survey of the genetics knowledge of nurses working in UK hospices. The response rate was poor (29%), suggesting that the subject area was of low importance and relevance to the nurses involved. Of those who did respond, most saw the issue as important but considered that genetics knowledge was part of the doctor's remit rather than their own and expressed lack of confidence in their ability to assess family history risk and low levels of knowledge about what to do with the information.

Discussing and assessing family history at end of life

It is important for health professionals in palliative care to raise the issue of family history with patients even if it has been addressed before. New insights and changed perspectives that the patient experiences as death approaches may lead to unresolved issues and concerns for their family. An ideal time to discuss the family history is on first meeting the patient when family members are also often present and it is appropriate to discuss family and carer issues. However, during an initial assessment there are usually multiple physical, psychological, social and spiritual issues, and overwhelming problems with symptoms often need to be addressed urgently. Health professionals may worry that raising yet another issue at this time will burden the patient. Difficult decisions and complex multiprofessional liaison about how the patient is going to manage in their current home environment will take precedence over asking about the family history.

Currently, for individuals from families with a significant history of cancer to benefit from accurate genetic risk assessment, genetic testing needs to be performed on a sample from the individual with cancer. There are concerns about carrying out the invasive procedure of collecting a blood sample in patients nearing the end of their life where the focus of all other aspects of care is on comfort, and indeed on the cessation of tests and measurements. The health professional in palliative care is well positioned to facilitate the collection of this sample. The information and consent process need to be adapted depending on the condition of the patient. It would not be relevant to discuss the implications of the genetic test for the patient who is close to death, but a simple outline of how the sample may be tested or stored for future use for their family can be comforting to patients at the end of life (Daniels et al., 2011). It is important to discuss how the genetic test results will be disclosed after the patient's death and to document clear instructions about which family member will be contacted with the results. Family members are often present or in regular contact with their dying relative, making these conversations easier. Close liaison with the clinical genetics service through this process is essential in order to ensure safe receipt and storage of the precious sample, timely dissemination of the results and follow-up of at-risk relatives if appropriate.

Looking to the future: opportunities of cancer risk assessment in the palliative care setting

As genetic testing becomes part of mainstream cancer care and patients are routinely tested at diagnosis to aid their individual treatment plans there will be less need for the collection of blood samples from dying patients. Nevertheless, it is important for health professionals in palliative care to remain cognisant of developments in cancer genetics so they can reiterate with authority and knowledge information given to patients and families by other treating teams. Palliative care health professionals are in the unusual position of having involvement with the patient and sometimes many of their family members at the same time, or within a concentrated time frame, when everybody's thoughts and feelings are focused on cancer. This provides an opportunity for clarifying what the family history of cancer means in terms of risk to family members. This may be reassuring to the patient and family, particularly if relatives are at no greater risk than the general population of developing the cancer (Lillie, 2006). Palliative care health professionals could seize the opportunity for more general health education about possible lifestyle and environmental risk factors associated with certain cancers. When relatives are facing the death of a family member, their own feelings and fears about cancer are heightened, opening up a 'teachable moment' (Quillin et al., 2008). Taking the opportunity to ensure that relatives are aware of their risk and the measures they can take to reduce this can help in the bereavement process (Lillie, 2008).

Summary

Ideally, a patient with cancer will have their family history assessed and genetic testing initiated soon after the diagnosis is confirmed. This may not happen for many reasons. Even if it is documented that the patient has been asked about their family history, end of life care provides a last chance to check the family history and, where appropriate, store DNA. It is the role of palliative care health professionals to seize this opportunity and to take action, offering health education about cancer risk factors to family members and seeking the advice of the clinical genetics services where necessary.

References

Ardern-Jones A, Kenen R, Eeles R 2005. Too much too soon? Patients and health professionals' views concerning the impact of genetic testing at the time of breast cancer diagnosis in women under the age of 40. *Eur J Cancer Care* **14**: 272–281.

CRUK (Cancer Research UK). *CancerStats: cancer statistics for the UK.* Available at: <http://www.cancerresearchuk.org/cancer-info/cancerstats> (last accessed 30 December 2012).

Daniels MS, Burzawa JK, Brandt AC, et al. 2011. A clinical perspective on genetic counseling and testing during end of life care for women with recurrent progressive ovarian cancer: opportunities and challenges. *Fam Cancer* **10**: 193–197.

Lanceley A, Eagle Z, Ogden G, et al. 2012. Family history and women with ovarian cancer: is it asked and does it matter? *Int J Gynecol Cancer* **22**: 254–259.

Lillie AK 2006. Exploring cancer genetics and care of the family: an evolving challenge for palliative care. *Int J Palliat Nurs* **12**: 70–74.

Lillie AK 2008. The missing discourse. How does the family history of cancer affect the care needs of palliative care patients? PhD thesis. University of Birmingham.

Metcalfe A, Pumphrey R, Clifford, C. 2010. Hospice nurses and genetics: implications for end-of-life care. *J Clin Nurs* **19**: 192–207.

Meyer LA, Anderson ME, Lacour RA, et al. 2010. Evaluating women with ovarian cancer for *BRCA1* and *BRCA2* mutations: missed opportunities. *Obstet Gynecol* **115**: 945–952.

Offit K 1998. *Clinical cancer genetics.* New York: Wiley-Liss.

Payne S, Seymour J, Ingleton C 2008. *Palliative care nursing: principles and evidence for practice*, 2nd edn. Maidenhead: Open University Press.

Quillin JM, Bodurtha JN, Smith TJ 2008. Genetics assessment at the end of life: suggestions for implementation in clinic and future research. *J Palliat Med* **11**: 451–458.

Quillin JM, Bodurtha JN, Siminoff LA, Smith TJ 2010. Exploring hereditary cancer among dying cancer patients- a cross-sectional study of hereditary risk and perceived awareness of DNA testing and banking. *J Genet Counsel* **19**: 497–525.

World Health Organization 2012. *WHO definition of palliative care.* Available at: <http://www.who.int/cancer/palliative/definition> (last accessed 30 December 2012).

A practical guide to setting up a cancer family history clinic in primary or secondary care

Chris Jacobs

Introduction to a practical guide to setting up a family history clinic in primary or secondary care

Identifying patients at risk of hereditary cancer, managing genetic risk and communicating genetic information to patients is now within the remit of all health professionals in cancer care. The model of the cancer family history clinic provides the opportunity to develop closer working practices between primary care, secondary-care cancer services and genetics services in order to enable a structure for systematic family history assessment and consistent and evidence-based cancer risk management for the benefit of patients and health services.

The service development projects that were set up as a result of the Department of Health White Paper (DoH, 2004) and described by Eeles et al. (2007) highlighted many of the benefits and challenges of mainstreaming genetics services in cancer risk assessment. The lessons learned from these projects formed the basis of a toolkit for incorporating genetics into mainstream services (Bennett et al., 2010) and are available on the NHS National Genetics and Genomics Education Centre website (<http://www.geneticseducation.nhs. uk/for-healthcare-educators/learning-outcome>). Scheuner et al. (2014) described the development, implementation and evaluation of a similar cancer genetics toolkit, demonstrating improvements in the quality of documented cancer family history and increased identification of patients at high risk by primary-care clinicians in the United States.

Across the southeast of England, a network of cancer family history clinics has been established with strong links between local health services and genetics. Clinical nurse specialists (CNS) in cancer care run these clinics with clinical governance and management provided by the local health services and specific genetics training, supervision and support provided by the regional genetics centre (RGC).

Drawing on the author's experience of working with these clinics for more than 10 years, this chapter focuses on the practical issues involved in setting up a cancer family history clinic in primary or secondary care. The learning objectives for Chapter 41 are:

- to be able to discuss the benefits of a cancer family history clinic for patients and local health services;

◆ to be able to identify the key elements involved in setting up a cancer family history clinic in primary or secondary care.

Collaborative working

As highlighted by Bennett et al. (2010), a key element of successfully integrating genetics into mainstream health services is collaborative working between health professionals in primary care, cancer care and genetics. The concept of working across disciplines is familiar to health professionals working in the field of cancer care where the multidisciplinary team (MDT) is a key part of clinical care. However, working across disciplines to achieve a collaborative partnership for the benefit of patients is not always straightforward, and a body of research has built up examining the interactions and dynamics of MDTs and specifically between different health professionals within MDTs (Lanceley et al., 2004; Devitt et al., 2010).

In order to analyse the key elements of working successfully across disciplines and organisations, it is important to identify the core concepts of successful collaboration. A systematic review of empirical studies in inter-professional collaboration identified two central elements: collaboration and the team. These two central elements involved developing mutual trust and respect through sharing, partnership, interdependency and symmetry in power relationships (D'Amour et al., 2005). Analysis of the theoretical frameworks for collaborative working identified that in order for collaboration to be successful it must serve the needs of the professionals as well as those of the client (San Martín-Rodríguez et al., 2005).

Benefits of a cancer family history clinic for patients and health professionals

Although awareness of cancer genetics amongst the general population has increased since the 1990s (Mogilner et al., 1998; Bluman et al., 1999), a recent study in the United States found that the level of knowledge about cancer genetics is still low, particularly amongst men and minority ethnic groups (Baer et al., 2010). A similar situation has been identified in the UK population (Genetic Alliance, 2012).

Individuals seek referral to cancer genetics services for many reasons, including finding out information about their risk, obtaining genetic testing, out of concern for their children and siblings, accessing screening, obtaining information about reducing the risk of cancer and reducing anxiety (Fraser et al., 2003). Despite expectations, genetic testing will not be an option for many at a lower risk of cancer, therefore local family history clinics provide an opportunity to discuss concerns and increase the availability of risk assessment.

National Institute for Health and Care Excellence (NICE) guidelines in the UK (NICE, 2013) recommend that when a person presents with symptoms or has concerns about relatives with cancer, a first- and second-degree family history should be taken in primary care (i.e. children, parents, aunts, uncles and grandparents) and a more extensive family history should be taken in secondary care (i.e. a third-degree family history including wider relatives such as cousins, great aunts and uncles and great grandparents).

A systematic review of the impact of cancer genetic risk assessment on patients at risk of familial breast cancer found that following genetic risk assessment, knowledge about breast cancer and genetics improved, risk perception was more accurate and breast cancer-related distress reduced (Hilgart et al., 2012). However, the studies reviewed only involved consultations with genetics health professionals. Further research is required to assess the best means of delivering risk assessment by other health professionals, in alternative settings and for different cancer types.

Systematically assessing risk using evidence-based risk assessment tools in a dedicated family history clinic enables trained staff to triage referral appropriately to screening and genetics services, benefitting both patients and health services. For patients, unnecessary screening and the associated risks are avoided. Managing those at lower risk in primary and secondary care avoids raising expectations that cannot be met as only those eligible for genetic testing or with complex family histories will be referred to genetics services. For health services, targeted referral facilitates the effective use of resources by moving well patients out of symptomatic clinics and avoiding the overloading of screening and genetics services.

Key elements involved in setting up a cancer family history clinic in primary or secondary care

Based on experience of setting up and overseeing cancer family history clinics in primary and secondary care, three of the themes identified by Bennett et al. (2010) as important for integrating genetics into mainstream services are also fundamental for successfully establishing a family history clinic: engagement of stakeholders in the planning and design of the service, collaboration with the RGC and access to ongoing cancer genetics education. Each of these elements will now be addressed drawing on experience and using practical examples to demonstrate implementation.

Engagement of stakeholders in the planning and design of the service

As highlighted by the experiences described in Chapters 38 and 39, involving stakeholders in the design and planning of the clinic from the outset is important for the sustainability of the service. In addition to seeking the engagement of individuals within the organisation, such as managers, senior clinicians and other colleagues, it is vital to engage stakeholders from outside the organisation in order to set up a robust and sustainable service that meets the needs of local patients and health professionals: for example, groups representing patients who will be referred to the clinic (such as local cancer support groups or lay representatives of cancer networks); health professionals who will refer to the clinic (such as GPs, practice nurses and cancer health professionals in related areas); health professionals whom the clinic will refer to (such as screening, genetics services and other local departments in related areas) and commissioners.

Prior to setting up a new clinic it is necessary to provide sound evidence of the clinical need and cost implications and to discuss this with managers. A robust business case needs to include details such as why the clinic is needed; the number of patients that will be seen; the number and level of staff that will be required; the financial costing of the clinic, including any costs involved in working collaboratively with other services such as screening and genetics; organisational needs, such as clinic rooms, computers, telephones and stationery, administrative and IT support and governance arrangements. Box 41.1 shows an extract from the service level agreement (SLA) between the primary care Breast Cancer Risk Assessment Service (BCRAS), based within Guy's and St Thomas' NHS Foundation Trust (GSTFT) in south London and the South East London (SEL) Breast Screening Service (SELBSS) based at King's College Hospital NHS Foundation Trust (KCHFT), demonstrating the division of responsibility across organisational boundaries.

Collaboration with genetics and screening services

Whichever model of cancer family history clinic is set up, it is extremely important that close links are established with the RGC. This provides a resource for the health professionals running the clinic, helps with the introduction and updating of evidence-based risk assessment tools and referral guidelines and ensures that pathways into genetic counselling and clinic protocols are consistent between the family history clinic and the RGC. At the very least the health professionals running the family history clinic will need access to genetics advice and second opinions because many family histories do not 'fit' into the guidelines. Good collaboration is beneficial for the RGC as well as the cancer units. For example, communication about changes to national guidelines or referral criteria for the RGC and negotiating about the timing for cancer patients undergoing genetic testing close to diagnosis or during treatment is much easier if there are clear lines of communication and consistent protocols across the region. Mutual respect and recognition of expertise is beneficial to all concerned.

The cancer family history clinics in southeast England have been set up as part of a network so that there is a coordinated approach to risk assessment, a communication pathway between the clinics and the RGC and a named genetic counsellor who is responsible for providing consistent advice, training, support and supervision to the health professionals in each clinic. Strong links and seamless referral pathways have also been developed with screening services. This has been particularly important in the primary-care clinics where these links were not already established. Figures 41.1 and 41.2 show examples of the cancer risk assessment forms for breast/ovarian and colorectal cancer that are used by the nurses running family history clinics in the south east of England to refer patients to the Guy's RGC or to request genetics advice.

Access to ongoing cancer genetics education

Genetics is a rapidly evolving field and it is essential to keep abreast of the changes. In order to meet the genetics competencies set out by the National Genetics and Genomics

Box 41.1 Extract from the service level agreement

1 Organisation of service

1.1 Outpatients

1.1.1 The BCRAS/GSTFT will provide and be responsible for all aspects of breast cancer risk assessment service provision for patients in Lambeth, Southwark and Lewisham (LSL) including:

- Setting up and running specialist nurse led clinics in the community and, if appropriate, in breast units at GSTFT and KCHFT.
- Organisation of appointments for the BCRAS.
- Ensuring clinicians at GSTFT, KCHFT and in primary care in LSL are aware of how to access the service.
- Ensuring clinicians at the SEL Breast Tumour Working Group are aware of how to access the service.
- Promoting the service to the public and to clinicians in LSL.
- Providing up-to-date patient information leaflets about cancer risk and general health awareness.

1.1.2 SEL Breast Screening Service will provide and be responsible for all aspects of breast screening service provision for patients in LSL, including:

- Breast screening as advised by the BCRAS/GSTFT and Guy's RGC (GSTFT) in line with NICE/NHSBSP high risk screening guidelines.
- Referral of patients requiring surgical management to a specialist breast treatment centre.
- Feedback on the outcome of screening for patients referred by the BCRAS/GSTFT and Guy's RGC (GSTFT).
- Ongoing evaluation of the Breast Screening Service.
- Database of moderate-risk cases and call/recall for those having high-risk screening.

1.1.3 Patients for whom genetics referral is indicated will be seen at Guy's RGC for genetic counselling/testing which is commissioned by Specialist Genetics Commissioning.

1.1.4 Eligible patients who are seen by Guy's RGC will be referred directly to the SELBSS for family history screening.

Extract reproduced with permission from the service level agreement (SLA) between the primary care Breast Cancer Risk Assessment Service (BCRAS), based within Guy's and St Thomas' NHS Foundation Trust (GSTFT) and the South East London Breast Screening Service (SELBSS) based at King's College Hospital NHS Foundation Trust (KCHFT).

Breast Cancer Family History Clinic

GP name:
Address:
Tel:

Patient details:
Name:
Address:
DOB:

Family tree

Is there Jewish and/or Polish ancestry? Yes ☐ (If Yes, indicate which side of family) No ☐

Notes:..
....
....

Breast cancer risk assessment   Near population ☐   Moderate ☐   High ☐

Screening

Eligible for surveillance within NICE guidelines Yes ☐   No ☐

Age at which mammograms to commence:·················Frequency of mammograms:··············

Mammogram arranged: Yes ☐   No ☐   Date of last mammogram:············

Breast awareness   discussed: Yes ☐   No ☐   Date of next mammogram:··········

Leaflets given   Breast awareness ☐   Risk level ☐   Screening ☐

Refer to Genetics   Yes ☐   No ☐

Discuss with Genetics   Yes ☐   No ☐

Signature..   Date................................
Print name...   Title.................................

NB. Please send completed family history of cancer form as well as family tree if possible

Figure 41.1 Example of a family history risk assessment/referral form used in the breast cancer family history clinics in southeast England.

Reproduced with permission of the Department of Clinical Genetics, Guy's Hospital, Copyright © 2013.

Bowel Cancer Family History Clinic

Family tree

GP name:
Address:
Tel:

Name of local clinic

Patient details:
Name:
Address:
DOB:
Hospital no:

Has anyone in Family had **Polyposis**? Yes ☐ (If Yes, then refer to Genetics)   No ☐

Notes...
....
....
....

Bowel cancer	Average ☐ Low-Moderate ☐ High-Moderate ☐ Refer to genetics ☐
risk assessment	

Screening

Eligible for screening: Yes ☐   No ☐   From age ....

Colonoscopy arranged: Yes ☐   No ☐   Date of colonoscopy.................

Frequency of colonoscopy...

Bowel awareness/diet discussed: Yes ☐   No ☐

Leaflets given
          Bowel awareness ☐   Risk level ☐   Screening ☐

Refer to Genetics	Yes ☐	No ☐
Discuss with Genetics	Yes ☐	No ☐

Signature.. Date...
Print name... Title..

NB.Please send completed family history of cancer form as well as family tree if possible

Figure 41.2 Example of a family history risk assessment/referral form used in the colorectal cancer family history clinics in southeast of England.

Education Centre (Burke et al., 2005; Burke, 2009; Kirk et al., 2011), health professionals running cancer family history clinics require initial genetics training and ongoing continuous professional development. Educational tools and training packages can be accessed via the website of the National Genetics and Genomics Education Centre (<http://www.geneticseducation.nhs.uk/>).

Nurses working in family history clinics in southeast England are encouraged to attend a locally run validated cancer genetics module and are trained and supervised by a genetic counsellor until they have been assessed as competent to safely assess cancer risk and communicate this to patients. This involves the genetic counsellor sitting in with the nurse during the family history clinic consultations, providing education, advice, supervision and support. Once these competencies have been achieved, a named link genetic counsellor continues to be available to provide genetics advice and to ensure that the nurse is kept up to date with any changes relating to cancer risk assessment. The nurses running family history clinics are expected to attend free update sessions provided by the RGC at least once every 2 years. Box 41.2 shows guidelines for a family history consultation which can be used as an *aide-mémoire* for how to structure a family history consultation.

Box 41.2 Guidelines for a cancer family history clinic consultation

Outline the purpose of the consultation

- Explain how long the consultation will take (15–20 minutes).
- Establish the patient's expectations of the consultation.
- Explain the purpose of the consultation and outline what will happen.
  Ask about the patient's health
- Ask if patient has had any symptoms/health concerns.

Take the family history and draw a family tree

- Explain why you are taking the family history and what you need to know.
- Ask about children, siblings, parents and about other relatives who have had cancer; maternal and paternal sides of the family; whether relatives with cancer are alive; if a twin has had cancer, check whether or not they are identical. A three-generation family tree is required.
- Ask about other types of cancer/other major illnesses in the family.
- In breast or breast/ovarian families, ask about ethnic origin (e.g. Jewish/Polish) and explain why you are asking.
- In bowel cancer families, ask if family members have had multiple bowel polyps/polyposis.

Box 41.2 Guidelines for a cancer family history clinic consultation *(continued)*

Work out whether or not the cancer risk is increased

- ◆ Explain the population risk of the cancers in the family.
- ◆ Ask for the patient's perception of their risk and note how they talk about their risk.
- ◆ Explain that you will look at both sides of the family separately.
- ◆ Explain that most cancer is not 'inherited'.
- ◆ Use tools provided by the RGC to assess risk and provide screening and referral advice.
- ◆ Tailor the risk communication to the individual, explaining the risk in a way the patient understands and in context for themselves and their family.
- ◆ Explain which cancers in the family do not influence the risk.
- ◆ If you are unsure, explain that you will discuss with genetics and get back to them.
- ◆ Provide the patient with an information leaflet about their risk level.

Explain the screening plan

- ◆ Outline the screening plan, explain what is involved in screening, the benefits and limitations and provide the patient with an information leaflet about screening.
- ◆ Explain that the screening plan could change if the family history changes or if genetic testing takes place.
- ◆ Discuss symptom awareness and general health education.

Refer to genetics if appropriate

- ◆ Explain why you would like to refer to genetics and what is involved, for example 'Your cancer family history could be hereditary, therefore it may be helpful for you to see a genetics doctor or genetic counsellor, who will explain more about what the family history means for you and your family and what you can do about it'.
- ◆ Help the patient to prepare for the genetics appointment by advising them to take along details about family members, for example name, date of birth, type of cancer, age at diagnosis, date and place of treatment, date of death, medical letters/death certificates etc.
- ◆ The decision to be referred to genetics is the patient's (if they are eligible).

Closing

- ◆ Check if the patient has any questions.
- ◆ Advise the patient to go to their GP if they have symptoms and to contact the family history clinic if they have questions/concerns in the future or their family history changes.

Summary

Cancer family history clinics provide patients with an opportunity to address concerns about developing cancer, to gain understanding of the implications of their family history and to access the risk management options that are appropriate for them. Triaging patients in a dedicated clinic enables those with a cancer family history to be managed appropriately without overwhelming specialist services. There are challenges to setting up any new service, and changes to the NHS will require clinical commissioning groups to set priorities in healthcare and base decisions regarding commissioning new services on sophisticated and robust evidence (Robinson et al., 2011). Experience of setting up and maintaining a network of cancer family history clinics in southeast England shows the key elements to be engaging stakeholders from the outset, working collaboratively with genetics and screening services and ensuring that staff running the clinics have access to ongoing genetics education.

References

Baer HJ, Brawarsky P, Murray MF, Haas JS 2010. Familial risk of cancer and knowledge and use of genetic testing. *J Gen Intern Med* **25**: 717–724.

Bennett C, Burke S, Burton H, Farndon P. 2010. A toolkit for incorporating genetics into mainstream medical services: learning from service development pilots in England. *BMC Health Serv Res* **10**: 125.

Bluman LG, Rimer BK, Berry DA, et al. 1999. Attitudes, knowledge, and risk perceptions of women with breast and/or ovarian cancer considering testing for *BRCA1* and *BRCA2*. *J Clin Oncol* **17**: 1040–1046.

Burke S 2009. Developing a curriculum statement based on clinical practice: genetics in primary care. *Br J Gen Pract* **59**: 99–103.

Burke S, Stone A, Martyn M, Thomas H, Farndon P 2005. *Genetics education for GP registrars.* Birmingham: Centre for Education in Medical Genetics, University of Birmingham.

D'Amour D, Ferrada-Videla M, San Martin Rodriguez L, Beaulieu M-D 2005. The conceptual basis for interprofessional collaboration: core concepts and theoretical frameworks. *J Interprof Care* **19**: 116–131.

Devitt B, Philip J, McLachlan SA 2010. Team dynamics, decision making, and attitudes toward multidisciplinary cancer meetings: health professionals' perspectives. *J Oncol Pract* **6**: e17–e20.

DoH (Department of Health) 2004. *Our inheritance, our future. Realising the potential of genetics in the NHS.* London: The Stationery Office.

Eeles R, Purland G, Maher J, Evans D 2007. Delivering cancer genetics services—new ways of working. *Fam Cancer* **6**: 163–167.

Fraser L, Bramald S, Chapman C, et al. 2003. What motivates interest in attending a familial cancer genetics clinic? *Fam Cancer* **2**: 159–168.

Genetic Alliance UK 2012. *Identifying family risk of cancer: why is this more difficult for ethnic minority communities and what would help?* London: Genetic Alliance UK. Available at: <http://www.geneticalliance.org.uk/docs/ethnicity-and-access-web-copy.pdf> (last accessed 11 February 2014).

Hilgart JS, Coles B, Iredale R 2012. Cancer genetic risk assessment for individuals at risk of familial breast cancer. *Cochrane Database Syst Rev* **2**: CD003721.

Kirk M, Calzone K, Arimori N, Tonkin E 2011. Genetics–genomics competencies and nursing regulation. *J Nurs Scholar* **43**: 107–116.

Lanceley A, Jacobs I, Menon U, Savage J, Warburton F 2004. The multidisciplinary team meeting: an ethnographic study. *Int J Gynecol Cancer* **14**: 2061.

Mogilner A, Otten M, Cunningham JD, Brower ST 1998. Awareness and attitudes concerning *BRCA* gene testing. *Ann Surg Oncol* **5**: 607–612.

NICE (National Institute for Health and Care Excellence) 2013. *Familial breast cancer: classification and care of people at risk of familial breast cancer and management of breast cancer and related risks in people with a family history of breast cancer.* NICE Clinical Guideline 164. London: National Institute for Health and Care Excellence.

Robinson S, Dickinson H, Williams I, Freeman T, Rumbold B, Spence K 2011. *Setting priorities in health.* London: Nuffield Trust.

San Martín-Rodríguez L, Beaulieu M-D, D'Amour D, Ferrada-Videla M 2005. The determinants of successful collaboration: a review of theoretical and empirical studies. *J Interprof Care* **19**: 132–147.

Scheuner MT, Hamilton AB, Peredo J, et al. 2014. A cancer genetics toolkit improves access to genetic services through documentation and use of the family history by primary-care clinicians. *Genet Med* **16**: 60–69.

Chapter 42

Managing cancer family history in primary, secondary and palliative care. Summary

Patricia Webb and Lorraine Robinson

Introduction to section 9 summary

The topics covered in Section 9 are arguably among the most important for health professionals and patients. The implementation of family history risk assessment in different sectors of the healthcare service, from primary to palliative care, is addressed with helpful tips on how to set up a cancer family history clinic and pitfalls to avoid.

Chapter 37. Managing cancer family history in primary, secondary and palliative care. Introduction

Ten years ago an average GP saw one patient a month who had concerns about their cancer family history and only a small proportion of patients with a cancer family history required referral for a genetic assessment. At that time, therefore, there was insufficient demand for GPs to gain the knowledge and skills required to assess and explain familial cancer risk.

A report about the organisation of cancer genetics services, led to recommendations for systematic family history risk assessment in secondary care and closer working between cancer units and clinical genetics services. The importance of cancer family history has been referred to in several sets of National Institute for Health and Care Excellence (NICE) guidelines between 2004 and 2013. A review of the outcome of the pilot projects set up as a result of a Department of Health White Paper in 2004 identified several key elements required for implementing cancer risk assessment in mainstream healthcare (Bennett et al., 2010).

Surveillance is not appropriate for all patients with a cancer family history and cancer units do not have the capacity or resources to manage all patients who have concerns. Chapter 37 considers the benefits and disadvantages of the various models for managing the growing demand for cancer risk assessment in primary and secondary care. The choice of model will be subject to availability of skilled personnel, financial resources and the needs of the local population. The population profile is particularly important and is now very much a part of GP and secondary care service planning.

Guided activity for Chapter 37

◆ Review how cancer family history is managed in your clinical area. Are you confident that all patients are asked about their cancer family history? If not, think about the optimal time and way to do this for your client group and service. Identify which model might fit with your local population needs, staffing and financial resources.

Further resource for Chapter 37

Eeles R, Purland G, Mather J, Evans D 2007. Delivering cancer genetics services- new ways of working. *Fam Cancer* 6: 163–167.

Chapters 38–40. Managing cancer family history in primary, secondary and palliative care

The experiences discussed in these three chapters highlight why it is important for health professionals in primary, secondary and palliative care who work with patients with cancer and at risk of cancer to develop a sound understanding of cancer genetics issues and to ensure they are working within the competencies set out by the National Genetics and Genomics Education Centre (see Chapters 2–6).

Guided activity for Chapters 38–40

◆ Reflecting on the experiences described in Chapters 38–40, consider what worked and what did not. Try and relate that to your own practice and identify what would be required to implement an effective and sustainable cancer family history clinic in your area.

Further resources for Chapters 38–40

Lillie AK 2006. Exploring cancer genetics and care of the family: an evolving challenge for palliative care. *Int J Palliat Nurs* 12: 70–74.

McAllister M, O'Malley K, Hopwood P, et al. 2002. Management of women with a family history of breast cancer in the North West Region of England: training for implementing a vision of the future. *J Med Genet* 39: 531–535.

Chapter 41. A practical guide to setting up a cancer family history clinic in primary or secondary care

Establishing the infrastructure for managing a family history requires skills, knowledge and time. Chapter 41 provides the basis for beginning to think about establishing an effective and sustainable cancer family history clinic and to consider the challenges of this within the financial constraints of the NHS. Three key elements are identified and discussed: engagement of stakeholders in the planning and design of the service, collaboration with genetics and screening services and access to ongoing genetics education for health professionals undertaking cancer risk assessment in order to enable them to meet the required level of competence and confidence.

Guided activities for Chapter 41

- Identify who the stakeholders would be if you were to set up a clinic within your service. Would this involve working across professional or organisational boundaries? Consider the potential problems with engaging each of these stakeholders and how these issues might be overcome.

- Identify how your service might link in with genetics and screening services. Who are the key personnel? How might you be able to gain access to them? What training, supervision/support might they be able to provide? What other resources are available?

- Map out a draft business case, identifying what current service provision is available, the needs of the local client group, what service you would like to provide, how this would improve the current service, what guidelines if any would support the proposal (e.g. NICE guidelines), how many patients might be involved, what level of staffing/training/administration/IT support/health service facilities/funding would be required, what promotion of the service would be required, what governance arrangements would be needed and how the service could be evaluated.

- Discuss your ideas and initial plans with your colleagues and line manager and identify who in your organisation might be able to help you to develop the business plan and take this forward.

Further resource for Chapter 41

National Genetics and Genomics Education Centre. Guidance for developing services involving genetics. Available at: <http://www.geneticseducation.nhs.uk/for-practitioners-62/a-toolkit-for-developing-services-involving-genetics> (last accessed 27 August 2013).

Reference

Bennett C, Burke S, Burton H, Farndon P 2010. A toolkit for incorporating genetics into mainstream medical services: learning from service development pilots in England. *BMC Health Serv Res* **10**: 125.

Index

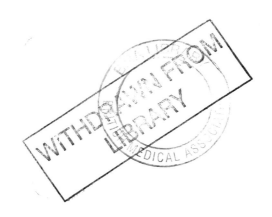